The
Complete
Illustrated
Book
of

# YOGA

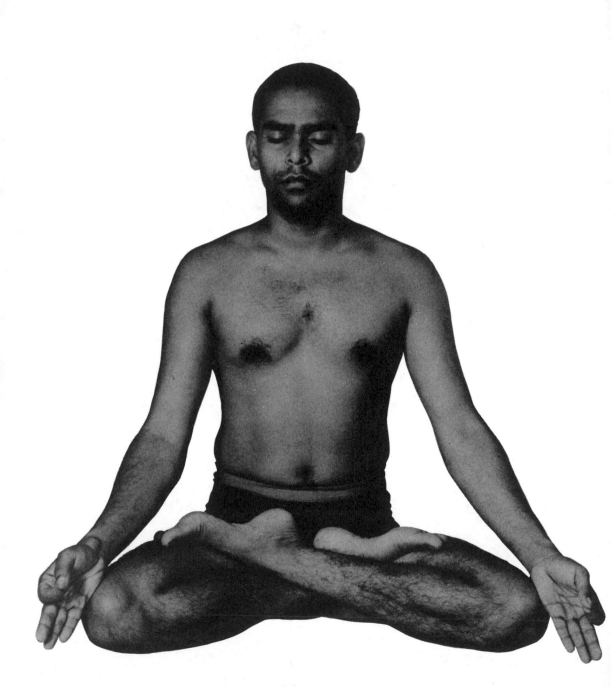

# The
# Complete
# Illustrated
# Book
# of
# YOGA

Swami Vishnu-devananda

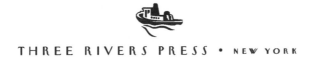

THREE RIVERS PRESS • NEW YORK

Dedicated to my Master Swami Sivananda

Published by Three Rivers Press, New York, New York.
Member of the Crown Publishing Group.

Random House, Inc. New York, Toronto, London, Sydney, Auckland
www.randomhouse.com

THREE RIVERS PRESS is a registered trademark and the
Three Rivers Press colophon is a trademark of Random House, Inc.

Previously published by the Julian Press, Inc., in 1960 and by Harmony Books in 1988.

Printed in the United States of America

Library of Congress Cataloging-in-Publication Data is available upon request.

ISBN 0-517-88431-3

18 19

# CONTENTS

# Charts

# PREFACE TO THE 1988 EDITION

OM SRI GANESHAYA NAMAH
OM SARAVANABHAVAYA NAMAH
OM AIM SARASWATYAI NAMAH
OM NAMO BHAGAVATE SIVANANDAYA
OM HAMAH SIVAYA
OM NAMO NARAYANAYA

As I write this preface to the new edition of *The Complete Illustrated Book of Yoga*, humanity is plunging deeper and deeper into crisis, yet a bright future awaits. The transition between the 20th and 21st centuries may bring us to an unprecedented technological paradise. The door is opening to an age of supercomputers to help organize our complicated society and modified ecology; superconductors to minimize energy waste; and robots to perform work not fit for humans, thereby increasing our leisure time and life spans. New medical solutions will possibly arise to control AIDS and eliminate other terrible diseases. A time may come soon when we will be growing vegetables in space stations as well as in our houses, or we may find ourselves migrating to other planets, as the ancients migrated to new worlds.

Yet, we are still unable to deal with our minds. The world crisis is but a reflection of the chaotic state of the collective consciousness. The most positive action we can perform to contribute to the momentous task of bringing our planet back into balance is to start changing ourselves.

Positive, focused thoughts are much more powerful than negative, confused thoughts. No external technology can control surging emotions and imaginations. No type of alcohol, drugs (whether tranquilizers, sleeping pills, or wake-up pills), or other such instruments can hope to offer a long-term solution to epidemic mental weakness. These chemicals destroy not only the bodies and minds of the users, but also those of their offspring, creating genetic disturbances and unbalancing the mental vibration. Real peace comes only to those who can control the body and mind with proper self-discipline.

This book is presented as an offering to each individual to make the simple willful decision to live a divine life in harmony with the inextricable laws of nature. If there is the will and the desire to realize limitless spiritual potential, then the practical methods of Yoga self-discipline and mind control outlined herein will prove invaluable.

I have titled this book *The Complete Illustrated Book of Yoga* because Yoga is a complete science of self-discipline. Yoga balances, harmonizes, purifies, and strengthens the Body, Mind, and Soul of the practitioner. It shows the way to perfect Health, perfect mind control, and perfect peace with one's Self, the world, nature, and God. Millions of people have begun to practice Yoga through the application of the simple time-tested techniques presented in this book. Though the scientific terms and examples used to explain the theory of Yoga have been designed for the modern reader, I have been religiously true to the ancient teachings of Hatha Yoga, as well as other forms, such as Kundalini Yoga, Raja Yoga, and Jnana Yoga. I have invented nothing new, only presented this perfect science of self-development in a form comprehensible for an analytic-minded era.

The Yogi sees life as a triangle. Birth is the first point of this life triangle. Its upward line represents the growth period; the top dot, youth; the downward line, decay. The last point is death, but the base line of the triangle is life hereafter, which ends in birth again. The growth period, known as the "anabolic process," reaches a plateau at about the age of 18 or 20 years. During the "youthful" period of life the rate of cell rejuvenation exceeds or equals cell decay. In a normal person, the body maintains this healthy, youthful state until about 30 years of age. At around the age of 35, the decaying or "catabolic process" begins to predominate, the anabolic process decreases, and the body machine starts its decline. This process later results in the state termed "old age" with its accompanying ills and despair, both physical and mental.

Yogis, however, say that we were not born merely to be subject to pain and suffering, disease and death. There is a far greater purpose to life. But the spiritual investigation of life's purpose requires a keen intellect and strong will, the products of a healthy body and mind.

For this reason, the ancient sages developed an integral system to ward off or retard the decaying or catabolic process, and to keep the physical and mental faculties strong. By closely observing the life-style and needs of the modern men and women of this planet I have synthesized the ancient wisdom of Yoga into five basic principles, which can be easily incorporated into everyone's own pattern of life. These principles are: (1) proper exercise; (2) proper breathing; (3) proper relaxation; (4) proper diet; and (5) positive thinking (deep philosophy) and meditation.

*Proper exercise* acts as a lubrication system to the joints, muscles, ligaments, tendons, and so forth, by increasing circulation and flexibility. Yogic exercise can be compared to no other system in its complete overhauling of the entire being. A Yoga Asana (or Posture) is meant to be held for some time (the term "Asana" means steady pose). Performed slowly and consciously, the Asanas not only produce physical benefits, but are mental exercises in concentration and meditation.

Yoga exercise focuses first on the health of the spine. The spinal column houses the center of the nervous system, the telegraphic system of the body. As a direct extension of the brain, the healthy spine aids in the health of the whole body. By maintaining the spine's flexibility and strength through proper exercise, circulation is increased, the nerves are ensured their supply of nutrients and oxygen, and the body retains its youthful state. As a Chinese proverb states, "Truly a flexible back makes a long life."

Asanas work on the internal machinery of the whole body, especially on such key pressure points as the Chinese acupuncture areas. Stimulation of these points increases the flow of nerve energy, or Prana (Sanskrit) or Chi (Chinese). The Asanas also affect the deeper and more subtle parts of the body. The internal organs receive massage and stimulation through the various movements of the Asanas and are toned into functioning more efficiently. As Yoga postures are always practiced with deep breathing, relaxation, and concentration, the Asanas also help to develop mental control. The mind that is unsteady by nature and constantly agitated by sensory inputs becomes withdrawn and detached from the objects of the senses, freed from distractions, and slowly brought under control (see Chapter 4).

*Proper breathing* connects the body to its battery, the Solar Plexus, where tremendous potential energy is stored. When tapped through specific Yoga breathing techniques (Pranayama), this energy is released for physical and mental rejuvenation.

Most people use only a fraction of their lung capacity for breathing. They breathe shallowly, using a small part of the rib cage. Their shoulders are hunched, they have painful tension in the upper part of the back and neck, and they suffer from a lack of oxygen. These people become tired easily and don't know why.

What the unfortunate majority of us need these days is a breathing program that can help us at our desks, stoves, and machines. Tension and even depression may be overcome by proper diaphragmatic breathing.

By far the most important benefit of good breathing is concentrating the Prana, or nerve energy, which increases our vital energy level. Control of the Prana leads to control of the mind.

All diseases of the body can be destroyed at the root by regulating the Prana; this is the secret knowledge of healing. Acupuncturists, shiatsu, faith healing, doctors with healing touch, and so forth, are all examples of the development of a high degree of conscious or unconscious control of the Prana. In ordinary breathing we extract very little Prana, but when we concentrate and consciously regulate our breathing, we are able to store a greater amount in our various nerve centers and brain. One who has abundant Prana radiates vitality and strength, which can be felt by those with whom he comes in contact (see Chapter 8).

*Proper relaxation* cools down the system, as the radiator does for a car. Relaxation is Nature's way of recharging the body. When the body and mind are continually overworked, their efficiency diminishes. In order to regulate and balance the work of the body and mind, it is necessary to learn to economize the energy produced by our body, which is the main purpose of learning how to relax.

Modern social life, food, work, and even so-called entertainments, such as rock 'n' roll dancing, all make it difficult for modern people to relax. More of our energy is spent in keeping our muscles in continual readiness for work than in actual useful work done. Even while resting, the average person expends much energy through needless physical and mental tension. Thus, most of the body's energy is wasted.

Remember that in the course of one day our body usually produces all the substances and energy necessary for the next. But often all these are consumed within a few minutes by bad moods, anger, injury, or irritation that reaches a high degree of intensity.

During relaxation there is practically no Prana being consumed. Although a little is spent maintaining the basic metabolic activities, the remaining portion is stored and conserved. In order to achieve perfect relaxation, three levels of relaxation—physical, mental, and spiritual—must be attained. No relaxation is complete until all three are reached (see Chapter 6).

*Proper diet* provides fuel for the body. The Yogic diet is a vegetarian one, consisting of pure, simple, natural foods that are easily digested and assimilated and that promote health. One should have a certain knowledge of dietetics in order to balance the diet. The body's nutritional requirements fall into five categories: protein, carbohydrates, minerals, fats, and vitamins. Eating nonprocessed foods directly from nature (preferably organic, free from chemicals and pesticides) will help ensure a better supply of these nutritional needs, since processing, refining, and overcooking destroy much of the food value.

There is a cycle in Nature known as the "food cycle" or "food chain." The sun is the source of energy for all life on our planet. Vegetarians eat at the top of this food chain, since they eat plants that derive their nutrients directly from the sun.

The Yogic attitude toward diet is to "eat to live, not live to eat." The Yogi considers, using both his knowledge of nutrition and his internal experience, which foods can be consumed in what minimum quantity with the most positive effect on the body and mind, and with the least negative impact on the environment and least pain to other beings. When one has a vision of world unity, the hunger of others, the suffering of animals, and the condition of the environment are all part of dietary considerations. One of the first ways to take responsibility for the planet is by eating with consideration.

Fasting is also a part of the Yogic dietary regime. Fasting plus rest is Nature's universal prescription for all ailments, from fevers to broken limbs. Along with prayer, it is recommended by all religions for purification, self-discipline, and self-control (see Chapter 7).

*Positive thinking* (deep philosophy) and *meditation* put you in control. The intellect is purified. The lower nature is brought under conscious control through steadiness and concentration of mind.

Yoga gives a sublime practical philosophy. As the great Yoga Master H. H. Swami Sivananda says, "The only basis of true and lasting unity of all humanity is the religion of the heart. Religion of the heart is the religion of love." And, "Samadhi [super-conscious state] is blissful union with the supreme Self. It leads to the direct intuitive realization of the infinite. It is an inner divine experience which is beyond the reach of speech and mind. You will have to realize this yourself through deep meditation. The senses, the mind and the intellect cease functioning. There is neither time nor causation here."

(If you want an understanding of the practical techniques for meditation, my book *Meditation and Mantras* may help.)

Yoga is a life of self-discipline built upon the tenets of simple living and high thinking. Please do not discount the value of the combined approach to Yoga self-culture. If you follow these five points, which compose a true holistic approach to our whole system of body, mind, and soul, you will gain strength and balance to face this decisive world era. When body, mind, and soul are healthy and harmonious, the higher mind can easily triumph over the vicious instinctive lower mind. Obstacles become stepping stones to success, and life is a school for the development of character, compassion, and realization of the Divine All-pervading Self. You will gain a new angle of vision of health and positivity. If you can heal your own body and mind, you will be capable of healing and taking care of the planet. I pray that you will practice the time-tested ancient techniques and philosophy presented in this book, and that you will attain Health, Happiness, and Eternal Peace. May Lord bless you. Thy Own Self. **OM TAT SAT**

**SWAMI VISHNU-DEVANANDA**
*Sivananda Ashram Yoga Camp*
*Val-Morin, Quebec*
*Canada*
*June 1, 1988*

*The Complete Illustrated Book of Yoga*

# 1

# PHILOSOPHY AND AIM
# OF YOGA

Man, not satisfied with modern inventions and knowledge of the ever-unfolding mysteries of nature, tirelessly seeks a goal beyond. As he observes nature's miracles through the mysterious atom, the mother of all things; through the stars and planets which, though unlimited, are floating, separating, and crashing into each other in that vast space and time beyond, his intellect refuses to work.

This tired intellect, wandering through the galaxies in space and in which our planet is only a minute speck, comes back laden with disappointment and shame.

Man is no longer satisfied with his intellect, the reasoning machine that brings no answers to his questions, "What is the purpose of life?" "Who am I?" "Where will I go?" "Is physical death the end of everything?" and the like. This intellect man boasts about, supposedly knowing everything, returns to its plane unable to discover the end of the galaxies, the biggest thing he can comprehend, and the forms of electrons, the smallest he can approximate through his reason. Either above or below these two magnitudes his intellect cannot penetrate through an unknown law.

It is but foolishness to search for truth with an instrument as limited as the intellect, to attempt to measure the unknown fathoms of the eternal question of the purpose of life.

Yet we cannot forever ignore the truth, if there is a truth. In fact, there are a few who have already transcended the limitation of space and time and can see the past, present, and future without this tiny intellect. These persons are called seers or saints and they have a scientifically devised method of binding truth that can satisfy the intellect although their knowledge is above it. Looking deceptively simple, their method is very difficult for untrained and impure minds. They use the same dissipated rays of the mind that the majority of mankind uses for external observation and feeling, and focus them on the dark inner recesses of the heart; in turn, the one-pointed rays of the mind illumine the dark corners of the unknown.

As long as one's wandering mind moves externally toward objects, one cannot come face to face with truth or God.

The answers for transcendental questions come to the seers and saints not from intellectual study or from laboratory experiments, but from the unknown, unlimited source of wisdom and knowledge gained during their silent hours of contemplation when the mind and intellect cease to function. For real knowledge of God or truth and answers for all such questions come only when the mind and senses are still and steady.

The question now arises: what is the use of such knowledge? Does God exist? Is there a life after death? What is the purpose of life? For without some purpose, we would not take the trouble to find the answers to such questions.

The few who discover truth declare that it will take away all our miseries. When man realizes truth, he comes face to face with something which is, by its own nature, eternally pure and perfect. All our misery comes from fear of death and disease and from unfulfilled desires. When man realizes truth and/or his real nature, he will discover that he is immortal. Therefore he never dies and has no fear of death. When he knows that he is perfect and full, he will have no more vain desires to be satisfied. So by removing the fear of death through understanding of his real nature, by knowing that the "Kingdom of Heaven" is within, man enjoys perfect bliss even while in his physical body.

The goal of life is to achieve, while still alive, a state free from death, pain, sorrow, old age, disease, and rebirth. To remove these afflictions, every religion has its tenets. Many practitioners of religions blindly follow their leaders without knowing the purpose of life and religion and are satisfied by mere belief without practice, just as the religious heads of many faiths ask the people to follow the leaders blindly. This act of the blind leading the blind has turned many sincere seekers from their real path for lack of belief in theoretical knowledge.

All the founders of religions saw God; they all saw their own souls, they all saw eternity as their future. What they saw, they preached. They gave methods to reach this state of experience or knowledge where everyone could see the nature of his eternal and immortal soul. The modern religious followers and teachers, more busy preaching than practicing, argue that such experiences were possible only for the founders of religion; no man can become really spiritual until he has reached the perception of those teachers. Every man needs to experience truth within himself; only then all his doubts will vanish and all his miseries disappear. Christ said, "If ye continue in my word, then are ye my disciples indeed; And ye shall know the truth, and the truth shall make you free." St. John 8:31, 32.

The science of Yoga gives a practical and scientifically prepared method of finding truth in religion. As every science has its own method of investigation, so also the science of Yoga has its own method and declares that truth can be experienced. The truth can be experienced only when one transcends the senses and when the mind and intellect cease to function.

The Yogic teacher does not stop to prove his theory as he advances it, nor does he try to demonstrate to or argue with his class; his teaching is authoritative, as he himself experienced what was taught to him by his own teacher. The truth he teaches is an accepted truth and those who are ready for it will intuitively recognize it. On the other hand, no arguments or discussions can bring truth to those who are not yet ready or evolved enough to receive it.

The teacher knows that much of his teaching is but the planting of seeds and that, for every idea the student understands, there will be a hundred that will come into his conscious recognition only after his mind is ready to understand and accept it. This does not mean that every Yoga teacher insists that his students accept his teachings blindly. He knows that at first the student cannot accept everything and so he insists that the student accept only that portion of the truth which he can prove to himself by his own experiments. The student is taught that before he can reach a deeper understanding, he must develop and unfold through service, devotion, and a moral life. As the student moves along the path of Yoga, he becomes aware of many new things that his teacher has already taught him theoretically. To a certain extent a student is advised to follow the teachings until he is able to experience truth within himself. In the beginning, he will profit by the advice and experience of the teachers who have traveled the path before him. For every man must learn through his own experiences. Walking along this path, he will see signs left behind as guideposts by those gone before him at each stage of the journey and in turn, he will leave his own road marks for those who will follow behind. A real student will not follow blindly but will take advantage of these signs until he reaches the goal without losing his way through this rough and difficult path.

The following anecdote illustrates the point: Once a teacher in India went to a holy river for a purification bath with many of his devoted followers. As it is the custom to bring a small vessel to carry holy water from the sacred river after the bath, the saint had brought one. Arriving at the river's sandy bank, the saint dug a hole, buried the vessel, and piled a heap of sand over it as a landmark. His followers had not seen what he was doing but noticed that he had made a pile of sand. Assuming this to be a part of the ceremony, they made similar heaps all over the river bank. When the teacher finished his bath, he looked for his vessel. Instead of finding one heap he saw the vast river bank littered with similar heaps. Astonished, he asked the reason for all these sand heaps. Hearing that they had tried to imitate him, the saint was wonderstruck over the foolishness of his followers who imitated him blindly. Needless to say, it took considerable time to find the saint's buried vessel.

Today we can see such followers in every religion, people who blindly follow their leaders without bothering to search for truth. Yoga philosophy and its teachers do not call for such blind faith, but ask the student to be patient and many things that appear vague at first will become clear as he progresses.

There are various forms of Yoga through which to attain universal consciousness, or oneness with the Supreme Being. Yoga is a science by which the individual approaches truth. The aim of all Yoga practice is to achieve truth wherein the individual soul identifies itself with the supreme soul or God. To achieve this, it has to transcend different vehicles or bodies of the soul, which bring individual or self-consciousness.

In fact, spirit * or pure consciousness in man is whole, without division, infinite in its nature, inactive and unchanging . . . the same spirit is found in everything . . . from mineral to man.

For spirit or pure consciousness projects the mind and matter, its creative power forms the veiling agent of the consciousness and creates forms out of formless spirit, infinite into finite as self-consciousness or individuality.

Spirit or pure consciousness never changes and it is the same spirit that radiates forth from mineral to man. As ascent is made on the

* The words "spirit" and "soul" are used in this text interchangeably and contain the same meaning.

scale of evolution from mineral to man, the spirit as pure consciousness varies in expression. In the mineral kingdom, spirit manifests itself as the lowest form of sentiency where consciousness is scarcely evident. It has been proved to a certain extent by modern scientists that life can be created from minerals and experimentation is being continued.

The first scientist to create life out of an inanimate object was Andrew Cross, who experimented with rocks. In 1837, he tried to make crystals by electrically heating a piece of iron oxide with hydrochloric acid and silicate of potash. Little white pimples appeared on the rock and after twenty-six days grew to be exact replicas of insects. Two days later, they crawled. Cross wrote, "I have never in word, thought, or deed given anyone a right to suppose that I considered them (insects) as a creation. I have never dreamed of any theory to account for their appearance. It was a matter of chance."

Another scientist, Morely Martin, who died in 1838, claimed to have recreated life from the oldest types of rock, Azoic. He heated the substance until it was reduced to cinders, and then subjected it to a number of operations until minute crystals were formed, which he named "primordial protoplasm." Finally, he magnified these crystals about three thousand times and those who peered through the eyepiece perceived thousands of minute fish wriggling in them.

There is no reason why life should not be created from such apparently lifeless matter as rock and metal. According to Yoga philosophy, there is no lifeless matter, for everything is consciousness itself. Scientists tell us that inside the tiniest particles of atoms is incredible movement. If there is movement, there must be some kind of energy to cause it, and that energy is the basis of all life.

The old philosophy of the Yogis that man, animals, birds, fishes, trees, earth, rocks, and elements are one is a theory gradually becoming accepted in the scientific world of the twentieth century.

The sentiency is more developed and can be seen in crystals that grow with definite forms and shapes. In the second stage of evolution above the mineral world, namely the plant kingdom, the development of consciousness is greater in degree than in the minerals, even though they also belong to the subconscious level. This is further developed in the animal world with its various psychic functions of the mind, where consciousness is more centralized. At last, with the further development of the intellect and other psychic functions such as cognition, perception, will, and knowledge, man is considered to be the highest in creation and highest in the scale of evolution.

From the above, it looks as though the soul were developing or evolving from mineral to man, but in fact soul is the same through these various changing phenomena of evolution. Spirit remains the same whether in mineral kingdom or in man. Behind this changing form of consciousness there is changeless, formless spirit, which is not affected or changed in any way through its expression or sentiency, but is veiled in various stages of its development.

How can the development of the spirit be explained if it is not changing from mineral to man? The seeming development of the soul is due to the development of the body and mind in which it is enclosed and by which it is more or less veiled. The consciousness is not able to throw its rays outside when enclosed with a black screen in the minerals.

When we study the plants and animals we notice that, owing to the nature of the body and development to some degree of the mind, the spirit expresses in a better way than in minerals. Here the light of consciousness is seen through the colored glasses of the lower mind.

Though the spirit in man is less contracted or veiled by the mind and body, there is still a veil that separates the spirit or consciousness from its full expression. Here man lives on a self-conscious plane. Animals live on a subconscious plane without any self-awareness. The self-consciousness in man is higher than subconsciousness. Universal consciousness is above self-consciousness and is the highest state of awareness where man feels and identifies with his real self or God-self.

As the mind develops, the veil covering the soul becomes thinner and finally disappears altogether. In this state, the soul realizes its immortality and its identification with the Supreme Being. This is the aim of all Yoga and this is the purpose of all religions. Yoga is a scientific way to bring about this evolution wherein there is no duality, no subject or object, wherein the knower, the knowledge, and the known are fused into one.

This can be achieved only when man transcends completely the limitation of body and mind that veils his pure consciousness or divinity. In order to transcend the body and mind so that he can use these instruments in his march toward the goal, the Yogi follows a rigorous discipline of body and mind. He goes into a detailed study of the vehicles in which the soul or consciousness is enclosed. A clear study and knowledge of these bodies or vehicles by which the spirit expresses are essential before we can take up the subject of spirit.

Man is far more complex than is generally assumed. Not only is he a physical body and a soul, but he is pure spirit with several vehicles or bodies for his expression. These vehicles of the soul, being of different degrees and density (the physical body being the grossest and the most perishable), manifest on such different planes as the physical, the astral, and others.

The causal body is the subtlest of the three bodies. Though man possesses all three bodies, he works mainly with the physical body. To a very small extent he works with his astral body, especially during the dream state and during meditation by Yoga students.

In the following chapters, we shall deal separately with the different bodies, their functions, qualifications, and other aspects of the vehicles, such as how they can be controlled and kept in a healthy condition so that we may utilize them for our particular needs at any particular time of our evolution.

After attaining a thorough knowledge and control of the three bodies, the individual takes to self-introspection or inquiry, "Who am I?"

Modern psychology has not taught this process of self-introspection by which one comes face to face with truth or God; where one knows there is neither pain nor sorrow, superiority or inferiority, or any individuality and separation.

This knowledge brings a feeling of oneness with the whole world and no longer does man see himself as man, but identical with the Supreme Being. This experience is beyond ordinary understanding. It brings the peace to which the Bible refers as "the peace that passeth all understanding." This knowledge is the end of all knowledge or Vedanta. There is no distinction between knower, knowledge, and known. In this state there is nothing to know, as the spirit or real man is knowledge itself and there is nothing external for him to know.

If you know how long it takes to get even theoretical knowledge of Vedanta, which puzzles even the ethnologically advanced man of today, then you can imagine how hard it is to experience these greatest truths: "Man is God," "I am God," "I am everywhere," and "I am the Self of all." The whole Yoga and Vedanta philosophy is based upon the theory of oneness, which can be attained by gradual perfection through reincarnation.

Although the followers of the various religions will not believe this truth of oneness of the soul, some of the great prophets such as Jesus proclaimed, "I and my Father are one," "I am in ye, you are in Me," "I am He." Most followers do not even understand the meaning of such great wisdom and they condemn the theories of reincarnation and evolution of the consciousness or soul. It is clearly stated in the

Bible in St. John 3:3–7, "Jesus answered and said unto him, "Verily, verily, I say unto thee, except a man be born again, he cannot see the Kingdom of God."

Nicodemus saith unto him, "How can a man be born when he is old? Can he enter the second time into his mother's womb, and be born?"

Jesus answered, "Verily, verily, I say unto thee, except a man be born of water and of the Spirit, he cannot enter into the Kingdom of God. That which is born of the flesh is flesh and that which is born of the Spirit is Spirit. Marvel not that I said unto thee, 'Ye must be born again.'"

If the theory of reincarnation and law of action and reaction are not accepted, then how can we explain the miseries and pains of this world? In every religion and in every age we see people suffering from disease, old age, and poverty. In every country there are people who are strong or weak, healthy or sick, and prosperous or poor irrespective of their beliefs in God and their religions. There are some whose lives seem to prosper and who apparently do not believe in a Supreme Being; yet there are many other good people who are religious and who are less fortunate.

If God is merciful, then how can He allow one man to suffer and another to have joy in the very same place and house, if both accept Him as the Almighty? Surely He cannot show favor to one and disfavor to another, if He is merciful and loving. Nor can we accept the theory that man goes eternally to hell or heaven, without any mercy from the all-merciful God. If an earthly father forgives his wicked son, then why not the Supreme Father who is all-loving, if He exists?

Our life on this planet may last one hundred years, of which some fifty are spent in sleep and dreams. Part of the time goes into infancy, which is almost a subconscious state. When disease and old age come, man's mental state deteriorates and, torn between fear and hope, he is almost living on a dream plane.

There is little time for man to understand his Father and evolve to a higher state of being. Before the majority of people are even able to believe in God, they are dead. Are we to believe then that because they could not bring themselves to lead a higher life in the short period of one life span, they are eternally doomed to suffer in hell? Is there then no chance for them to attain salvation?

Again it is too simple to assume that God is a man-making factory who manufactures new souls daily, which He sends to earth for suffering and pain, and finally dispatches to hell or heaven in an eternal cycle.

If there is no rebirth, what is the purpose of all knowledge and its institutions, such as libraries and laboratories, churches and temples? Why can we not spend our time as do animals or bushmen, without all this modern civilization? Why do we want to bring peace to the world and remove suffering through our effort, will, power, sympathy, and service? If there is no rebirth on earth after leaving the physical body, then why not annihilate the whole human race and its civilization with the new horror bombs? If there were no rebirth, man would not lose anything if the world were annihilated by a global war. No more souls would come to the earth; God could rest from His labors as he could not send new souls to an earth polluted by radiation, thus excluding an existence for man, animals, and plants. To answer these questions, we have to accept the law of *karma* or of action and reaction and of rebirth if we are rational beings.

Every soul learns in life through trial and error and corrects his mistakes as he progresses along the way. Every action, whether good or bad, bears fruit and man's future life and condition depend upon what he does at the present moment. Through sufferings he learns more with each birth, in each life cycle. As he learns more, he wants to know more about his existence, about God, and about the purpose of life. But this thinking comes to him only as he gradually evolves from the lower level of a life philosophy of eating, drinking, and merry-making.

Yoga philosophy holds not only the answer to all man's problems, but also offers a scientific way to transcend his problems and suffering. Moreover, Yoga philosophy does not quarrel with any religion or faith and can be practiced by anyone who is sincere and willing to search for the truth. There is no vague doctrine involved. Even comparatively little effort will bring immense returns of knowledge, strength, and peace.

# 2

# MAN, HIS THREE BODIES, AND THEIR FUNCTIONS

The spirit contains within it all potentialities and as man progresses he unfolds new powers and new qualities in his life.

Man can manifest and function upon several planes according to his evolution. The majority of people of this age can manifest only on the lower planes. Although every man, no matter how undeveloped, potentially possesses all the higher principles, the higher planes are utilized by a few advanced persons only.

Though the physical body is the lowest in the scale and the crudest manifestation of man, it is man's most essential principle for his growth in his present stage of development. The body, being the temple of the living spirit, should be carefully tended in order to make it a perfect instrument.

As we look around, we note that the physical bodies of different men show different degrees of development. Some are strong, others are weak; some are lean, while some are fat. It is the duty of each developed man to train his body to the highest degree of perfection so that it may be used to pursue the spiritual purpose.

One of the important teachings in Yoga philosophy is how to care for the body under the intelligent control of the mind. The sage, Patanjali, in his *Yoga Aphorisms,* defines Yoga as "a suspension of the modifications of the thinking principle which is obtainable through different methods such as controlling the vital breath and steady pose, both of which are intimately connected with the mind."

This connection is proved by our daily experiences. When one is absorbed in deep thought, breathing slows down. Suspension of the mental activity increases in proportion to the slowing down of the breath; in cases of asphyxia, mental activity ceases altogether until respiration is restored. Complete disappearance of the mind takes place with the death of the body.

These considerations prove that mind, vital breath, and the body are interdependent. Mind and body are the instruments through which we get all experiences.

There are various modes of Yogic practice whereby the mental modifications and the vital breath are brought under control, and God is realized in different ways. The prerequisites of all Yoga are morality, a spiritual disposition, and regular practice of Yogic exercises. One form of Yoga, Hatha Yoga, gives first attention to the physical body, which is the vehicle of the spirit's existence and activity. Purity of the mind is not possible without purity of the body in which it functions, and by which it is affected. So preference is given in Yoga philosophy to the mobilization of the body and the control of the vital breath.

We can divide Yoga as follows:

1. Directions for the purification of the body inside and outside.
2. Practice of postures.
3. Practice of *Mudras* and *Bandhas,* which are similar to the postures and produce a sort of electrical current or force, called *kundalini shakti* (Serpent Power).
4. Control of vital breath through Yogic breathing.
5. Stilling of the mind and its modifications by cutting off the sense perception.
6. Progression in mental control or concentration.
7. Meditation on various nerve centers, which makes the mind steady like a candle flame in a sheltered place.
8. The last stage, the superconsciousness, when the little ego "I" merges with the Supreme Ego or God.

The first three processes are to train the gross physical body. The next three steps, breathing, stilling the mind, and concentration, are to strengthen and control the second vehicle of the spirit, the astral body. Meditation, the seventh process, is used to transcend both the physical body and the astral body. Here the spirit operates in the causal body, the subtlest of the vehicles. In this body, spirit can express clearly and know its powers and potentialities because here the ego and mind function only to a limited degree.

In the final stage, there is no more bondage for the spirit. Here the spirit, as pure consciousness, has full expression as it has transcended all limitations and barriers of its vehicles of the bodies and mind. In this state, spirit or soul unites with God or the universal spirit.

Spirit or soul as such is the whole without any division. Mind and bodies, being the active power of the spirit which springs from it and brings individual consciousness, are parts of that whole. Thus consciousness or spirit, while remaining unchanged in one aspect, changes in another aspect into active power, manifesting as mind and body. In the final stage, the spirit becomes again aware of its real nature through the negation of the veiling principle, the mind-body.

We will now proceed to analyze the various bodies in which spirit operates.

The human organism consists of different and distinct parts, more or less indissolubly connected. *Stula*, the gross, *sukshma*, the subtle, and *karana*, the causal, are the names given to those which constitute different bodies of the pure Spirit or *Atman*. The first is the visible dense body containing particles of matter taken from the earth or physical plane, the lowest in our five-fold world system.

The matter of this plane too, like that of the other four, is of five grades, the three lower consisting of what is known as solid, liquid, and gaseous matter respectively. Of the remaining two, the higher consists of the atomic part of the physical plane, and the rest is etheric substance differing in density.

The visible part of the body is divided into two sheaths known as the *annamaya kosha*, the food sheath, and *pranamaya kosha*, or vital sheath. The *annamaya kosha* is formed of solid, liquid, and gaseous matter, while the vital sheath consists of the etheric particles and atoms, and is also the part in which the life principle in man primarily expresses itself. Though these sheaths are as a rule separable from each other, they are separated only in exceptional cases such as under chloroform or during a mesmeric trance, where partial and temporary severance between the two may occur.

The *pranamaya kosha* or vital sheath is similar to the form of the food sheath and is, therefore, spoken of as an etheric double. The two *koshas* finally part company and become disintegrated only at the so-called death state.

During sleep, the spirit leaves the food sheath, passing into the subtle body and resting in itself without any contact with the physical body, though both bodies are connected.

The etheric sheath or *pranamaya sharira* is not as well known as the physical body, although closely connected with it, and is its exact counterpart in appearance. This etheric or vital sheath has been known to people through the ages, giving rise to many superstitions and investigations. Composed of matter of a finer quality than that of our physical body, the vital sheath is its exact counterpart and may be separated from it under certain conditions. Ordinarily, separation is very difficult, but in persons with some degree of spiritual development owing to psychic function, the etheric body may be detached and often goes on long journeys.

This body continues to exist for some time after the death of the person to whom it belonged. It is visible to living persons under certain conditions. Commonly known as ghost, spirit, etc., it is invisible, but readily visible to those with clairvoyant powers. There is now ample proof that under favorable conditions the vital sheath of a dying person may be seen by friends and relations, and others close to him, the mental condition of the observer having, of course, much to do with it. The clairvoyant can see this sheath, counterpart of the physical body, rising from the physical body as the hour of death approaches. It is seen hovering over the physical body, to which it is bound by a slender thread. When the thread snaps, the person is dead and the soul passes on, carrying the other bodies with it.

It must be remembered that this sheath is but a finer grade of matter of the physical body, and merely a vehicle of the soul. In the post-mortem condition, as well as during sleep, the *jiva* or individual does not function on the physical plane called *bhu loka*, but spends his time on the next higher, the astral plane, *bhuvar loka*, whose matter is of course finer.

Of the vehicles or bodies used on this plane, two are grouped together under the name *sukshma sharira*, or astral body. One of these is made up of the five grades of matter of that plane, and it is in this vehicle that man's emotional nature has its play.

The other vehicle that lingers with it is composed of the matter of the gross lower subplanes of the *swar loka* or the fire plane; through it man exercises his ratiocinative faculty, as the two vehicles work together until they finally separate. They are known as one body under the name of *sukshma sharira, manomaya kosha,* or mental sheath. The final separation between the two occurs when the individual has dwelt in the *bhuvar loka* and the next plane for such a time as the nature of his last physical life warrants, and the moment for the dissolution of the emotional vehicle arises. Then it passes on to the *swar loka*, the next plane, the surviving part being the true mental vehicle.

After his stay in *swar loka* for such a period as he is entitled by his unblemished or virtuous physical life, man's mental vehicle also breaks up and he retires to the next plane, *maharloka*, situated in the three higher subplanes of the *agni* in its causal body.

This vehicle is comparatively permanent; its formation took place millions of years ago when the creature passed from the purely animal state to become a man. Since then it has been growing more or less, along with its physical body, which operates on the physical plane. Another name for this vehicle is *vijnanamaya kosha*, the body of knowledge par excellence, or intellectual sheath.

A vital distinction exists between the knowledge that the individual acquires through this intellectual sheath and that acquired through the lower *manomaya kosha*, the astral body. The knowledge gained by the latter is the product of a tedious and complicated process of reasoning that is apt to err, and this margin of error is increased by distortions arising from the action of the emotions on the reasoning process. This accounts for the division of the mind into a pure and impure state.

These three bodies are explained by His Holiness Swami Sivananda in the book *First Lessons in Vedanta*. "Ice represents a physical body, water represents the subtle body, and the steam represents the *karana sharira* or the seed body."

The physical body is composed of five elements, namely earth, water, air, fire, and space. Made of chyle, blood, flesh, fat, bone, marrow, etc., it is called *deha* in Sanskrit, because it decays in old age and has several stages of existence, which are birth, growth, change, decay, and death.

The subtle or astral body is made of nineteen elements, which are five organs of action, five vital airs, five organs of knowledge, and the four mental principles called mind, intellect, subconscious, and the ego. The astral body is a means of experiencing pleasure and pain. It is dissolved only when man reaches his final liberation wherein he becomes one with God.

The seed body is known as the *karana sharira* or causal body. The beginningless indescribable ignorance is called the causal body, because it is the cause of both the gross and subtle bodies.

Five sheaths cover the soul or the spirit. Just as a pillowcase covers a pillow, so the soul is covered by body, vital air, mind, intellect, and the causal body. These five sheaths are known as *annamaya kosha*, the food sheath; *pranamaya kosha*, the vital sheath; *manomaya kosha*, the mental sheath; *vijnanamaya kosha*, the intellectual sheath; and *anandamaya kosha*, the blissful sheath.

The *annamaya kosha* or the food sheath in the gross physical body is made of five elements: earth, water, fire, air, and space or ether. Made of food, it will finally become food again; for after the body is buried, it becomes food power for plants and animals.

The vital sheath is made of vital airs and five organs of action. The mental sheath is composed of the mind, subconscious, and five organs of knowledge, called *jnana indriyas* in Sanskrit. The intellectual sheath consists of intellect and ego, working with the five organs of knowledge or the sense organs of knowledge. The last one is the bliss sheath, because through it the individual soul experiences the effects of a good deed. When we sleep, we know joy, bliss, calmness, and peace, which are obtained through this sheath. By doing good actions, we experience joy.

The three attributes of the bliss sheath are known as *priya,* which is the joy experienced when looking at an object. Next is *moda,* the great joy felt when possessing the object one likes, and the *pramoda,* the greatest joy experienced after enjoyment of the object one likes.

These five sheaths are divided into three bodies, the physical, astral, and causal. The physical has only one sheath, the food sheath. The astral has three sheaths, the vital, mental, and intellectual, and the causal body has the last one, the blissful sheath.

In the waking state, when man functions with his physical body, all five sheaths are functioning. In the dream state the physical body never works, so man works with the four sheaths, which are the vital, mental, intellectual, and blissful. In deep sleep state he functions with one sheath only, the blissful sheath, or the *anandamaya kosha.*

Existence, birth, growth, change, decay, and death are the qualifications of the physical body. Hunger, thirst, heat, and cold are the qualifications of the vital sheath. Thinking, doubting, anger, lust, exhilaration, depression, delusion, etc., are the workings of the mental sheath. Discrimination and decisions are the functions of the intellectual sheath, and experience of happiness is the function of the *anandamaya kosha* or blissful sheath.

These different bodies and various sheaths cannot be understood by those whose minds are wrapped in material sheaths and who think that everything is only a chemical reaction of the brain. But no one can deny the existence of the subtler bodies of the soul, which operate in various bodies in various mental conditions.

In the next chapters we shall deal with practical and scientific ways to control the bodies or vehicles of the pure spirit.

The science of Yoga dates from the so-called prehistoric times, when man led a natural life and was not under the spell of modern civilization. The sages of India, seeing that each and every person must face death, disease, and old age, directed their attention toward finding a remedy for these conditions. Compared to primitive man, we are physical and mental wrecks, hence the need for us to practice Yoga is urgent.

Yoga science has two aspects: physical and spiritual. To a Yogi, health means absence of disease and of old age, for old age and death are the inevitable results of disease. Yoga aims to remove the root-cause of all diseases, not to treat its symptoms as medical science generally attempts to do.

It preaches a sane and natural manner of living which, if followed, will benefit everybody. Close to nature, it advocates a return to natural life in preference to the artificial living habits that we have developed. Yogic exercises were practiced by the ancients to perfect their bodies.

The casual observer who has seen the care, time, and attention that the Yogi bestows upon his body generally jumps to the conclusion that the Yogic philosophy is merely a form of physical culture expressed by "standing on one's head."

Far from this, Yoga philosophy teaches that real man is not his body, but that the immortal I, of which each human being is conscious to some degree according to his mental evolution, is not the body but merely occupies and uses the body as an instrument. It is written in the *srimad Bhagavad Gita* that the body is likened to a suit of clothing, which the spirit puts on and takes off from time to time as the old suit becomes worn. This fleshy covering is essential to man's manifestation and growth in this particular stage of his development. Though the Yogi gives great care and attention to the physical body, he goes beyond this point and brings the body under the control of the mind, both of which he finally uses for his final higher spiritual pursuits.

Saints of yore in India not only knew about the visible physical body and its functions but went beyond the physical plane and operated with subtler bodies. Their knowledge of mind and of its mysteries and functions is now recognized throughout East and West by those who deal with such subjects. Modern psychology of the mind is nothing compared to the ancients' understanding of it. Today's psychologists and scientists do not clearly understand the difference between the spirit, mind, and body. No one, of course, can really understand mind and soul as long as he experiments on the outside, not turning inward and stilling all his thoughts to watch his own mind and soul.

# 3

# YOGIC CLEANING OF THE PHYSICAL BODY

As we have seen, the expression of the spirit increases in proportion to the development of the body and mind in which it is encased. Therefor, Yoga prescribes methods to train and develop the physical body and mind. The highly trained body must first of all be strong and healthy. The goal of all Yogic teaching is how to concentrate the mind, how to discover its hidden facets, and how to awaken the inner spiritual faculties.

As we go deeper into Yoga, we find that it teaches that mind is only the body's finer part and both interact and each acts upon the other.

When one is angry, the emotions of the mind affect the body, which makes the eyes red, the fists clench, and the face fierce-looking. However, with most of mankind the mind is very little developed and is entirely under the control of the body. Even a superficial analysis will reveal that we have, in fact, very little command over the mind because the body exerts a powerful control over it.

By learning to control the body we can easily train the mind. The following facts prove the interdependence of the body and mind and their reactions upon each other.

By treating the body with modern shock therapy, mental symptoms are relieved. This was accidentally discovered by a psychiatrist who noted in certain patients a disappearance of mental symptoms, when they had suffered typhoid fever. The cause of this cure was revealed during experiments ten years later, when mental patients were injected with various fever-producing organisms. During the experiments, spectacular results were obtained when patients suffering from a syphilitic mental derangement were inoculated with malaria. Out of these and other experiments came shock therapy.

Disappearance of symptoms of mental disease was also noted when patients were injected with various substances, such as milk and foreign blood, which stimulate a strong reaction on the part of the body. This, in turn, helps to remove mental tension, showing clearly that body and mind are interconnected.

In order to gain control of body and mind, we must first have the help of certain physical exercises. After the body is sufficiently controlled, we can start training the mind. With the training of the mind, concentration power increases and we will be able to manipulate the internal forces and to find the basic unit from which the whole world is made.

The end and aim of science is to discover this unit from which all this manifold universe is being manufactured, the one intelligence that becomes many.

Part of the Yogic discipline is physical exercises, although the major part is mental. In Yoga, control of the body starts with cleaning processes known as *kriyas,* the first step to eliminate poisonous substances accumulated in the system.

The body is constantly throwing off waste materials through its mechanisms. Kidneys eliminate uric acid and other waste products, which come through the blood. Sweat glands remove waste materials through perspiration, which contains poisons. We throw away impurities of the body through various openings by means of perspiration, urine, excretion, and breathing. But for this excretory system, the body would be loaded with disease-carrying poisons.

Yoga pays great attention to removing waste materials which our organs are not able to throw off. In some cases, Yogic cleaning even assists nature in removing waste products.

We clean our skin daily, which keeps the pores of the skin open and free from dirt. Again, everybody brushes his teeth. But Yogic cleaning goes a little farther and cleans some of the important parts of the body that are generally neglected. These cleaning processes are scientific and hygienic and remove ailments caused by improper attention to these portions of the body.

Six *kriyas* are meant for cleaning the respiratory system, food pipe, stomach, eyes, and the lower colon. These exercises are specially prescribed for those who are flabby and phlegmatic. The names of these six *kriyas* are *dhauti, basti, neti, nauli, tratak,* and *kapalabhati,* or cleaning the stomach, cleaning the colon, cleaning the nasal passage, cleaning the abdominal organs, gazing exercise for the eyes, and cleaning the respiratory organs.

Dhauti is divided into four: (1) *antar-dhauti,* internal washing; (2) *danta-dhauti,* cleaning of the teeth; (3) *hrid-dhauti,* cleaning of the throat; (4) *moola-sodhana,* cleaning of the rectum.

Again, *antar-dhauti* or internal washing is divided into four parts: (a) wind purification; (b) water purification; (c) *agni-sara,* fire purification; (d) cloth purification.

## WIND PURIFICATION

This *dhauti* is a difficult process and is practiced only under the guidance of an expert. Moreover, to swallow air to the stomach by closing the epiglottis is a matter of training. Here the Yogi trains himself to close his epiglottis and, with a sudden push, he pushes a little volume of air to the stomach. He rests for a second and repeats the same process until his stomach is filled with air. Then slowly he belches the air along with the foul gases from the stomach.

## WATER PURIFICATION

Drink a large quantity of salt water and shake the abdominal portions. Contract the stomach and put the fingers at the root of the tongue and tickle until the water is vomited. The Sanskrit name for this process is *kunjar kriya.*

## AGNI SARA

The student sits with crossed legs and inhales deeply. Then with a forced exhalation he empties the lungs as much as possible. After the exhalation, he keeps the breath out for a few moments without inhaling. In this condition, his diaphragm is raised naturally to the thoracic cavity and he can manipulate the abdominal muscles. Again, as long as his diaphragm is in the raised position, he pumps the abdominal muscles inward and outward in a quick succession. In each round, when he empties his lungs, he pumps fifteen to twenty times without inhaling. This is one round. A student can practice ten rounds daily.

This exercise stimulates the liver, spleen, kidneys, and pancreas, reduces the abdominal fat, and removes constipation.

### CLOTH PURIFICATION

The alimentary canal is a long tube that extends from mouth to anus. It is made up of the mouth, pharynx, esophagus, stomach, small intestine, and large intestine. The greater part of the alimentary canal lies in the abdominal portion of the ventral cavity.

This cleaning process is very essential to remove mucus and other waste products from the esophagus and stomach. The general structural plan of the digestive tube is:

1. A lining of mucous membrane, in which there are numerous glands.
2. A submucous layer of loose connective tissue into which glands may penetrate from the mucous membrane and in which the main blood vessels are located.
3. Layers of smooth muscular tissue.
4. An outer layer, which is fibrous in nature.

The stomach is the most dilated portion of the digestive tube. It succeeds the esophagus. The inner surface of the stomach is thrown into folds called rugae, when the organ is empty. This is due to the looseness of the submucous layer and the action of the muscles. These inner linings of the stomach are covered with a coating of food products and waste materials from the food. Especially when there is accumulation of dirt on the stomach walls, there will be a feeling of sluggishness of the stomach and loss of appetite.

Acute indigestion usually follows the intake of substances that are obnoxious to the stomach. Consumption of too great quantities of food or a wrong diet may irritate the stomach lining or these substances may decompose in the stomach and thus initiate acute dyspepsia. A frequent cause is the taking of food that has begun to decompose, particularly in hot weather. Another common cause is the use of alcohol. The lining of such a stomach is swollen and reddened, covered with much mucus and, in some cases, there may be hemorrhage.

In mild cases, the symptoms are indigestion and an uncomfortable feeling in the abdomen, headache, depression, nausea, belching, and vomiting. Vomiting is nature's way to eliminate unwanted food and mucus from the stomach.

Dyspepsia is another common disease from which many persons suffer. Dyspepsia means difficult or painful digestion. The outstanding symptom of dyspepsia is abdominal discomfort or pain. The intensity of the sensation may vary in degree from a slight feeling of heaviness to agonizing pain almost beyond endurance. This occurs usually after meals. Again nature's remedy, vomiting, may sometimes give relief.

Another condition of the stomach, called gastroptosis, or falling of the stomach, is not uncommon. It occurs more often in women than in men. Small amounts of food satiate persons having gastroptosis and they have little desire for food after the first mouthful. This is apparently due to the inability of the food and secretions to get out of the stomach into the small intestine. Because of the stagnation and pressure caused by the drag of the stomach, the duodenum, the first part of the small intestine, becomes dilated. When substances are absorbed from the duodenum they may be poisonous, bringing on headache, dizziness, nausea, and lack of appetite.

The stomach is one of the major organs that may cause various diseases if it is not kept clean and healthy. Therefore, some of the Yogic cleaning practices are a practical help to keep it in good condition.

The cloth purification is practiced in the following way. Take a fine piece of muslin cloth, three inches wide and fifteen feet long. The borders should be well stitched and no pieces of loose thread should be hanging from its sides. Wash it clean with soap before use. Dip it in tepid salt water. Squeeze out the water and swallow one end of it little by little. On the first day, swallow only one foot of the length. Keep it there for a few seconds and then take it out very slowly. On the next day, swallow a little more, retain it a few minutes, then take it out slowly. Thus little by little you can swallow the whole length, being careful to catch the end firmly with the hands. Retain it for about two minutes and then remove it. Do not be hasty. Do not injure your throat by rough treatment. When this *kriya* is over, drink a cup of milk. This is a sort of lubrication for the throat. This exercise should be done with an empty stomach, preferably in the morning.

You need not practice this every day. Once in four days or once a week is sufficient. This exercise cannot do any harm at all, if gradually practiced. Everyone will feel a little vomiting sensation on the first two or three attempts. As soon as the *kriya* is over, wash the cloth with soap and dry it.

This is an excellent exercise for those who are flabby and have a phlegmatic constitution. Gradual, steady practice cures gastritis,

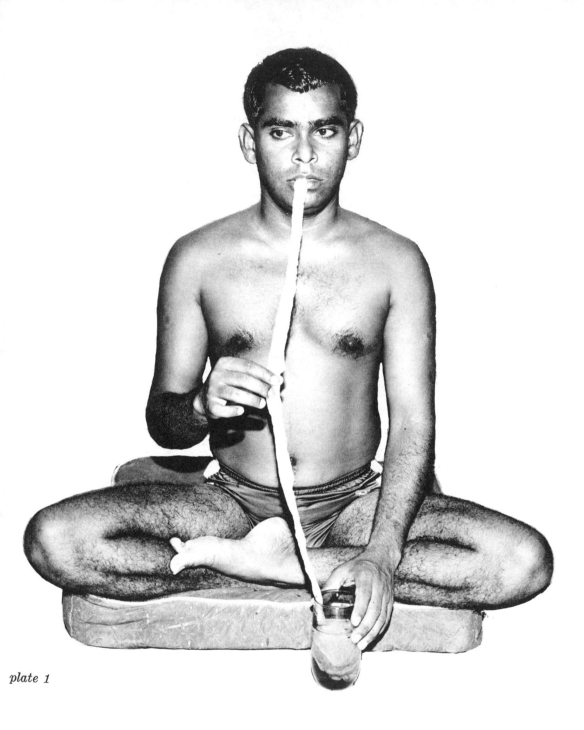

plate 1

dyspepsia, diseases of the stomach and spleen, disorders of phlegm and bile.

To get the cloth moving slowly without any difficulty, gulp down a little salt water along with the cloth. This will lubricate the esophagus and throat and enable the cloth to move smoothly.

To be on the safe side, always practice this cleaning in the early morning with empty stomach, preferably under the guidance of an able teacher.

## DANTA DHAUTI

*Danta dhauti* is cleaning of the teeth, which is commonly done by civilized man. Along with cleaning of the teeth, it is essential to give gum massage, which strengthens the gums and squeezes out the impure matter from the gum pores.

## HRID DHAUTI

For cleaning the tongue and root of the throat, join together the index, middle and ring fingers and insert them into the throat. Rub well the root of the tongue, wash it again, and repeat the process several times. Mouth washes and gargles with salt water are also essential to keep the throat free of infection.

There are general inflammations of the throat, associated with redness, swelling, and excessive discharge of mucus from many different causes. The most common causes are exposure to cold, an extension of inflammation from the tonsils or nose, use of tobacco, excessive exposure to dust, smoke, and irritating fumes; atmospheric conditions may cause irritation of the throat.

There may be severe pain associated with swelling and inflammation of the throat, including pain in the ears because of blocking of the tubes that lead from the nose to the ears. *Hrid dhauti* should be practiced daily with cleaning of the teeth and tongue.

With the thumb of the right hand, rub the depression in the forehead near the bridge of the nose. By this practice, diseases arising from derangements of phlegmatic humors are cured. These exercises purify the nervous system and clairvoyance is induced. They cure various abdominal diseases, enlarged spleen, some skin diseases, and disorders of phlegm and bile.

## KARNA DHAUTI (EAR CLEANING)

Various disturbances affect the canal up to the point of the eardrum. Under such circumstances, it is necessary to remove the infection and to prevent its recurrence by the use of proper cleaning. The wax of the ear is easiest removed, when it becomes hardened, by the use of a syringe with slightly warm water or with a piece of cotton. This need not be done often. Too frequent syringing may be harmful. Never put anything in the external ear such as wires, toothpicks, or ear spoons, as the tissues are most delicate and may be seriously harmed by such practice.

## MOOLA SODHANA (RECTUM IRRIGATION)

*Moola sodhana,* cleaning the lower colon with water, will be explained in the practice of *bhasthi.*

## NETI (NASAL CLEANING)

*Neti* is cleansing of the nasal passage of the respiratory system. The nose and pharynx establish connection between the respiratory system and the exterior. A part of the pharynx is used in common by the respiratory and digestive systems.

The respiratory system consists of the larynx, trachea, bronchi, and lungs. Its function is to permit air to come in close contact with the circulating blood so that gaseous exchanges can occur.

When we inhale air we also inhale dust particles and germs. To prevent this foreign matter from entering the lungs, nature has designed a filtering system. In the nostrils the tough hairs first filter the gross dust particles and prevent them from entering into the lungs. Secondly, the mucous membrane is ciliated and the cilia remove particles and germs from the air as it passes.

The cilia act together to remove fluids or particles that come in contact with the ciliated surface. The air is warmed and moistened as it passes through the nasal cavity and comes in contact with the mucous membrane.

The most important of the structures in the nose, from the point of view of disease, is the mucous membrane or tissue that lines the cavities. It is one of the most sensitive tissues in the body, and when bruised or hurt in any way it may give a person considerable trouble. It is common to incur minor infections, particularly in the hair follicles or in the roots of the hairs in the nose.

It is now generally well known that common pus-forming germs, such as staphylococcus and streptococcus, are widespread and easily get into the human body whenever they come in contact with a tissue that has been damaged. They may set up an infection that eventually may spread throughout the entire body.

To assist nature in cleaning such foreign matter in the nasal passage and the mucous membrane, string, water, and air are used by Yogis. These not only remove foreign matter, but prevent catching colds and keep the olfactory nerve in a healthy condition.

Before going into the technique, a small description of the structure of the nasal passage and pharynx will help the student to practice this cleaning in a scientific way. Although the nose and pharynx are not really parts of the respiratory system proper, they will be so considered here for convenience.

The pharynx is divided into parts; some of these are common to the digestive and respiratory system. The larynx, in addition to being a passageway for air, is used for the production of voice. Thus many organs that play a part in respiration serve other functions as well.

The nasal cavity is divided into two nasal fossae by the nasal septum. The roof of the nasal cavity is made up chiefly by the cribriform plate of the ethmoid bone. The floor is composed of the palatal processes of the maxillae and the horizontal processes of the palate bone. The walls of the nasal cavity are covered with periosteum and mucous membrane.

The next important thing to be noted here during the cleaning process is the pharynx. The pharynx is common to the respiratory and digestive systems in a part of its extent. It is a vertical tubular passage that extends from the base of the skull above to the beginning of the esophagus below. Anteriorly, it communicates with the nasal cavity; beneath this, with the oral cavity; and below this with the laryngeal cavity.

This communication between the nasal cavity and the oral cavity of the pharynx helps in cleaning this portion with a piece of special string. Half the string is hard enough to push through the nasal cavity until it touches the root of the throat. With the help of the fingers, the string is pulled out through the mouth. As the thread comes

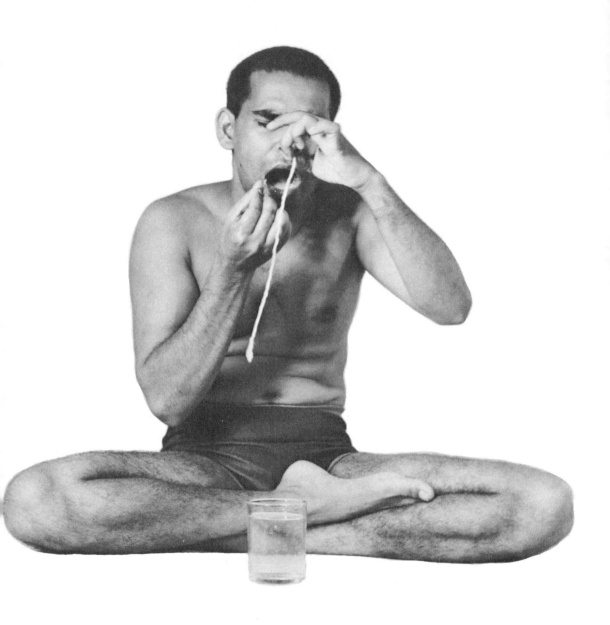

plate 2

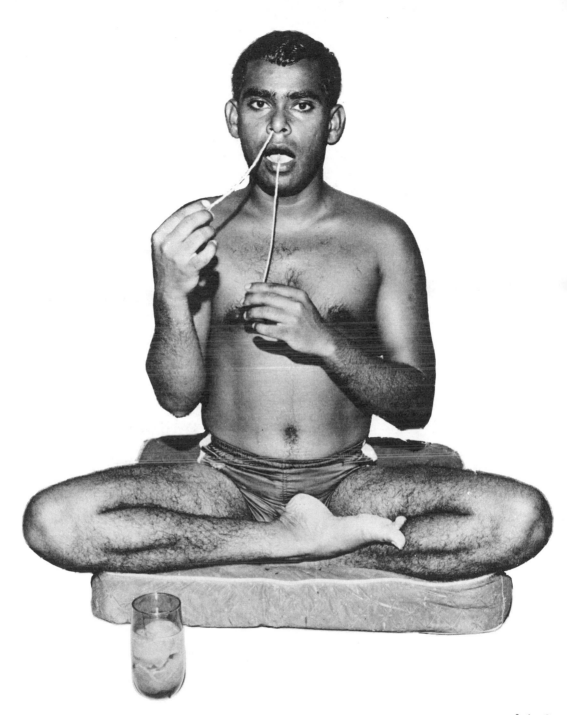

plate 3

out through the nasal passage, pharynx, and mouth, the other half of the string is soft enough to absorb and clean various foreign particles accumulated in its way. This is called thread *neti* or thread-cleaning technique.

If this special string cannot be obtained, then a rubber catheter, readily available at any drug store, can be used. The string or the catheter must be sterilized before use and should be thoroughly cleaned afterward. The string should be dipped in lukewarm salt water before insertion.

Take the stiff portion of the string first and bend it in a bowlike shape and, using the index finger and thumb, insert it into the right nostril first, a few inches inside, then withdraw it; then insert in the same manner into the left nostril.

It is common to sneeze violently for the first few days, but gradually the sneezing will subside as progress is made. It will be easier to insert the string as far as possible toward the throat. When the string is felt to be at the root of the tongue, with the index finger and thumb pull the end through the mouth and out until the whole string passes from the nostril. A few days' practice, with the help of a teacher, will perfect this technique.

There is another easy method of cleaning the nostrils that can be practiced without any difficulty. This is done with lukewarm salt water. To a glass of lukewarm water add a teaspoonful of common salt and stir well.

With the use of a nasal douche, which is available at any drug store, pour a small portion of the salt water through one nostril, closing the other with the thumb. Raise the head and allow the water to flow down to the throat and out of the mouth. Do not try to inhale the water as it brings an unpleasant sensation. Just allow it to flow to the mouth naturally, by keeping the head raised, then spit it out.

At this point, a small quantity of water will remain in the nasal passage, which must be blown out immediately by a forced expiration.

This process should be repeated three times with each nostril.

By practicing this, we can eliminate the very common disease, the common cold. Breathing becomes easier, hence it is preferable to do the breathing exercises after this cleaning. Besides removing foreign matter from the nasal passage and the throat, it also helps to strengthen the eyes because there is a stimulation of the blood vessels of the eyes and nose by this cleaning.

TRATAK (GAZING EXERCISE)

*Tratak* is steady gazing at a particular point or object without winking. Though this is one of the six purificatory exercises, it is mainly intended for developing concentration and mental focusing. It is very useful for students of Hatha Yoga, Jnana Yoga, Bhakti Yoga, and Raja Yoga. This practice helps also to improve eyesight.

On the following pages are shown three variations of the *Tratakam* technique:

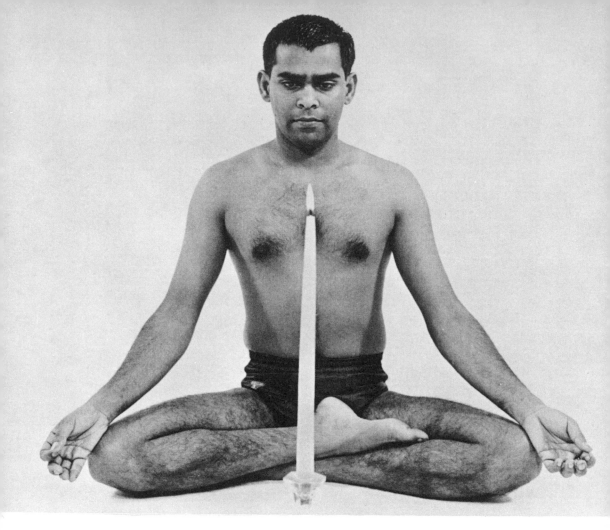

*plate 4*

## Technique:

### VARIATION 1

Keep a candle flame three to four feet away from your body. The level of your eyes and the candle flame should be in a horizontal line. Sit erect, keeping the spine straight and the body relaxed.

For one minute look upon the flame with a steady gaze and without winking. After a minute, close the eyes, relax the eye muscles, and visualize the flame between the eyebrows for a minute. Then again gaze with open eyes on the flame for awhile and then relax and close the eyes. This may be continued for five to six minutes. Gradually increase the period of gazing from one to three minutes, spending equal time relaxing the eyes. This exercise stimulates the nerve centers, brings concentration, and strengthens the eyes. Start doing it gradually.

# Technique: **Tratakam** [gazing exercise]

### VARIATION 2 : BHRUMADHYA DRISHTI [FRONTAL GAZING]

Advanced students start concentration by directing and turning the half-closed eyes toward the space between the eyebrows, which is also known as the third eye. By directing the gaze at this point the olfactory nerves and optic nerves are stimulated and, in turn, the autonomic nervous system and central nervous system are awakened. Done slowly, this exercise has a soothing effect on the cranial nerves and enables the mind to become one-pointed. Advanced students will find this exercise very useful as a breathing exercise and to awaken the *kundalini sakthi*. However, one should avoid too much strain on the eye muscles. Prolonged practice without the guidance of a teacher may affect the eye muscles as well as the nervous system. The same caution should also be taken in nasal gazing. In the beginning, practice for a minute or two and gradually increase to ten minutes, without strain.

*plate 5*

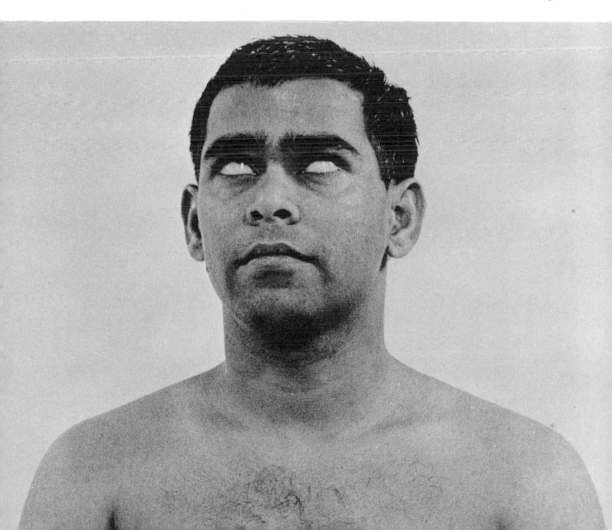

# Technique: **Tratakam** [gazing exercise]

## VARIATION 3 : NASAGRA DRISHTI [NASAL GAZE]

Sit in a comfortable position with body relaxed and gaze at the tip of the nose for one or two minutes. Avoid too much strain during practice; if you feel any pain or tiredness, close the eyes and relax the eye muscles. Repeat practice and relaxation a few times. This strengthens the eye muscles and increases concentration power by fixing all the attention toward the tip of the nose and through it to the central nervous system. In the frontal gaze the eyeballs are turned upward, and in the nasal gaze the eyeballs are turned toward the tip of the nose. Some people will find the nasal gaze easier than the frontal; to some the reverse will be the case. Choose any of the gazing exercises, according to your teacher's advice.

*plate 6*

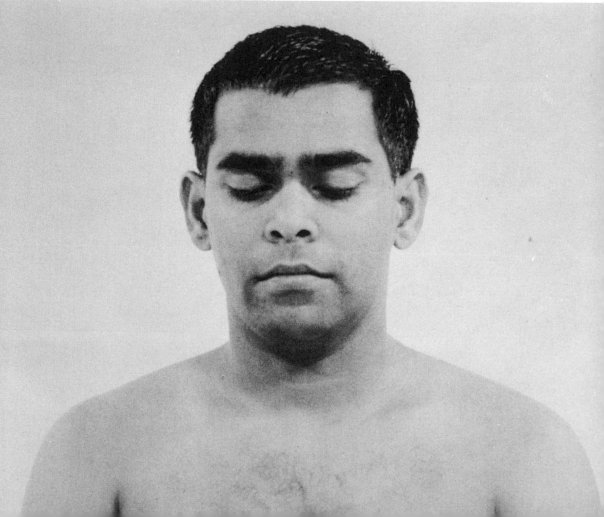

KAPALABHATI (DIAPHRAGMATIC BREATHING)

*Kapalabhati* is an exercise for the purification of the nasal passage and lungs. Though this is one of the six purificatory exercises, it is a variety of *pranayama* (breathing exercises).

This is especially used to control the movements of the diaphragm and to remove spasm in bronchial tubes. Consequently, persons suffering from asthma will find this very helpful. It also aids in curing consumption, removes impurities of the blood, and tones up the circulatory and respiratory systems.

*Kapalabhati* is the best exercise to stimulate every tissue of the body. After and during the practice, a peculiar vibration and joy can be felt, especially in the spinal centers. When the vital nerve current is stimulated through this exercise, the entire spine will be like a live wire and one can feel the movement of the nerve current.

Great quantities of carbon dioxide gas are eliminated. Intake of oxygen makes the blood richer and renews the body tissues. Moreover, the constant movements of the diaphragm up and down act as a stimulant to the stomach, liver, and pancreas.

Before learning some of the higher breathing exercises such as *bhastrika pranayama*, it is very important to master *kapalabhati*; *bhastrika* breathing is considered to be the best breathing exercise for awakening the spiritual power after the purification of the *nadis* or nerves.

TECHNIQUE. After taking a comfortable sitting position, preferably the lotus pose, take a few deep breaths. See that the diaphragm is moving properly. (Movement of the diaphragm is explained in the chapter on breathing exercises.) During inhalation, the diaphragm descends and the abdomen is pushed out. During exhalation, the diaphragm pushes the lungs up and the abdomen goes toward the spine. This constant up-and-down movement of the diaphragm throws the air in and out. Here more attention is focused on exhalation than inhalation.

Sudden contraction of the abdominal muscles raises the diaphragm and in turn a volume of air is forced out of the lungs. This is an inward stroke of the abdomen. As soon as the air is thrown out, relax the abdominal muscles, which in turn allows the diaphragm to descend. As the diaphragm comes down, a volume of air automatically rushes in. Here, inhalation is passive and exhalation active.

Start one round of this exercise with ten or fifteen expulsions. At the end of ten expulsions, take a deep inhalation and hold the air as long as possible. This will add its oxygen value and bring a peculiar, pleasant vibration throughout the body, as though you are bathing every tissue of the body with energy. A few days' practice will convince you of its wonderful, stimulating sensation.

Practice three rounds in the beginning, each round consisting of ten expulsions, and gradually increase the number of rounds to five or six. After a few weeks' practice, increase the expulsion to twenty or twenty-five. Between successive rounds, normal respiration is allowed to give the needed rest.

*plate 7*

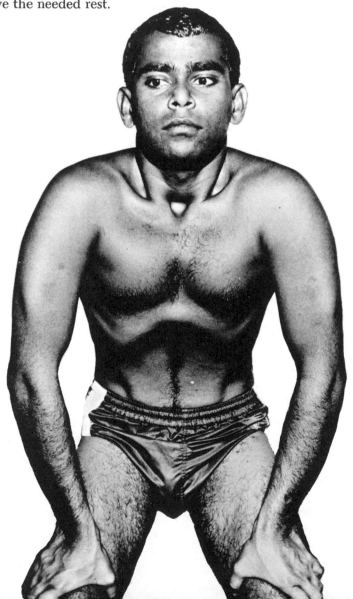

During the practice, concentrate on the solar plexus and eventually the nervous system will become spiritually active. This will be manifested by a throbbing sensation in the spine and a lightness throughout the entire body.

## UDDIYANA BANDHA AND NAULI
## (ABDOMINAL CONTRACTION)

*Uddiyana bandha* and *nauli* are exercises to strengthen the abdominal muscles and to remove sluggishness of the stomach, intestines, and liver. The muscles of the abdominal wall protect the abdominal viscera and assist in regulating the thoracic pressure in breathing. These muscles aid in micturition or emptying the bladder and defecation or emptying the bowels. There are six pairs of muscles in the abdominal wall.

In man, owing to his upright position, the pressure of the weight of the abdominal viscera falls on the ventral part of the line of attachment of the abdominal wall to the pelvis. As he stands, any weak places in this portion of the wall will be subjected to strain.

The places that are weak are known as the abdominal inguinal ring, the subcutaneous inguinal ring and the umbilicus, and the femoral ring. These weak places are generally the seat of hernia, owing to the pressure of the abdominal viscera. A rupture may occur in any of these places, which is called hernia, or the ring through which protrusion of an organ takes place. When the loss of tone in the abdominal muscles occurs, any act that increases the pressure within the abdomen, such as coughing or lifting, may bring abdominal hernia.

If the pelvis and vertebral column are fixed, the abdominal muscles assist in expiration by compressing the lower part of the thorax. If the pelvis alone is fixed, the thorax is bent directly forward and the muscles of both sides act together. If the muscles of one side contract, the trunk is bent toward that side and rotated toward the other side. Therefore, the action of the abdominal muscles depends on the point of fixation and actions change by fixing the muscles as stated above. This can be verified by trying the above described movements.

*Uddiyana bandha* and *nauli* are the best exercises for strengthening the abdominal muscles that assist in elimination of waste products. Moreover, manipulation of these muscles increases circulation.

TECHNIQUE. To practice *uddiyana bandha,* first of all one has to empty the lungs by a strong and forcible expiration. When the lungs are empty, the diaphragm rises naturally to the thoracic cavity. Now there is no interference by the diaphragm; during this time, draw up the intestines and the navel toward the back, so that the abdomen rests against the back of the body high in the thoracic cavity. This can be practiced in either a sitting or a standing position. While standing, place your hands firmly on the thighs, keep the legs apart, and bend your trunk slightly forward. Do not attempt to hold the abdomen too long in this position. Keep the abdomen in this position as long as you can hold the breath comfortably outside without inhaling. This can be repeated five to eight times with brief intervals.

*plate 8*

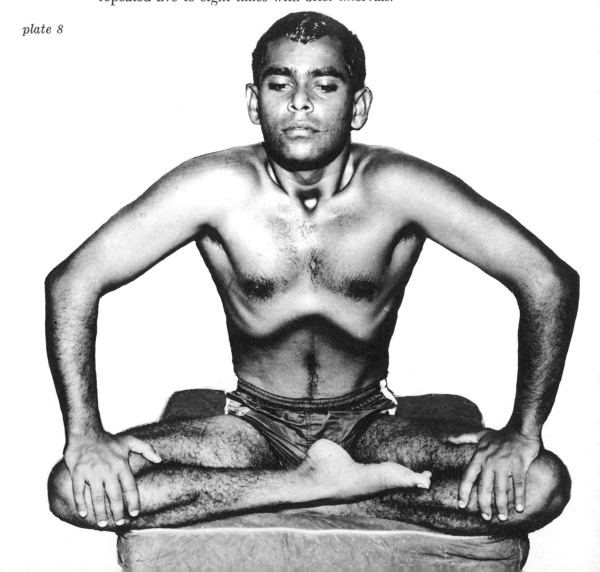

## NAULI KRIYA (MANIPULATION OF THE ABDOMINAL MUSCLES)

When the student is able to do the *uddiyana bandha* or abdominal contraction perfectly, then only is it possible to practice this exercise. For beginners, it takes some time to master this, as various abdominal muscles have to be brought under control. This is intended for regenerating, invigorating, and stimulating the abdominal viscera and the gastrointestinal or alimentary system.

TECHNIQUE. Here also the same technique of *uddiyana bandha* should be applied. While standing, practice *uddiyana* abdominal contraction first; while in this position, allow the center of the abdomen to be free by contracting the left and right sides of the abdomen. This position will bring the abdominal muscles in a vertical line. This is *madhyama nauli* (central contraction).

After mastering the central *nauli*, the next step is to get control over the left and right muscles of the abdomen separately. This is known as *vamu* and *dakshina nauli* (left and right contraction). The technique is the same as the central one, except that one has to apply more pressure on the thighs with the hands. If the left side is contracted, then the left hand presses on the thigh, the trunk bending slightly forward and to the left. The opposite applies to the right side.

All these processes of *uddiyana*, central, left, and right *nauli* are called churning or rotating of the abdominal muscles. This churning of the abdominal muscles is done in a quick succession of manipulating the abdominal muscles from the central *nauli* to the left and then to the right with *uddiyana bandha*. All the above processes combined bring wonderful control over the abdominal muscles.

The success of these exercises depends on the abdominal muscles. Before practicing *uddiyana* and *nauli*, one has to lose excess fat by other Yogic exercises mentioned in this book.

It is an interesting study to see the two types of abdomen. In some cases abdominal muscles are very tight, whether there is fat or not. Those who have this type of abdomen find it very difficult to practice this until they loosen their muscles. In the second group, persons who have rather loose muscles can control them in a short time.

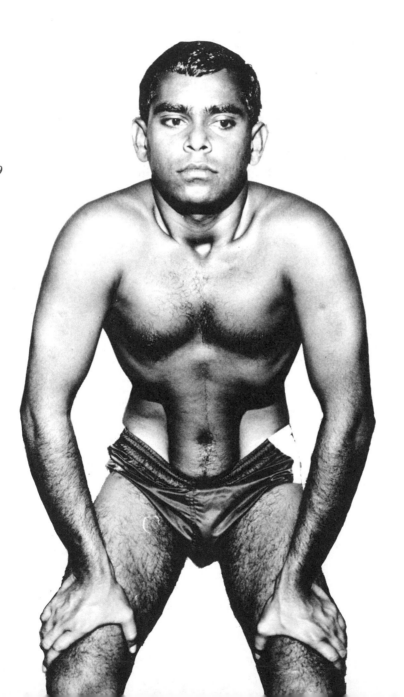

*plate 9*

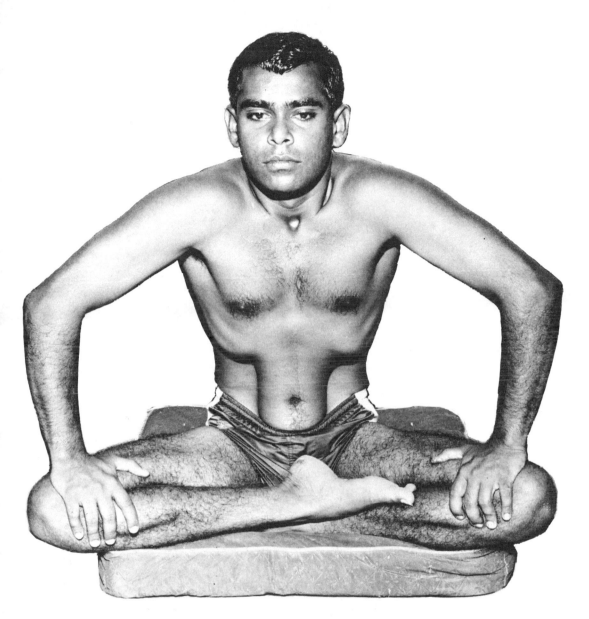

*plate 10*

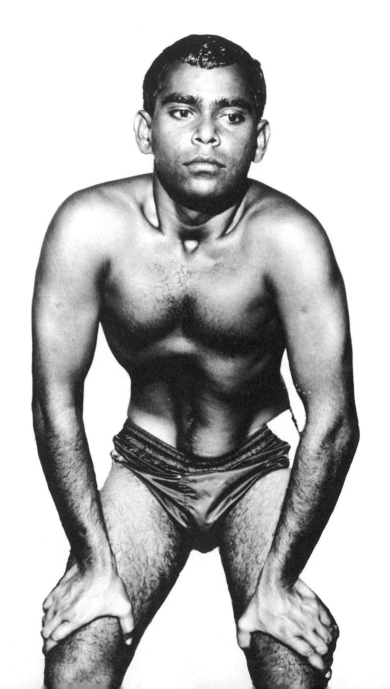

*plate 11*

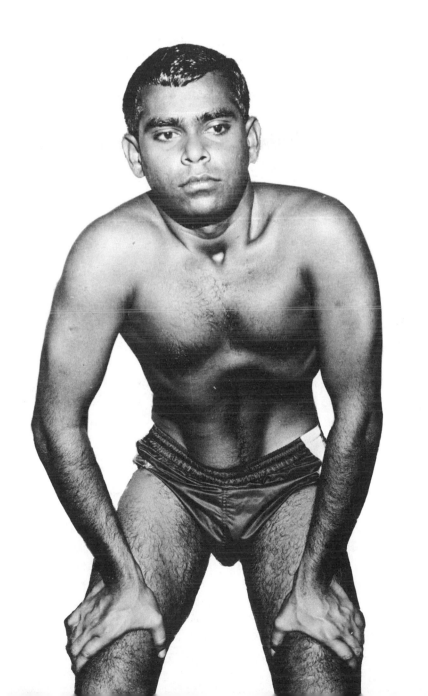

plate 12

BASTI (CLEANING OF THE LOWER INTESTINES)

The large intestine is divided into the cecum, ascending colon, transverse, descending, and sigmoid colon and rectum.

The cecum is a pouch hanging downward at the junction of the ileum and colon. The appendix is attached to the cecum. The ascending colon extends from the cecum to the underside of the liver, where it bends and becomes the transverse colon. The transverse colon crosses the abdomen, bends, and becomes the descending colon. Between the descending colon and the rectum is the sigmoid colon. The rectum begins from the end of the sigmoid colon and the canal continues beyond the rectum proper as the anal canal.

Mass movements occur in the colon. These are secondary to the peristaltic waves in the small bowel. In man the pelvic colon becomes filled with feces from below upward; the rectum remains empty until just before evacuation. It takes about twenty-four hours for waste material to reach the rectum.

The products of digestion are practically absorbed by the time food has reached the end of the small intestine or ileocecal sphincter. However, if an individual eats large quantities of fruits and green vegetables, much of the unabsorbed food reaches the large intestine. A small amount of this may be absorbed by the large intestine and the rest passes out with the feces.

The absorption of any food substance by the large intestine is much slower than by the small intestine. After giving an enema, a certain amount may in some cases enter backward into the small intestine and become absorbed. Persons with constipation and other intestinal ailments are advised to practice cleaning of the lower colon by a natural method, known as *basti*.

TECHNIQUE.    The *basti* process of cleaning is done by creating a vacuum in the intestines by which water is drawn to the lower colon. We all know the purpose of an enema and how it is operated. The difference between the enema and *basti* is that the former is caused by water pressure, and the latter by creating a natural vacuum without any external means. The vacuum is created by the *nauli kriya* through the central manipulation of the abdominal muscles as described elsewhere in this book.

Sitting in a tub of water and practicing *nauli* creates a vacuum by which water is drawn to the large intestine. To keep the sphincter muscles open, insert a small tube about four inches in length into the rectum. As soon as the water is drawn, the tube should be removed and then, with a few abdominal churnings (*nauli*), the water is thrown out from the large intestine with mucus and other waste products.

This cleaning strengthens the abdominal muscles, cures urinary and digestive disorders, and chronic constipation.

From the moment of birth until death, the question of the daily bowel movement is very important. Chronic constipation might produce various ailments and, therefore, it should be checked. Causes of constipation are:

1. Failure to pay attention to the desire for bowel movement.
2. Lack of enough residual material to form stool to excite activity.
3. Lack of sufficient vegetables and fruits in the food.
4. Lack of fluid by not drinking sufficient water.
5. Muscles necessary for expelling the bowel contents are too weak to act.
6. The habitual use of purgatives is a frequent cause of constipation. Owing to irritation, the colon becomes contracted and tight or the colon becomes too weak by overstimulation. The laxative medicines of today, which come in such tempting forms as candy and chocolates, should be avoided altogether. Frequent use of such laxatives by children is the main source of stubborn constipation in later years.

Individuals resort to different methods to relieve constipation. Just as the colon can be abused with laxatives, so can it be abused by irritating enemas.

In the practice of *basti* or Yogic cleaning of the bowels, there is no such irritation. Here water is drawn to the colon by the vacuum created by the abdominal contraction; hence there is no damage or overfilling with water. Moreover, it is absolutely natural.

The *basti* cleaning may be practiced once in a week or twice monthly.

This is the last exercise in Yogic cleaning. With these Yogic cleaning processes, we can eliminate almost all the poisons from our bodies.

Now we shall proceed to the second stage in Yoga practice, that of the Yogic exercises.

# 4

# DIFFERENCES BETWEEN YOGIC EXERCISES AND PHYSICAL CULTURE

The previous chapter dealt scientifically with an elaborate cleaning process of the various systems. The Yogi regards the physical body as an instrument for his journey toward perfection.

There are numerous modern physical culture systems designed to develop the muscles. Physical culturists develop them by mechanical movements and exercises. Yogic exercises not only develop the body, but also broaden the mental faculties. Moreover, the Yogi acquires mastery over the involuntary muscles of his organism.

The fundamental difference between Yogic exercises and ordinary physical exercises is that physical culture emphasizes violent movements of the muscles, whereas Yogic exercises oppose violent muscle movements as they produce large quantities of lactic acid in the muscle fibers, thus causing fatigue. The effect of this acid and the fatigue it causes is neutralized by the alkali in the muscle fibers, as well as by the inhaling of oxygen.

It is on this theory that modern physical culturists work. They try to increase the intake of oxygen so that fatigue may be lessened while working. Although their theory seems sound enough, the founders of the Yoga system for many centuries possessed a knowledge superior to all modern theories. The Yoga system is not new; it had been taught for many centuries before the modern systems were conceived.

Muscular development of the body does not necessarily mean a healthy body, as is commonly assumed, for health is a state when all organs function perfectly under the intelligent control of the mind.

Rapid movement of the muscles causes a tremendous strain on the heart. In the Yogic system, all movements are slow and gradual with proper breathing and relaxation. Carbon dioxide and other metabolites are produced by active muscles. A moderate excess of these substances stimulates the heart to beat more strongly, so exercises produce their own essential heart stimulant.

During exercise, more blood is returned to the heart than during rest. This is due to an increased venous return, which the contracting skeletal muscles introduce into the flow of blood. The pressure on the vessels by the contracting muscles pushes the blood along and the venous valves prevent the backward flow. The blood must move on toward the heart when pushed by the active muscles; as a result, the heart is better filled, which in turn stretches the fibers. When the fibers are stretched they contract more forcibly, which means a stronger heartbeat and more blood being pumped out. The more forceful contraction owing to stretching of the muscles was discoved by the physiologist Starling and is called Starling's law of the heart.

The heart, the most important organ, starts beating in the embryo even before nerves have grown out to it and it continues working until the last moment of man's life. Therefore, it is advisable to avoid strenuous exercises that put extra strain upon it.

The main purpose of exercise is to increase the circulation and the intake of oxygen. This can be achieved by simple movements of the spine and various joints of the body, with deep breathing but without violent movement of the muscles.

As the exercises are meant for increasing circulation through the motion of skeletal muscles and to increase the intake of the oxygen, let us take a hasty glance at the function of the muscles in heavy and moderate exercises like Yogic exercises.

When muscles contract glycogen breaks down to lactic acid and additional energy is released. This energy is used for the reforming of organic phosphates from inorganic phosphates and/or organic compounds. One-fifth of the lactic acid so produced is oxidized to carbon dioxide and water, energy again being released. This last batch of energy is utilized in the reformation of glycogen from the remaining four-fifths of the lactic acid. Fatigue is the result of the muscles' inability to get enough oxygen to oxidize a sufficient amount of the lactic acid formed. When too much lactic acid accumulates, the muscles become temporarily unable to contract. During the strenuous exercises, for instance, we are unable—even though respiration is deeper and faster—to breathe in sufficient oxygen to meet muscular demands. An oxygen debt is created. This debt is the difference between the amount of oxygen actually needed by the active muscles and what is actually received. Thus, after the completion of the exercise, we continue to breathe deeper and faster than we do ordinarily at rest, in order to repay the oxygen debt.

What happens in moderate exercise? With the beginning of moderate exercise like housework, walking at moderate speed, etc., the skeletal muscles become more active than before. A series of events occurs which results in a greater flow of blood carrying an increased supply of oxygen and fuel to the active muscles. As muscle activity increases, muscle metabolism does likewise. The increased metabolism means greater heat production. The warming of the muscles lowers their viscosity and increases the efficiency of the work they perform. Body temperature probably will not rise appreciably. The warmed blood leaving the muscles will shortly reach the heat-lowering center in the hypothalamus. Reflex dilation of skin vessels will allow more heat loss by radiation, balancing the increased heat production.

The increased muscle metabolism will also mean a greater output of carbon dioxide, resulting from the increased oxidation of glucose. Increased amounts of carbon dioxide will diffuse into the smaller blood vessels of the muscle fibers causing the walls of these vessels to relax. Their consequent dilation will allow more blood to flow more quickly through the skeletal muscles.

The increased amount of carbon dioxide in the blood will not only exert local action but will, in its travels, help to coordinate the general responses of the circulatory and respiratory systems with the demands placed upon them. Upon reaching the heart, the carbon dioxide directly stimulates the cardiac muscle to stronger contractions. The more forceful beat of the muscle will result in an increased output of blood per beat.

The increased carbon dioxide concentration in the blood flowing through the medulla of the brain directly stimulates the respiratory center. In turn, the respiratory center responds with an increase in the frequency of the impulses it rhythmically discharges. The greater number of impulses which eventually reach the diaphragm and intercostal muscles induce stronger than usual contractions. Thus breathing becomes deeper.

Stimulation of the vasoconstrictor center sends impulses along vasoconstrictor nerves to the arterioles of the abdominal cavity. Construction of the many arterioles in this region significantly increases the peripheral resistance and the general arterial blood pressure rises. Constriction of these blood vessels also serves to shunt blood from the abdominal organs to the skeletal muscles whose vessels are dilated. The increased number and force of skeletal muscle contractions squeeze down upon the veins more vigorously and thus help to pump blood back to the heart more quickly. The respiratory pump also aids in this; deeper breathing means greater fluctuation of the pressures within the thoracic and abdominal cavities. The alternating expansions and compressions of the large veins in these cavities will be increased in force and more blood will be forced onward to the heart.

The increased return of blood to the heart stretches the heart muscle, increasing its force of contraction and, thereby, its output per beat. The faster heart rate plus the stronger contractions of the cardiac muscle increase the cardiac output per minute and this, in turn, aids in producing the rise in blood pressure. Faster and deeper breathing ventilates the lungs more thoroughly. A greater amount of carbon dioxide is thus removed in the expired air, which prevents its concentration from rising too high in the blood because too much carbon dioxide can increase the acidity of the blood to a dangerous extent.

During exercise the active muscles oxidize more glucose and do it more rapidly than before, because of the increased temperature in them. This tends to deplete the blood sugar concentration. Since the sugar in the blood is in equilibrium with the glycogen in the liver, a fall in blood sugar concentration causes more glycogen to break down into glucose, which is released into the blood. As the muscles drain more glucose from the blood, more is poured into it from the liver. Some of the lactic acid formed in the breakdown of glucose also gets into the blood, is carried to the liver, and is there converted to glycogen. There is an adequate mechanism, then, for supplying fuel to the active muscle. In moderate exercise the oxygen supply can keep pace with the oxygen used and no oxygen debt results. The only residual effects will be a depletion of the carbohydrate reservation and a need for more protein to be used in rebuilding the cells that broke down in activity.

As we prepare to take strenuous exercise, there usually is a mental and emotional warming up. The memories and emotion caused by previous experiences, especially if the exercise involves competition of one sort or another, stir up the nervous system to an increased "tone." This helps to ready the body for the demands soon to be placed upon it. The subjective feelings may induce autonomic effects; a quickened pulse, faster breathing, and dilation of the pupils are not uncommon at times like this.

The many changes previously described for moderate exercise take place in strenuous exercise, too. You might imagine there would be even more, but where differences occur they are mainly differences in degree rather than in kind. The heart rate is faster, blood pressure higher, respiration faster and deeper, and circulation time more rapid than in moderate exercise.

Adrenaline may be released from the adrenal medulla and aid in the respiratory and circulatory changes. It would also favor the release of glucose from liver glycogen and delay fatigue of skeletal muscles.

The greatest limiting factor for the maintenance of severe exertion is the oxygen supply. Even though the spleen is stimulated to contract and discharge red blood cells into the blood, the intake of oxygen cannot meet the muscular demands for it, consequently, lactic acid is accumulated in muscle and in blood. Without sufficient oxygen to reconvert, fatigue sets in. There is a limit to the size of the oxygen debt that an individual can incur and here is where the Yogi emphasizes slow-motion exercises.

In the laboratory the usual and best all-round method for measuring efficiency is to have the subject breathe in air from the atmosphere and to expire it into a portable bag during the time he is doing work. A set of valves in the tube connecting the mouthpiece with the bag is used for this method of breathing and collection. After the test period, the gas volume is measured and its contents are analyzed for the respiratory gases. It can then be calculated that a certain amount of oxygen was consumed. It is known that oxidation involving a unit of oxygen can perform a definite amount of work. By dividing this value into the work done (which is measured indirectly), experts arrive at the efficiency.

What factors modify or influence the efficiency of a muscular act? There are five important ones—the initial stretch of the muscles, temperature, the viscosity of the muscles, the speed performance, and fatigue.

It has been noted that stretching a muscle before it contracts enables it to contract more forcibly. A stretched muscle can, therefore, perform more work than one only normally relaxed.

It has been proved that more work is done in lifting moderately heavy weights than in lifting lighter or heavier ones. Thus, moderately loading a muscle is the most efficient way of getting the most work done. When not stretched enough, the muscle is not very efficient.

By viscosity is meant internal friction, the friction resulting when molecules rub against the framework of the muscles fiber during contraction and retard the contraction process. Part of the energy developed during contraction must be used in overcoming this internal resistance. Viscosity thus decreases efficiency. It has been shown that when a muscle contracts slowly, less energy is required to perform a given amount of work than when it contracts rapidly. The greater the rapidity of contraction, the faster the fluid protoplasm flows through the structural framework of the muscle fiber and the more friction develops. Although viscosity is wasteful of efficiency, it is really an inherent factor of safety. It acts as a brake to prevent muscles from responding so fast as to tear themselves apart.

From what has just been said about viscosity, it must be apparent that there is some optimal speed of muscular contraction which is most efficient. Too great a speed of contraction results in little work, because of increased internal friction and consequent lowered efficiency. Too slow a speed, on the other hand, although it permits a large amount of work to be done, results in the expenditure of much energy in maintaining the contracted state; efficiency is again low. A moderate speed of performance is, therefore, most efficient. It is now being recognized that driving a man at his work to the point of exhaustion is not practical, with regard to the health of the individual, or with respect to getting more and better work done.

Much of the increased efficiency is due to the increase in co-ordination and sureness of performance that training develops. These effects depend upon the central nervous system.

The untrained subject will stumble, both mentally and physically, more often than the trained. The increased confidence that better performance brings with it, plus the increased coordination, will result in economical and efficient activity in which the Yogic exercises are performed.

Though not all of you have the desire to emulate the prowess of the trained Yogi, you can, knowing that it is largely a matter of training, increase your own efficiency for, perhaps, less strenuous tasks we have to do. Moderate and consistent Yogic exercises, aside from making you feel better and relaxed, can help your body to become more adequate for the demands placed upon it. Moreover, a well-trained body helps a great deal to train the mind, which is the main purpose of all Yoga, in order to attain complete freedom and immortality, which is the aim of all religions of the world.

By properly following the Yogic exercises, we can check the accumulation of toxic acids and can eliminate them if already over-accumulated in the blood itself. The following is an extract from a medical journal: "The chief killer is a disease known as arteriosclerosis or hardening of the arteries. The arteries become stiffened; their inner walls are lined with a coating of calcium. Sometimes they clog and crack and the person then dies of a stroke. Or they overwork the heart by trying to force blood through tubes narrowed due to calcium deposits and cause heart failure."

It now becomes clear that Yogic exercises can help to increase circulation and keep arteries elastic.

Not long ago, a physician made a study of three hundred men and women who had long been victims of chronic fatigue. Some had come to him suspecting that the root of their trouble was infected teeth, low blood pressure, flat feet, or anemia. But practically none suspected what was really causing the fatigue. The doctor found the most common causes of fatigue were heart trouble, diabetes, kidney infections, and glandular disorders. Most of these symptoms could be easily removed with natural diet, relaxation, breathing, and Yogic exercises.

The elasticity of the muscles also plays an important part in keeping the body youthful. The abnormal accumulation of fat, which is evenly or unevenly distributed in the muscular system in relation to strenuous exercise or inactivity, results in the hardening of the body's muscular tissues.

Yogic exercises pay great attention to the spinal column and other joints. Moreover, they maintain an even supply of blood to every part of the body.

The elasticity of the arteries also plays an important role in preserving health for it maintains the pressure between beats of the heart. It keeps the blood flowing steadily. The flow of the blood would be intermittent with nonelastic arteries; a spurt would appear with each systole. With elastic arteries, the blood is forced steadily along the capillaries and veins.

Without a proper blood supply, the different tissues cannot be kept in good condition. For example, the application of a tight bandage interferes with the circulation of the blood, lowers the temperature of the part that is poorly supplied, and causes a swelling. In normal cases, severe symptoms like swelling may not appear, but the various tissues cannot be kept in a healthy condition and efficiency to carry out various activities alloted to them diminishes without proper circulation.

## MOBILIZATION OF THE JOINTS

If we study such animals as dogs and cats, we notice that they often stretch and contract their spines after awakening. Infants move their spines naturally in a variety of positions. Flexibility of the spine is lost as the body grows. The first indication of ossification of the bones is noted in the eighth week of intrauterine life. Long after birth, the final stages in the replacement of the cartilage by bone occurs. Bones continue to grow in circumference by the deposition of new bone from the deeper layers of the periosteum, on the external surface. The cessation of growth of bone occurs at about eighteen years of age in girls and soon after twenty in boys.

In addition to supporting the framework, the skeleton provides places of attachment for muscles, tendons, and ligaments. Above the pelvis are piled twenty-four vertebrae. The framework of the body not only stands, but bends, sways, and twists.

The movements are restricted for most persons, owing to biologic shortening of ligaments. The average individual can no longer touch the floor with his fingertips when his knees are straight, even at the age of twenty. This type of ligamentous stiffening can be kept at a minimum through Yogic exercises and the body will be as pliable as a child's, even at the age of eighty.

The bindings in man are known as ligaments, which are bands or sheets of fibrous tissues, connecting two or more bones, cartilages, or other structures. If posture and balance are good, the ligaments have a long and elastic life. If not, they cause discomfort, pain, and trouble. Therefore, it is essential that we examine the nature, function, and mobility of the spine and its ligaments that play a prominent role in Yogic postures.

As man grows older, his backbone stiffens because the ligaments become tighter. It must be remembered here that the ligamentous structures are continuous and if mobility is restricted in any area, the entire attachment is affected; this brings general immobility of the body.

Excessive stiffness can be due to different causes, but especially to faulty body alignment and poor balance, which cause shortening of the ligaments. Shortening of the ligaments in the vertebral column can be noticed in those who sit a good part of the time, such as students, office workers, writers, and artists. This is because persons in a sitting position thrust the head and neck forward and cause the spine to compensate by forming a round back.

When an individual resumes the erect position of the spine while either sitting, standing, or walking, there may be some severe pain in the neck radiating through the shoulders down to the arms. This may, in turn, bring headaches and scalp sensitivity. The pressure caused by the shortening of the ligaments at the base of the skull irritates the nerves that pass through the facial attachment. This nerve irritation is picked up to some degree by the peripheral nerve branches set off at the points of ligamentous shortening to the outermost extremities. Such aches and pains of the head, shoulders, and arms can be relieved by such Yoga postures as the fish pose and shoulderstand, which stretch the ligaments and permit free and easy movement of the head and neck, thus relieving the compression of the nerves and the sensitivity of the nerve branches.

For a lasting effect and a permanent stretching of these ligaments, a correct head and upper spine balance and flexibility are necessary, all of which can be accomplished by daily practice of the Yogic poses.

The facial ligaments consist of multiple layers of connective tissue composed of parallel bundles of fibers, woven in such a way as to be able to take enormous strains and stresses. These ligaments possess great strength; they are an indispensable part in our daily motions of walking, standing, and lifting. The facial attachments tend to shorten after a period of great activity followed by a period of inactivity.

This tendency of shortening can be seen in athletes, sportsmen, and dancers who, after a period of inactivity, undertake severe training, extensive stretching, and long limbering-up periods to regain their lost elasticity.

The Yogi gives great attention to the vertebral column and its ligaments, the pillar of the support of the trunk and cranium, which also protects the spinal cord and the roots of the spinal nerve. The spinal nerves emerge between the vertebrae.

Four definite curves are noticeable in the vertebral column, namely, cervical, thoracic, lumbar, and pelvic or sacral.

The primary curves present at birth are two, thoracic and sacral. The cervical curve develops as the child begins to hold up his head, between three and nine months. When the child begins to walk, the lumbar curve appears.

All four curves lend resilience and spring to the vertebral column, which are essential for walking and jumping. Improper positions may exaggerate the curves of the vertebral column. An increase in the thoracic curve is called kyphosis; in the lumbar curve, lordosis. A lateral curvature of the spine is called scoliosis. Owing to tuberculosis of the vertebrae, erosion of the bodies of the vertebrae may take place, resulting in abnormal curvature.

Yogic exercises are mainly designed to keep the proper curvature of the spine and to increase its flexibility by stretching the anterior and posterior longitudinal ligaments. The posterior longitudinal ligament extends from the epistropheus to the sacrum. All the discs and edges of the bodies of the vertebrae are attached by this ligament. A fifteen-year-old can easily touch his toes with the fingertips while keeping the knees straight. This flexibility of the spine lessens at thirty and continues to decline at forty until at sixty and over, any bending may be difficult and painful. In fact, stiffened ligaments will not stretch at all and the body is held at the base of the skull, throughout the spine, pelvis, and knees by ligaments that have lost their elasticity.

A Yoga practitioner, even at an advanced age, maintains flexible ligaments and spine. Some of the difficult Yogic exercises (shown in this book) demonstrate just to what degree the human body can be trained to maintain maximum pliability of the spine and the various joints.

## CONNECTION BETWEEN THE ENDOCRINE SYSTEM AND YOGA

Long before the modern scientists knew anything about the endocrine glands and their functions, the Yogis advocated exercises for these important endocrine glands. Yogis knew that the endocrine system affects the emotions of the mind, and vice versa.

These glands are also known as ductless glands, because they pass their secretions directly into the blood or lymph, instead of into excretory ducts. The endocrine glands are pancreas, thyroid, parathyroid, suprarenal, pituitary, and the gonads.

Full growth, differentiation, and function of the various parts of the body are possible only when there is a balanced activity of the internal secretion glands. Their secretions are called hormones (which means to excite or arouse) and their effect can be either immediate or delayed. They are relatively simple chemical substances, which must be either oxidized or excreted after they have exerted their specific

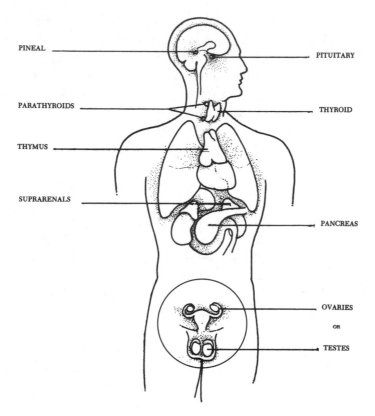

PINEAL

PITUITARY

PARATHYROIDS

THYROID

THYMUS

SUPRARENALS

PANCREAS

OVARIES

OR

TESTES

ENDOCRINE GLANDS

effects. If these secretions suffer, pathologic conditions in different parts of the body are rapidly established.

The thyroid gland is located in the anterior middle portion of the neck. It consists of two lateral lobes, which are united by a strip called the isthmus.

The thyroid gland helps to regulate functions such as the anabolic (growth and repair) processes and catabolic (waste) processes, mental development, and attainment of sexual maturity. The thyroid is one of the most powerful agencies set up by nature to protect the body against poisons.

There are two forms of hypothyroidism, exophthalmic goiter and adenomatous goiter. In the former the thyroid secretion is thought to be abnormal, which results in gastrointestinal disturbances, sleeplessness, nervousness, rapid pulse, palpitation, excessive perspiration, tremor, and loss of weight. The temperature does not rise above normal because increase in heat loss is brought about by more perspiration and dilation of the cutaneous blood vessels.

Whenever the thyroid becomes so enlarged that it causes a visible fullness in the neck it is called a goiter. There are several types of goiter, depending on different causes, and having differing. significance for our health. The goiter should be medically examined to determine its cause, and to decide if treatment is needed. Prevention is better than cure, so with the help of such Yogic exercises as *sarvangasan* (shoulderstand) and a proper diet, the thyroid can be kept in a healthy condition. One kind of simple goiter is due to an iodine deficiency in the intake of food and drink. This can be easily remedied by adjusting the diet.

According to medical authorities, the most damaging type of goiter is the relatively small gland with the rapidly developing evidence of toxicity. This disorder has been called exophthalmic because of its frequent association with bulging eyeballs. Experiments have proved that administration of large doses of thyroid can produce thyrotoxicosis in healthy persons. This toxic form of thyroid disorder is most common in persons between the ages of fifteen and forty, and is frequently associated with a nervous and emotional disposition. Often there is a correlation between a thyroid disease and an unstable nervous system.

When the thyroid hormone supply is inadequate for normal health, the rate of oxygen is reduced and the basal metabolism may be found as much as 40 per cent below the normal for a person's age, height, and weight. In the laboratories, the basal metabolism test is done by measuring a person's hourly oxygen consumption. Tests are usually extended over eight-minute or ten-minute periods, during which the person breathes through a rubber mouthpiece from a tank containing a measured amount of air. Carbon dioxide and excess moisture are absorbed as they are exhaled into the apparatus and a decrease in the amount of air in the tank is caused by the oxygen the person inhales.

An abnormally low basal metabolism may produce certain kinds of obesity, which can be prevented by the practice of thyroid Yogic exercises.

Extreme hypothyroidism in the adult is known as myxedema. This brings conditions such as a diminution of mental activity, slowness of speech and movement, a coarse, dry skin, and loss of hair. In adenomatous goiter, an increase of the normal secretions occurs and the symptoms of hypothyroidism appear after the gland has become enlarged.

The parathyroid glands lie on the posterior surface and are within the capsule of the thyroid gland. Their secretion regulates the calcium and phosphorus metabolisms, and helps to control the concentration of calcium and inorganic phosphate.

In hyperparathyroidism, the chief symptom in the human being is tetany, which may be due either to the removal of the parathyroid glands or to spontaneous development. This condition causes restlessness and tetanic spasm of the flexor muscles.

Yoga therapy aims through its various postures to restore the internal secretions of these glands to their normality. There are different exercises for the strengthening of different glands.

Mental emotions such as fear, sorrow, anger, jealousy, hatred, love, and envy have been noted to affect our bodies, especially the endocrine system and nervous system, according to their degree of intensity. In extreme sorrow or fear, even death may occur. These emotions are like shock waves affecting the nervous system and leading to the degeneration of the endocrine glands. The endocrine system is controlled by the sympathetic and vagus nerves. When the emotions are not very severe, they may not cause physical death, but definitely affect the nervous and endocrine systems.

An effect of emotional reaction is high blood pressure. During fear or anger, it is common to notice a faster heartbeat. Emotions affect the adrenal gland, which secretes extra doses of adrenalin. Adrenalin increases in the blood stream, accelerates the heartbeat, and raises the blood pressure. Such mental emotions constantly strain the heart, causing nervous disorders and heart ailments.

Yogic postures help to strengthen the endocrine system through exercise, and also bring the emotions under control through concentration and relaxation.


YOGA AND THE CELLS AND CIRCULATION

Now let us study Yogic exercises and their actions upon the minute cells of which the body is composed. The physical body is built of trillions of cells, each cell containing a miniature life and energy for a definite function. Individual lives are really only bits of some degree of intelligence enabling the cells to work properly. Though the cells function instinctively, they are subordinate to the control of man's central mind and readily obey orders, consciously or unconsciously.

Among living things, some animals consist of only one cell and are called unicellular; animals of more than one cell are called multicellular. Regardless of the number of cells, each has two main parts, the cytoplasm and the nucleus. The nucleus is the vital part of the cell and apparently the center for chemical activities necessary for its life.

A group of cells may be defined as a tissue. There are primarily four types of tissues. When various tissues of the body are put together in different ways, they form membranes and skin.

Considerable attention should be given to the skin as it is an important structure. There are various functions of the skin; it serves as a mechanical barrier to prevent injury to deeper tissues; bacteria cannot penetrate readily through the dead cells of the outer layer and it protects against invasion by foreign organisms. It also acts as a sense of touch. From the color of the skin the conditions of the body can be determined. For example, in hypertension or in any other condition in which the skin's blood vessels are dilated, it is red. In anemia it will be pale, owing to the lower number of red corpuscles. It may appear purple in heart diseases and pneumonia, owing to the improper oxygenation of the blood. The skin appears yellow because of increase in bilirubin in the blood when a patient suffers from jaundice.

Much information can be gleaned if one studies the color changes of the skin. An increased amount of blood flowing through the skin vessels will keep the skin in a healthy condition. Also it is very important to remember here that various cells of the body, which are used like building bricks, obtain their energy and nourishment through the blood stream. Without proper material these cells cannot carry out their proper work. Persons who are undernourished have not nearly the normal amount of blood cells and are consequently unable to have their systems function properly. The cells must have body-building material; there is only one way in which they can get this, and that is by means of nourishment from the food brought by the blood circulation, which is kept up easily through various Yogic movements and exercises.

# 5

# CONQUEST OF OLD AGE
# THROUGH YOGIC
# EXERCISES

In the previous chapters we dealt with the therapeutic values of Yogic practices. In this chapter we will deal with the technique of various poses, their benefits, and their action on muscles, joints, ligaments, and glands.

The physical body can be compared to an automobile. To run a motor car we need gas, electric current to ignite it, a cooling system, lubrication, and an intelligent driver to control its movements. This body has five similar needs to run in perfect order. We know that no motor car can run without the above-mentioned requirements; so also the physical body cannot run for a prolonged period without gas, electric current, a cooling system, lubrication, and a directing intelligence.

First of all the body draws its fuel or gas from the food we eat, the water we drink, the air we breathe, and a small amount from the radiation of the sun's rays. Most of the energy for the body we get from the air we breathe, and not, as is commonly assumed, from food and water.

Absorption of energy from the air will be dealt with in a later chapter (Breathing, Chapter 8).

The Solar Plexus is the storage battery in the body which supplies Pranic energy to the whole body (Pranic energy and the Solar Plexus are dealt within another chapter).

Now we need a cooling system for the physical body. No engine can run long without a cooling mechanism. So also, the physical body will not run for long periods without a cooling system. This can be achieved only by relaxation.

The next important point is the lubrication of the joints: this is achieved by various bodily movements. The nerve currents are the electricity in human beings and lack of nerve energy will definitely put the whole system out of order. Last, the body should be properly controlled by an intelligent driver, the mind. Prayer, devotion to one Supreme Being, sympathy, love, courage, discrimination between the real and the unreal, will train the mind as an intelligent driver.

In order to get the maximum benefit, the above-mentioned five requirements are utilized during practice.

We know that the modern physical exercises require more energy than Yogic exercises, as every violent movement burns up lots of it. Also, more lactic acids are formed in the muscle fibers by such quick movements; this is more tiresome to the muscles.

The slow movements of the joints during Yoga practice waste no energy. Deep breathing with mild retention during the practice allows for more oxygen absorption. Less lactic acid is produced and, as this is easily neutralized by the alkali, it avoids muscle fatigue.

Owing to twisting and other movements of various joints, blood vessels are pulled and stretched and blood is equally distributed to every part of the body. The stretched muscles and ligaments during the Yogic practice are immediately relaxed, carrying more energy to the muscle fibers. Just as water flows through an open tap, so energy flows into the relaxed muscles.

All Yogic exercises are based on the formula of stretching, relaxation, deep breathing, and increasing circulation and concentration.

## MEDITATIVE POSES

Yogic culture is divided into eight parts:
1. *Yama,* ethics
2. *Niyama,* religious observances
3. *Asana,* postures
4. *Pranayama,* breathing exercises
5. *Pratyahara,* withdrawal of senses from objects
6. *Dharana,* concentration
7. *Dhyana,* meditation
8. *Samadhi,* superconsciousness

There are 840,000 poses according to the Yoga *Shastras,* of which 84 are important. In this book all the main poses, with their variations, are given with detailed explanation.

*Asana* means posture. *Asanas* can be divided broadly into two main groups, meditative postures and cultural postures. There are four meditative poses: the lotus pose or *padmasan, siddhasan, swastikasan,* and *sukasan* or the easy, comfortable pose. There is another, known as *vajrasan,* which can be practiced by persons who cannot use any other position.

These meditative poses are very important when students sit for breathing exercises and meditation. One must be able to sit in any one of these four positions for one to two hours at a stretch without moving. First of all, an erect position of the spine will keep it in its natural curve. Secondly, training the body to sit for long periods without movements reduces its metabolic processes to a minimum. When the body is kept in a steady position for a long time, the mind becomes free from all physiologic disturbances caused by physical activities of the body. Moreover, a straight spine helps the students to concentrate because in the straight position there is a steady flow of nerve current or nerve energy through the body.

Advanced students can feel this movement of the nerve current through the spine, bringing them natural concentration without effort. This nerve energy can be increased and can be utilized for awakening the spiritual power in man through breathing exercises or *pranayama* and concentration. This will be dealt with in later chapters.

The steadier the pose, the more you will be able to concentrate and make the mind one-pointed. Select any one of the four postures you like and sit for fifteen minutes. Gradually increase the period to an hour or two. Always keep the head, neck, and trunk in one straight line.

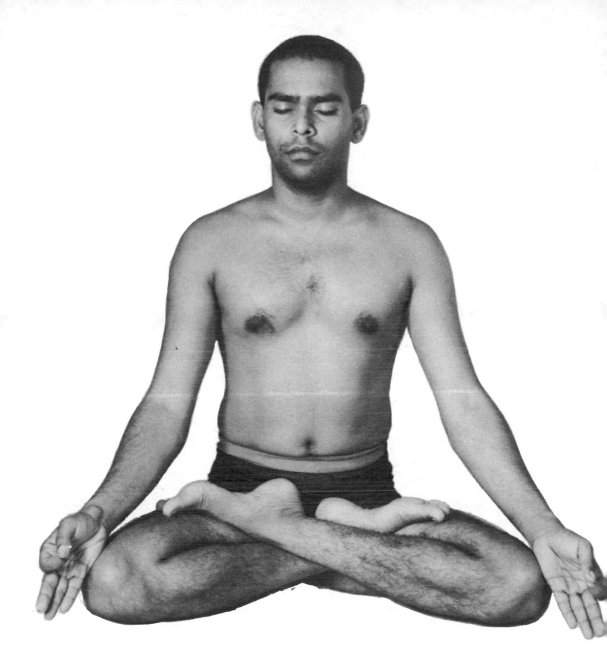

## Technique: **Padmasan** [lotus pose]

*plate 13*

Sit on a four-folded blanket and stretch the legs forward. Take hold of the right foot with the two hands, folding the leg at the knee and placing the foot on the left thigh. Similarly, fold the left leg and place it on the right thigh. Keep the body erect and place the hands between the heels, one over the other. If this is not suitable, you can keep the hands on the knees. The left knee or thigh should not be raised from the ground.

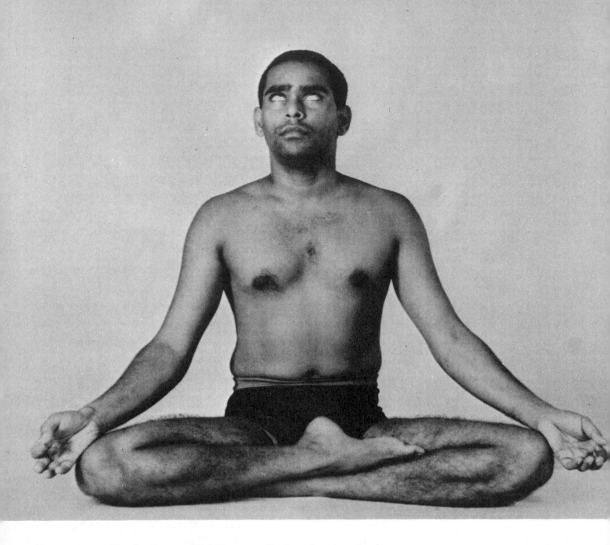

plate 14    Technique: **Siddhasan** [adept's pose]

*Siddha* means an adept in Sanskrit. Since great adepts used this *asana*, it bears the name *Siddhasan*. *Siddhas* (perfected Yogis) speak very highly of this *asana*. Young celibates and those who attempt to become established in celibacy should practice this *asana*.

Sit and stretch the legs forward. Bend the left leg at the knee and place the heel at the soft portion of the perineum, the space between the anus and the scrotum. Then fold the right leg and place the heel against the pubic bone or just above the genitals. The genitals should be arranged in such a manner that no pressure is felt. Keep the body erect and place the hands as in *padmasan*.

## Technique: **Mukthasan, or Guptasan**

Stretch the legs. Bend the right leg at the knee joint and keep the right heel against the pubic bone or just above the genitals. Now bend the left leg at the knee and keep the left heel above the right heel, close to the pubic bone. In this position there will not be any pressure at the perineum, and the genital organs are free from pressure. People who cannot practice *sidhasan* may find this exercise more comfortable.

*plate 15*

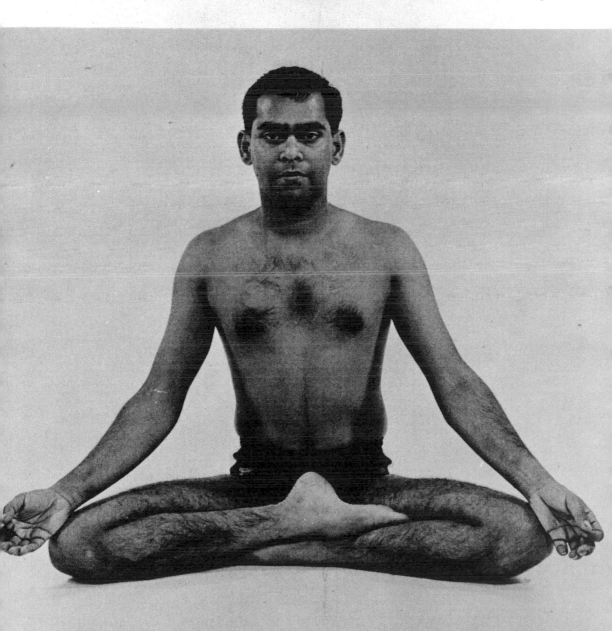

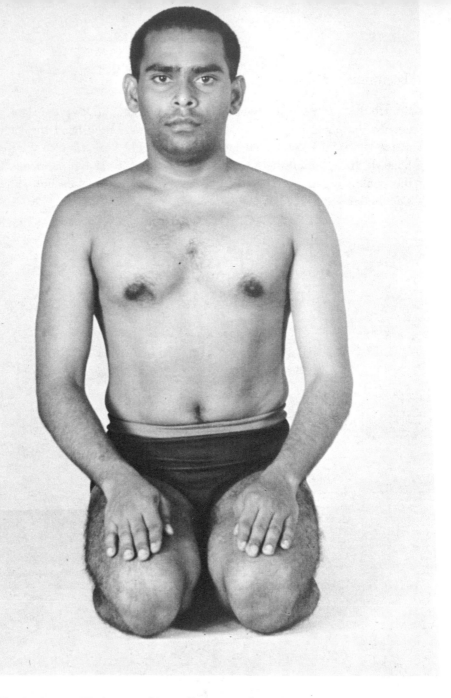

plate 16      Technique: **Vajrasan** [kneeling pose]

Kneel down. Sit on the heels with the spine erect.

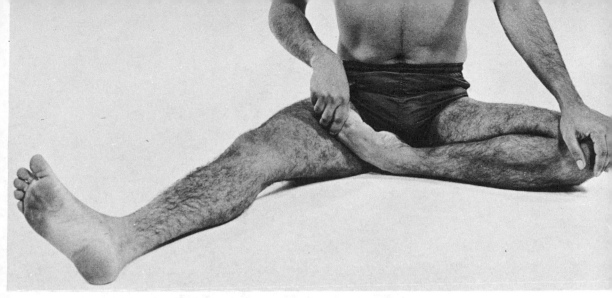

*plate 17*

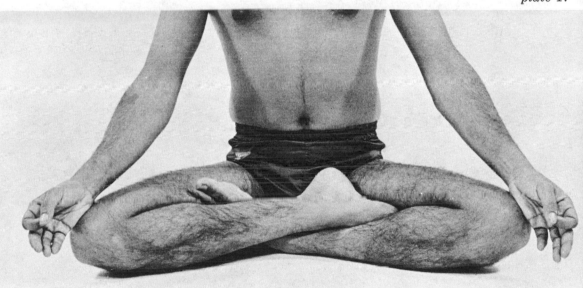

## Technique: **Swastikasan** [ankle lock pose]

*plate 18*

*Swastika* means a "prosperous" in Sanskrit. When this pose is performed, the ankle lock brings the appearance of the *swastika*.

Sit on the four-folded blanket. Stretch the legs in front of you. Bend the right leg at the knee and keep the heel against the groin of the left thigh so that the sole will be lying in close contact with the thigh. Similarly, bend the left leg and set it against the right groin. Insert the toes of the left foot between the right calf and thigh muscles. Now you will find the two feet between the calf and thigh muscles. This is very comfortable for meditation. Keep the hands as instructed in *padmasan*.

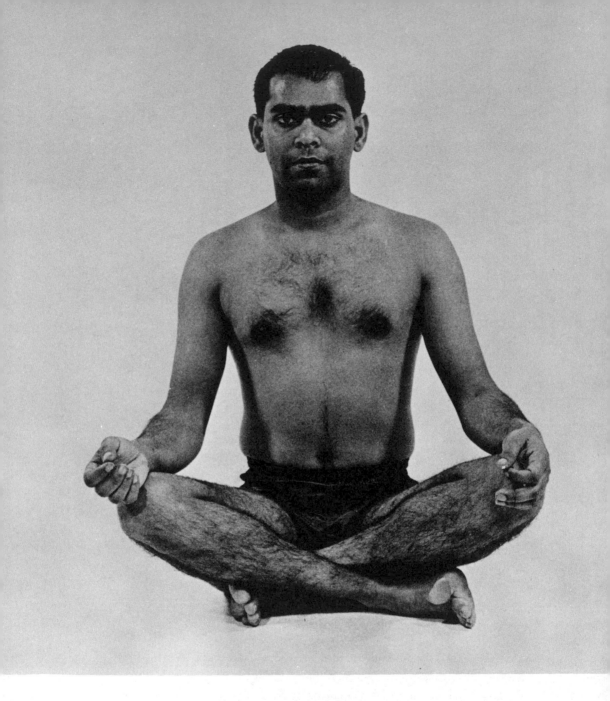

plate 19     **Technique: Sukhasan** [easy pose]

*Sukhasan* is an easy, comfortable sitting posture for *japa* and meditation, the important point being that the head, neck and trunk should be in a line without any curve. This is usually done in an ordinary cross-legged position. However, if necessary you may sit on a chair.

## SOORYA NAMASKAR OR SUN EXERCISE

This exercise is called *soorya namaskar* because it is practiced in the early morning facing the sun. The sun is considered to be the deity for health and long life. In ancient days, this exercise was a daily routine in the daily spiritual practices. One should practice this at least twelve times by repeating twelve names of the Lord Sun. This exercise is a combined process of Yoga *asanas* and breathing. It reduces abdominal fat, brings flexibility to the spine and limbs, and increases the breathing capacity; it is easier to practice *asanas* after doing *soorya namaskar*.

Before students practice the more complicated and difficult postures, the spine should acquire some flexibility. For a stiff person, the sun exercise is a boon to bring back lost flexibility.

There are twelve spinal positions, each stretching various ligaments and giving different movements to the vertebral column. The vertebral column is bent forward and backward alternately with deep breathing. Whenever the body is bent forward, the contraction of the abdomen and diaphragm throws out the breath. When the body bends backward, the chest expands and deep breathing occurs automatically. This way, flexibility increases and breathing is corrected; moreover, it mildly exercises the legs and arms, thus increasing the circulation.

On the following pages are shown each of the twelve positions making one full round of *soorya namaskar*. Repeat twelve times daily.

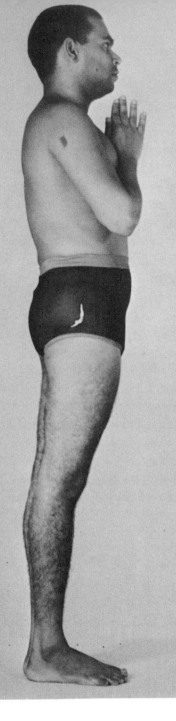

plate 20

**Technique: Soorya Namaskar**
**Position No. 1**

Face the sun. Fold the hands. Legs together, stand erect.

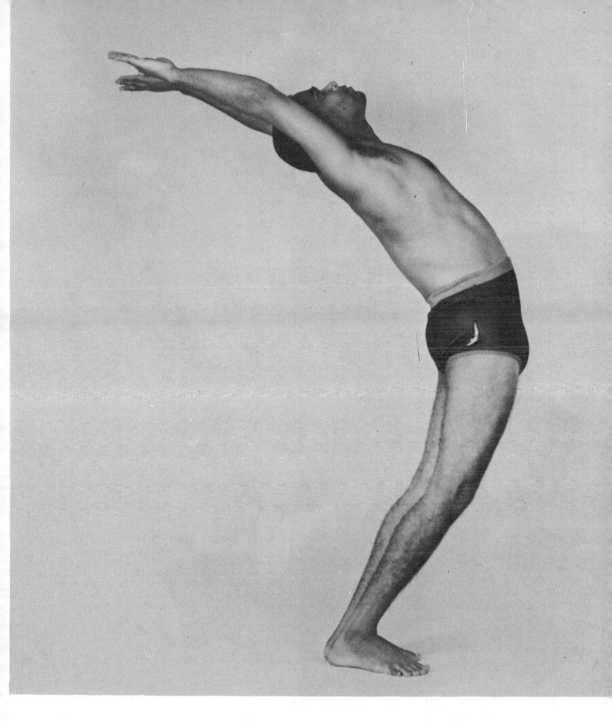

Technique: **Soorya Namaskar**
Position No. 2

Inhale and raise the arms. Bend backward.

plate 21

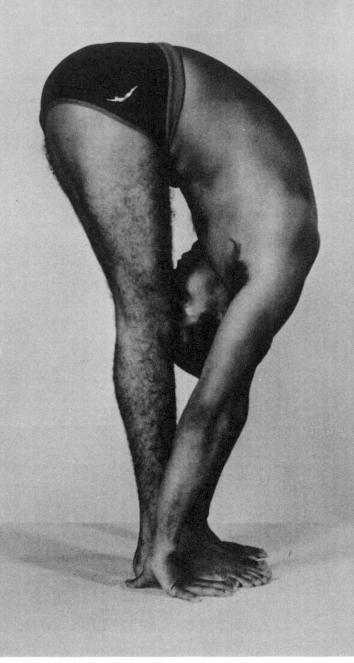

plate 22

Technique: **Soorya Namaskar**
Position No. 3

Exhale and bend forward till the hands are in line with the feet. Touch the knees with your head. In the beginning, the knees may be slightly bent until the head can touch them. After some practice, the knees should be straightened.

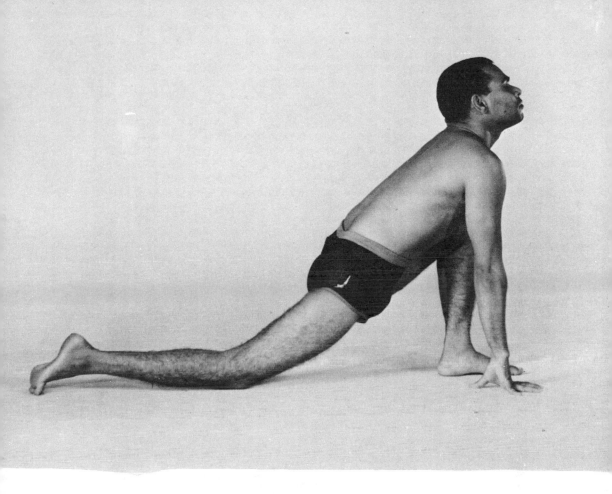

Technique: **Soorya Namaskar**                                   *plate 23*
Position No. 4

Inhale and move the right leg away from the body in a big backward step.
Keep the hands and left foot firmly on the ground, bending the head backward. The left knee should be between the hands.

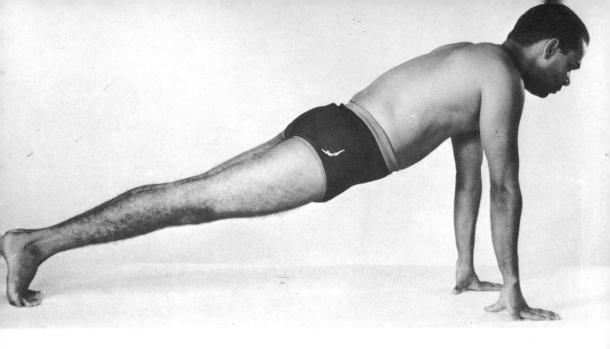

plate 24     Technique: **Soorya Namaskar**
Position No. 5

Inhale and hold the breath. Move the left leg from the body and, keeping both feet together and the knees off the floor, rest on the hands (arms straight) and keep the body in a straight line from head to foot.

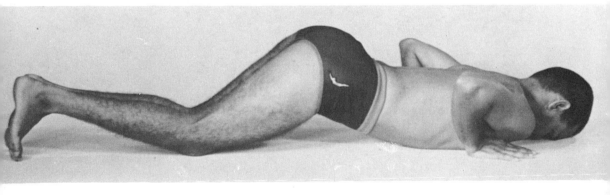

plate 25     Technique: **Soorya Namaskar**
Position No. 6

Exhale and lower the body to the floor. In this position, known as *sastanga namaskar* or eight-curved prostration, only eight portions of the body come in contact with the floor: two feet, two knees, two hands, chest, and forehead. The abdominal region is raised and, if possible, the nose is also kept off the floor, the forehead only touching it.

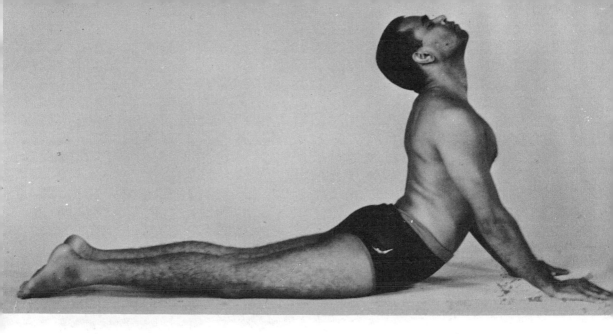

Technique: **Soorya Namaskar**
Position No. 7

*plate 26*

Inhale and bend backward as much as possible, bending the spine to the maximum.

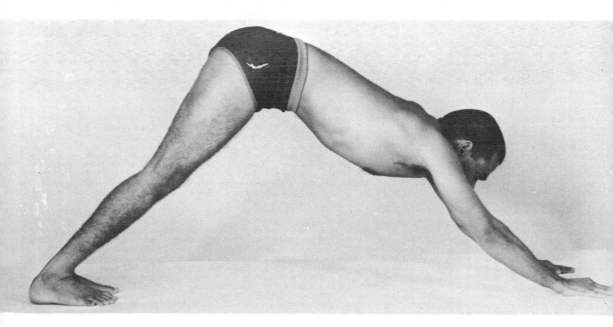

Technique: **Soorya Namaskar**
Position No. 8

*plate 27*

Exhale and lift the body. Keep the feet and heels flat on the floor.

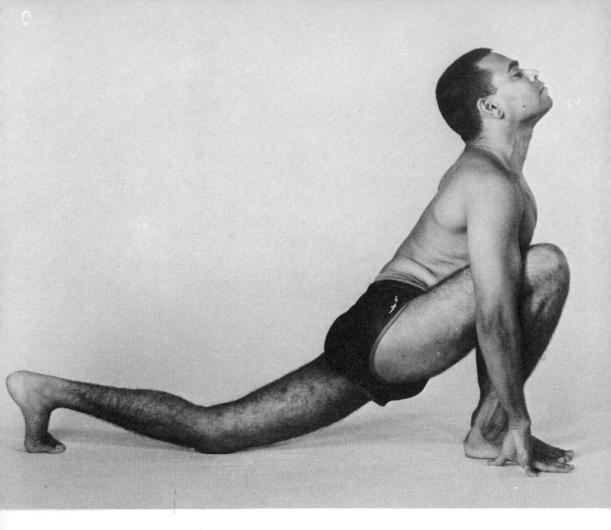

plate 28

Technique: **Soorya Namaskar**
Position No. 9

Inhale and bring the right foot along the level of the hands; left foot and knee should touch the ground. Look up, bending the spine slightly. (Same as Position No. 4.)

Technique: **Soorya Namaskar**
Position No. 10

Exhale and bring the left leg forward. Keep the knees straight and bring the head down to the knees as in the third position.

*plate 29*

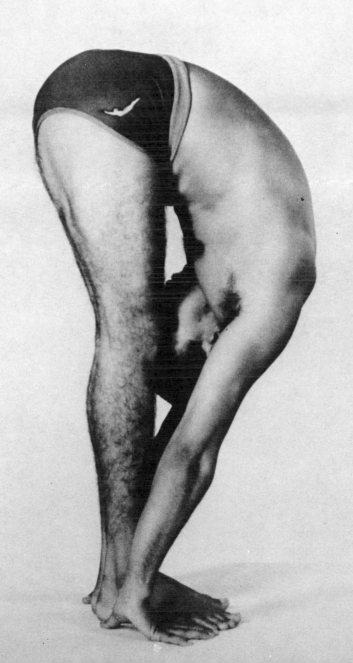

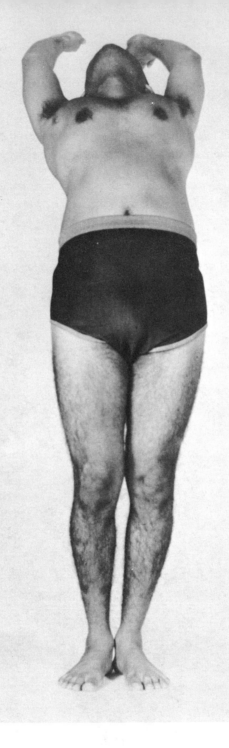

plate 30

Technique: **Soorya Namaskar**
Position No. 11

Raise the arms overhead and bend backward inhaling, as in Position No. 2.

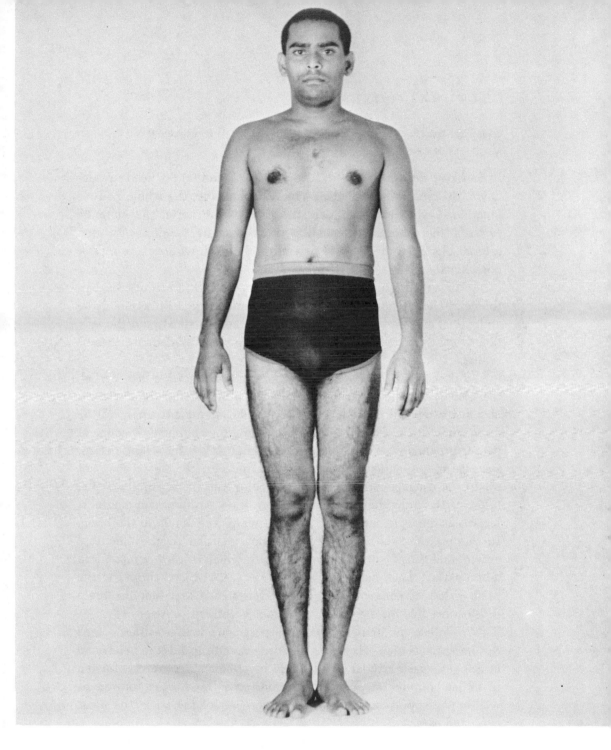

Technique: **Soorya Namaskar**
Position No. 12

Exhale, drop the arms, and relax.

*plate 31*

## CULTURAL POSES

### SIRSHASAN, THE HEADSTAND: ITS VARIATIONS AND BENEFITS

In Sanskrit, *siras* means head. As one has to stand on his head upside-down, this position is called *sirshasan*. In this pose, the whole body is inverted. Owing to gravitation, the arch of the aorta, the common carotids, the innominate, and the subclavian are flooded with rich arterial blood. In this pose alone can the brain draw a rich supply of pure blood.

In an upright position, gravity opposes the return of blood to the heart from regions below its level. Generally the contraction of the abdominal and limb muscles, the force of the heartbeat, and the suction from the respiratory movements keep up an adequate venous return.

If one stands upright in an unmoving position for a long period, the blood accumulates in the dependent parts and the right heart is not adequately filled. This brings an insufficient blood supply to the brain and the individual faints. Such fainting commonly occurs at parade grounds when the soldiers stand at attention for a long period. Because of stagnation in the abdominal vessels, the heart does not pump the usual amount of blood, lessening the blood supply to the brain. If the individual is kept in a horizontal position, consciousness returns as the usual amount of blood is pumped up again to the brain. In this position, the flow of blood is not retarded by the effects of gravity and thus favors filling of the heart, which in turn pumps up in a better way. Thus the first effect of a decreased blood supply to the brain is loss of consciousness. It is a well-known fact that the brain cells cannot live for more than ten minutes without oxygen.

We use the brain for many purposes and it is essential to feed this important organ. Therefore, no other exercise equals the headstand in bringing fresh arterial blood. Daily practice of this exercise for ten to fifteen minutes increases the memory and intellectual power, as well as the supply of blood to the upper part of the back, the neck, eyes, and ears.

Cerebral hemorrhage is the most frequent of all affections of the brain. It is caused by a thickening of the arterial coats. A sudden strain increases the pressure and may rupture one of the vessels, which is fatal. Persons with either high or low blood pressure should not attempt headstands.

Many veins are provided with valves that prevent the backward flow of blood. Varicose veins may occur in the lower extremities, owing to enlargement of veins. The walls of the veins stretch and the veins appear knotted. Interference with the return of blood from the lower limbs favors the development of varicose veins. During the headstand, the valves of the veins have ample rest, because the gravitational pull automatically carries the venous blood from the lower extremities to the heart, without the help of the valves.

In this position, various exercises are given for stretching the ligaments and muscles and to bring maximum flexibility to the spinal column.

In an inverted position, cervical and thoracic parts of the vertebral column get more pressure and the lumbar and sacral parts of the vertebral column and cartilages are relieved of the pressure. The headstand is also a good exercise for strengthening the vertebral column. This exercise is of particular benefit to those who need concentration power in their work, such as students, politicians, scientists, and writers.

plate 32

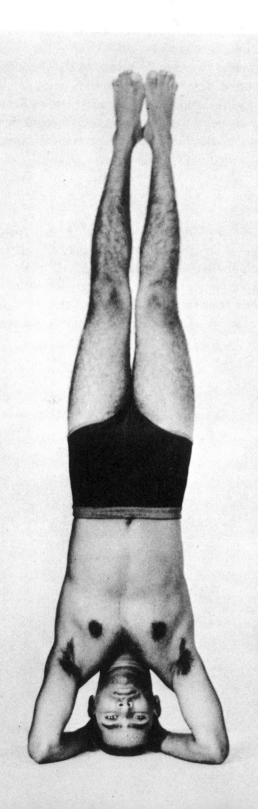

# Technique: **Sirshasan** [headstand]

The exercise is practiced with the help of the hands and arms. The whole weight of the head and trunk is placed on the interlocked hands and the elbows. The two elbows and interlocked fingers form the three points or tripod on which the body is balanced. The weight on the head is so little that it is not even felt. When the weight is divided equally between the elbows and the locked fingers, it is easy to balance.

Use a soft cushion or a four-folded blanket. Spread the blanket on the floor. Sit on your knees. By interweaving the fingers, make a fingerlock and keep it on the blanket so that the locked hands serve as a vertex and the two elbows as the base, enabling the forearms to balance the body. The top of the head may be supported from behind by the fingerlock while doing this *asana*.

Keep the top of your head on the blanket close to the fingerlock. The parietal (frontal) portion of the top of the head should be placed on the blanket and not the portion nearer to the forehead. This will help you to keep the spine erect in this *asana*. If the portion nearer to the forehead is used, the spine will suffer a curvature in balancing the whole body.

Now the knees are brought close to the body, and the toes are allowed to touch the ground for balancing. When the trunk is sufficiently thrown back, you can slowly remove the toes from the ground. Slowly raise the legs high up in the air till the whole body becomes erect. Stand in the *asana* for five seconds only and gradually increase the period to 15 minutes. By regularly practicing even five to ten minutes of headstand, the maximum benefits can be derived.

Always breathe through the nose only and never through the mouth. In the beginning, some persons will find it difficult to breathe through the nose, but after a few days this will change.

In learning the headstand in the above manner you will not need any help. You can learn the method of balancing by repeated attempts. Instead of a fingerlock method, you can keep the palms of your hands on the blanket, one on each side. You will find this easy. When you have learned to balance the whole body, you can take to the fingerlock method.

Lower the legs slowly to the floor to the original position. Lower the legs very, very slowly and avoid jerks. After completing the *asana*, stand erect for a minute or two. This will harmonize the blood circulation.

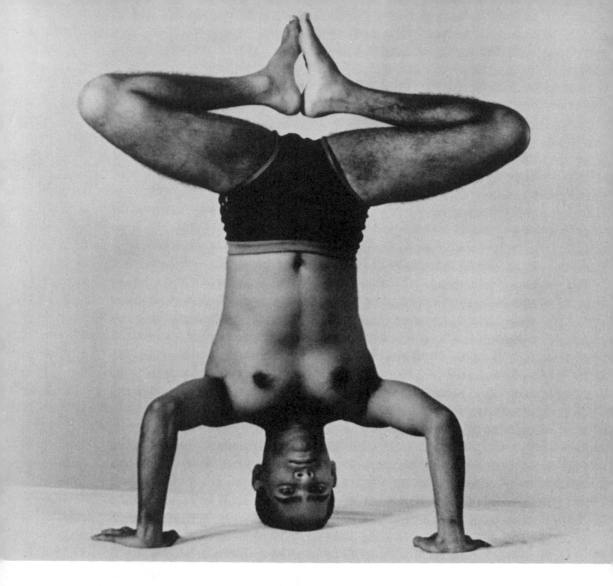

*plate 33*   Technique: **Sirshasan** [headstand]

VARIATION 2

In this position, the hands are kept separated and the head takes an equal
weight. This is designed to strengthen the muscles of the shoulders, superficial muscles of the back, and the muscles of the arms. By stretching the
thighs and keeping the soles of the feet together, the circulation of the
lower extremities is increased. This also stretches the veins and strengthens
the muscles of the thighs, legs, and feet.

# Technique: **Sirshasan** [headstand]

## VARIATION 3

The same benefit is derived as in Variation 2. This gives an extra stretching and twisting to muscles of the thighs and legs and squeezes the venous blood from the tired veins.

*plate 34*

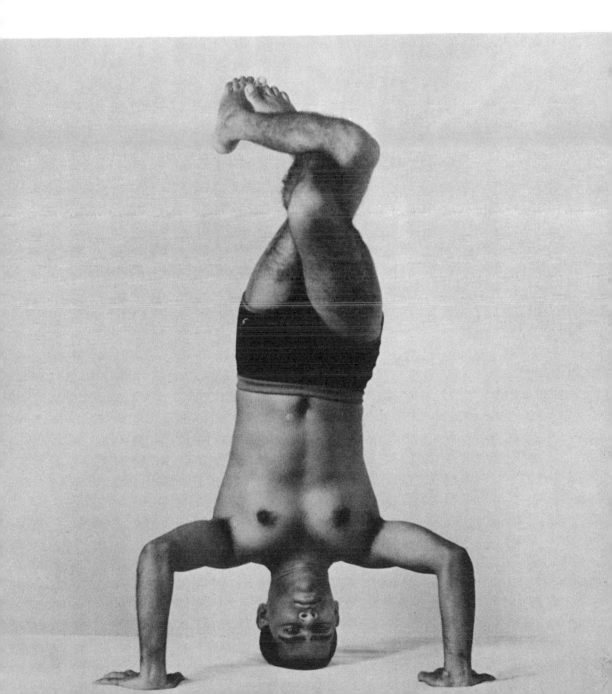

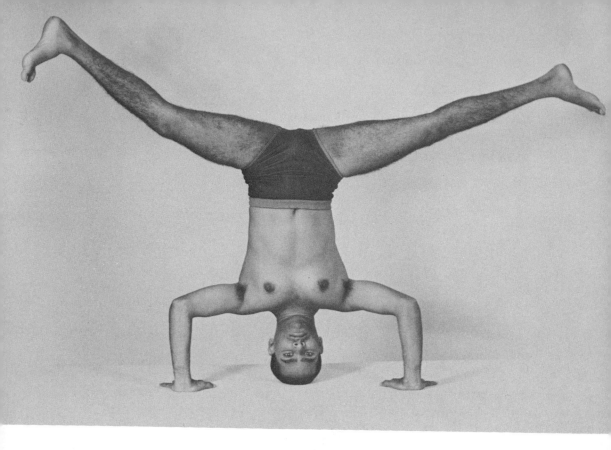

plate 35

## Technique: **Sirshasan** [headstand]

VARIATION 4

In this pose, the muscles of the thighs and legs, which are used for walking and standing, are given a maximum stretching.

## Technique: **Sirshasan** [headstand]

VARIATION 5

Here, the hands are folded in front of the head as a support. In this position, more pressure is put on the head. The cervical and thoracic portions of the vertebrae get immense pressure and the ligaments connected with the vertebral column are supplied with more arterial blood.

plate 36

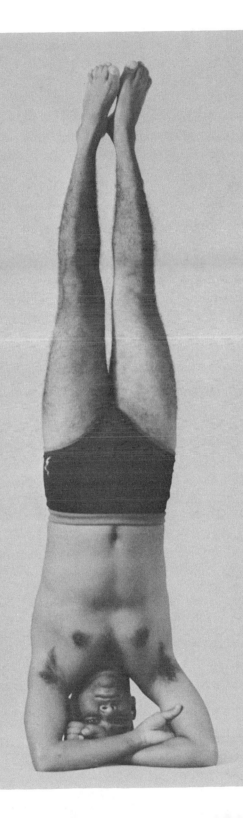

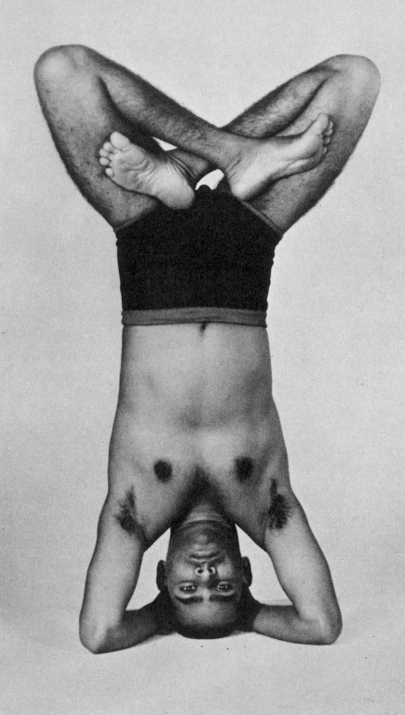

plate 37

# Technique: **Oordhwapadmasan** [headstand, lotus pose]

### VARIATION 1

After securing the balance in the headstand, advanced students take up this exercise to bring maximum flexibility to the ankle, knee, and hip joints.

Before trying to do this exercise, one should be able to sit in the lotus pose. The technique and benefits are the same as for the headstand. However, here we go further and while standing on the head, we lock the legs in *padmasan* or lotus pose. Do not attempt to start the headstand while sitting in *padmasan*.

There are three variations of this exercise to stretch the lumbar and sacral vertebrae and their ligaments. The lumbar and sacral parts of the vertebral column are twisted to both sides and bent as shown in the pictures. This is to be repeated at least three times. It will strengthen the ligaments and the vertebral column.

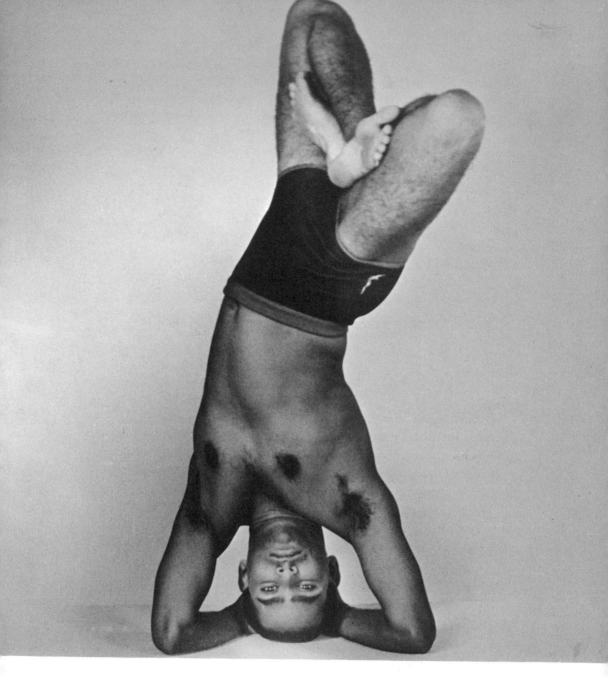

plate 38     Technique: **Oordhwapadmasan** [headstand, lotus pose]

VARIATION 2

Twisting of the spine in both directions should be practiced by advanced students. Generally we twist our bodies while sitting or standing. But in this pose the lumbar region is naturally relaxed, and therefore free rotation of the spine is possible.

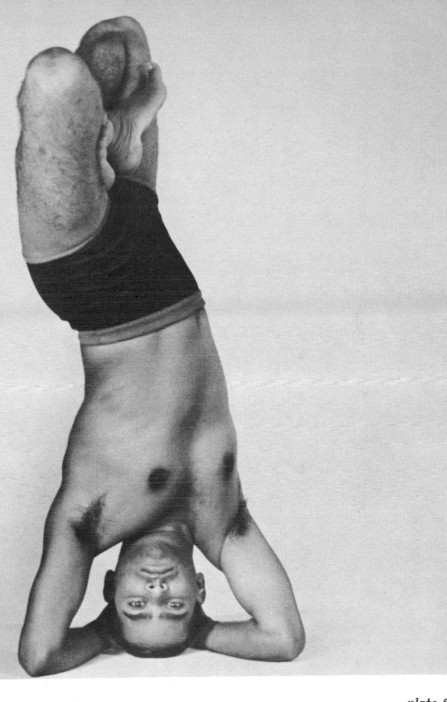

plate 39

plate 40

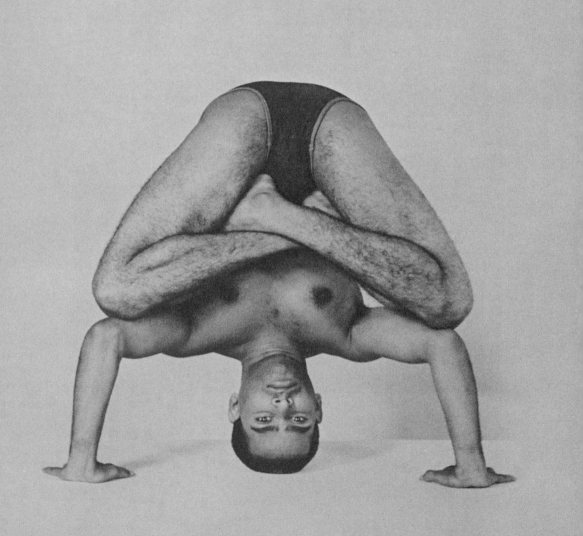

## Technique: **Oordhwapadmasan** [headstand, lotus pose]

VARIATIONS 3 AND 4

To complete the movement in *oordhwapadmasan,* the knees should be brought down, without unlocking the lotus pose, and touch the armpit. When the arms are kept separated the knees can be rested on the arms.    *plate 41*

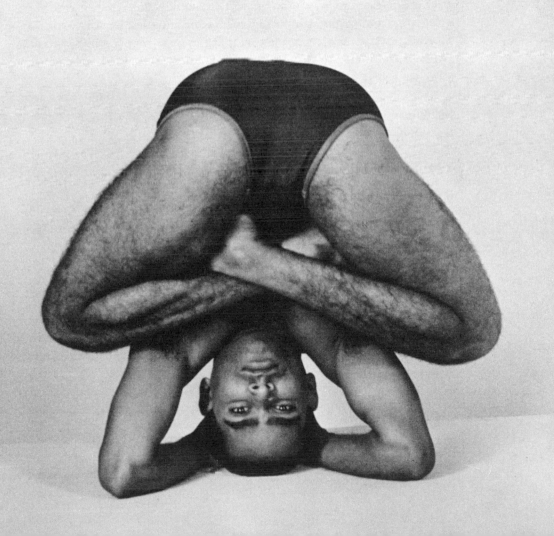

### SARVANGASAN, THE SHOULDERSTAND

This exercise is similar to the headstand. In headstand, circulation and concentration are directed to the brain, but in shoulderstand the concentration and circulation are directed to the thyroid and parathyroid. We have seen in the previous chapters what effect the thyroid and parathyroid secretions have on the body. The thyroid is the most important gland of the endocrine system, and this exercise gives it a rich supply of blood. Again it stretches the deltoid, supraspinatus, and infraspinatus of the shoulder muscles. The chin lock by the chin on the chest exerts an extra pressure on the thyroid through which its secretions are kept at par. This *asana* is a good substitute for modern thyroid treatment. The ligaments of the cervical region are especially stretched in this exercise.

There are many variations of the shoulderstand to increase the circulation and stretch various ligaments and muscles. *Sarvanga* means all parts, so the very name suggests that this pose is concerned with all parts of the body. It will also give a helping hand for persons with varicose veins.

Fifteen minutes is the maximum for this pose; starting time for beginners is one minute. Breathe normally through the nose. Some persons practice this for half an hour.

## Technique: **Sarvangasan** [shoulderstand]

### VARIATION 1

Spread a thick blanket on the floor. Lie flat on the back. Slowly raise the legs. Lift the trunk, hips, and legs to a vertical position. Rest the elbows firmly on the floor and support the back with both hands. Raise the legs till they become vertical. Press the chin against the chest. This is the chin lock.

While you perform this *asana*, the back of the neck, the posterior part of the head, and the shoulders should touch the floor. Breathe slowly and concentrate on the thyroid glands. Do not allow the body to shake to and fro. When the *asana* is over, lower the legs very slowly and smoothly. Avoid jerking. Do this *asana* very gracefully. In it the whole weight of the body is thrown on the shoulders. You can do this twice daily, morning and evening. To derive full benefit from this *asana*, the *matsyasan* should follow in sequence.

plate 42

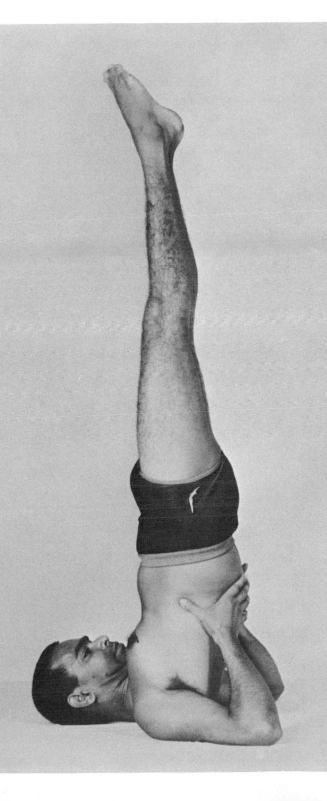

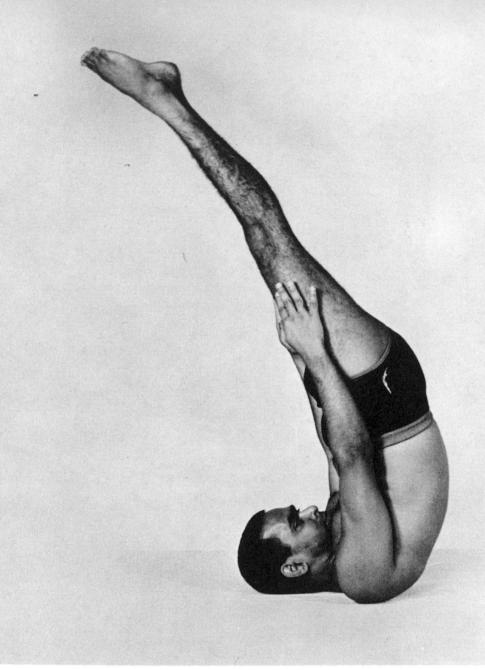

*plate 43*

## Technique: **Sarvangasan** [shoulderstand]

### VARIATION 2

In this position the hands that support the body are removed and kept vertically along the body. By removing the hands, the whole weight falls on the cervical region and shoulder muscles.

## Technique: **Sethu Bandhasan** [bridge pose]

From the shoulderstand (*sarvangasan*) position stretch the legs and slowly touch the flood with the legs. This is *sethu bandhasan*.

This is done after *sarvangasan* or shoulderstand, so that the thoracic and lumbar regions of the spine bend in the opposite direction.

*plate 44*

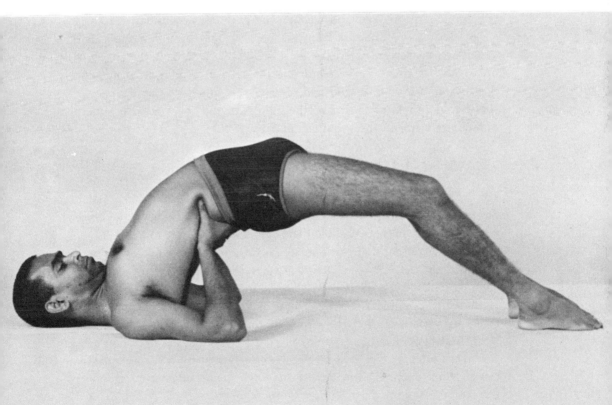

## EXERCISE FOR THE SHOULDER MUSCLES AND THE CERVICAL VERTEBRAE:

### MATSYASAN, FISH POSE

Owing to improper clothing, our bodily movement is generally restricted to a very limited area, especially the cervical region of the vertebrae and the shoulder muscles. Clothing supported by suspenders and shoulder straps pressing on the points of the shoulders tends to pull them downward and forward. It is a common deformity among students, together with other postural defects. It has been noted that the cut of most ready-made clothing causes pressure on the back of the neck and the tip of the shoulders, constantly pulling them.

Moreover, neckties, tightly buttoned shirt collars, and poorly cut jackets restrict movements of the cervical region and stop the free flow of circulation to the upper portion of the body. Women's tight foundation garments can cause considerable havoc wtih blood circulation, breathing, and movements of the sacral and lumbar region, which can produce headaches and weaken the abdominal muscles.

To remove stiffness from the cervical and lumbar regions and shoulder muscles and increase the circulation to these affected parts, *Matsyasan* or fish pose is invaluable. Moreover, this also strengthens the thyroid and parathyroid and relieves the congestion and cramp of the shoulder muscles caused by the shoulderstand. This exercise should immediately follow the shoulderstand.

## Technique: **Matsyasan** [fish pose]

For beginners: Lie on your back. Stretch the legs and keep the hands' palms down under the thighs. Raise the chest with the help of the elbows and, bending the neck as much as possible backward, rest on the top of the head.

For advanced students: Spread a blanket on the ground and sit on it with the legs stretched. Bend the right leg and place the heel on the left hip joint. Again bend the left leg and place the heel on the right hip joint. This is *padmasan* or foot lock. Then lie on the back. The *padmasan* should not be raised from the floor. Rest the elbows on the floor. Now lift the trunk and head. Rest the top of the head on the floor by bending the back and neck well. Then catch hold of the toes. This is *matsyasan*. Remain in this *asana* for two or three minutes. Those individuals who have difficulty performing *padmasan* may do the first form of *matsyasan*.

In this position, the chest is thrown open and so deep breathing through the nose should be practiced. This helps to remove the spasm from the bronchial tubes and thus relieves asthma.

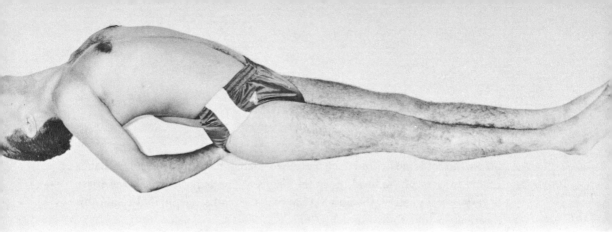

*plate 45, variation 1*

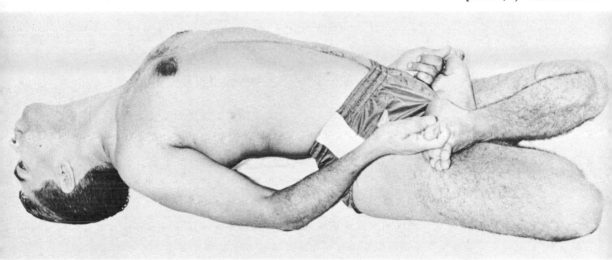

*plate 46, variation 2*

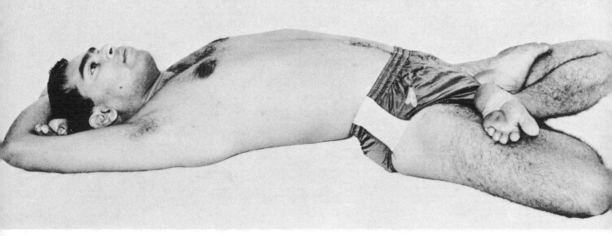

*plate 47, variation 3*

Technique: **Matsyasan** [fish position]

VARIATION 4

Sit in the lotus pose, and then lie down facing the floor. Keep the hands folded in front of the head. Keep the thighs as flat as possible. This exercise is very useful in strengthening the hip joints. Breathe deeply and retain this position for four to five minutes.

*plate 48*

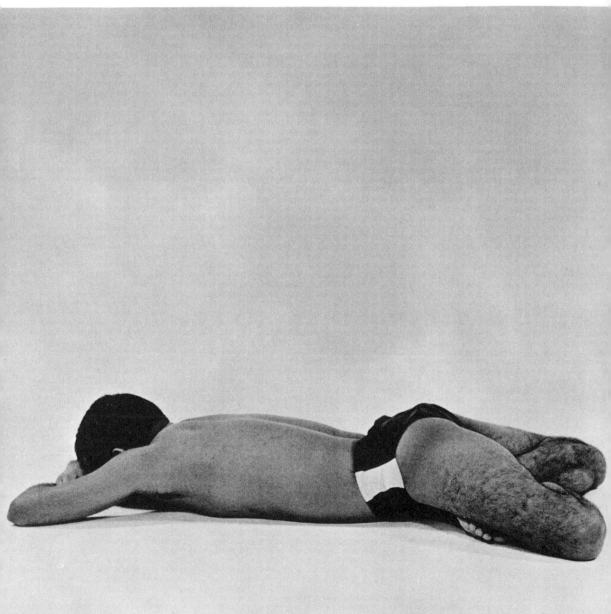

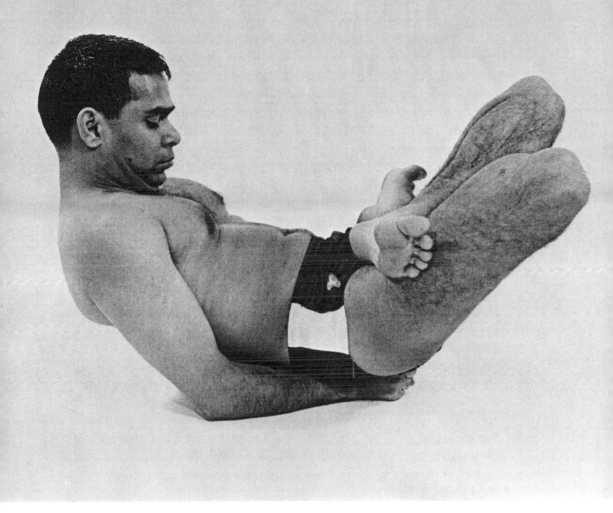

# Technique: **Tolangulasana** [balance pose]

*plate 49*

Sit in the lotus position, then place your elbows firmly on the floor and lift the buttocks, placing them upon the elbows. Lift the upper trunk and bend the head; press the chin with the chest. Hold your breath during the position. This exercise is very good for removing tension from the hip joint and the shoulder.

YOUTH AND FLEXIBILITY OF THE SPINE
THROUGH YOGA POSTURES

Good posture and a flexible spine are the cure of some evils, and certainly a preventive of many. In infancy, prevention has the greatest influence on the life expectancy of the baby though much can be done in later life to correct posture faults and a stiff backbone through continuous manipulations of the spinal column.

With a proper knowledge of the spine and its movements, the body can be trained to maintain its flexibility from early childhood until death.

All the benefits derived from the spinal movements cannot be explained in one book, but a careful study of the postures presented here will give an idea to what degree the human body can attain maximum flexibility of its spine and joints.

To determine a correct posture, the following test can be applied, the first part showing the ability to take an erect posture: The long axis of the trunk should continue the long axis of the head and neckline. To assist the observer in greater accuracy, a vertical line or thread may be dropped from the front of the ear to the forward part of the foot. In poor posture, the axis of the head, neck, and trunk will form a zigzag instead of a straight line.

Another method to estimate the extent of deformation is by standing the individual next to an upright pole. Three deviations from the correct posture are: (1) the gorilla type, in which the head is thrust forward, the chest sunken, and the abdomen protruding; (2) the round-back posture or type, where the hollow at the small of the back is obliterated; and (3) where the chest is pushed forward and upward and the lower spine overextended, forming a marked exaggeration of the natural lumbar curve.

By practice of the Yogic system, we not only retain the elasticity of youth and eliminate the abnormal growth of mineral deposits in the bones, but to a great degree we can also regain lost youth. The elasticity of the body further depends on the state of the blood vessels and the vertebral column; the gradual accumulation of sedimentary deposits, such as lime in the arterial and venous valves, owing to the impurities in the blood, gives rise to inelasticity in these parts. The faster these deposits accumulate, the quicker old age is upon us.

The Yogic manipulation of the spine can be divided broadly

into four categories: forward bending, backward bending, sideways movement, and twisting or the lateral movement of the spine.

FORWARD BENDING OF THE VERTEBRAE

Forward bending of the vertebrae can be divided into four categories:

1. Cervical forward bending
2. Thoracic forward bending
3. Lumbar forward bending
4. Sacral forward bending

Now let us go to different excrcises for various portions of the spine.

# YOGIC EXERCISES FOR CERVICAL REGION

## Technique: **Halasan** [plough pose]

### VARIATION 1

Lie flat on your back on the blanket. Keep the hands, palms down, near the thighs. Without bending the legs, slowly raise the hips and the lumbar part of the back also and bring down the legs until the toes touch the floor, beyond the head. Keep the knees straight and close together. The legs and thighs must be in one straight line. Press the chin against the chest; this will bend the cervical region and increase the circulation to that part. Breathe slowly through the nose.

     Remain in this pose as long as possible and go back to the original position lying flat. Repeat three to six times.

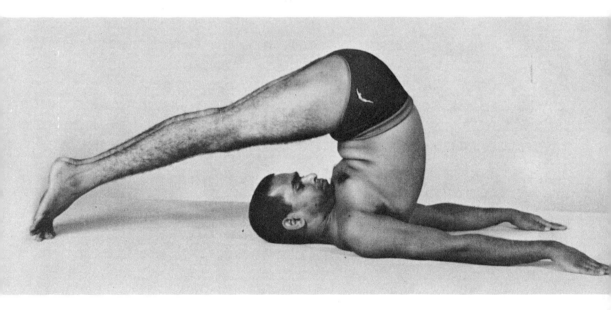

*plate 50*

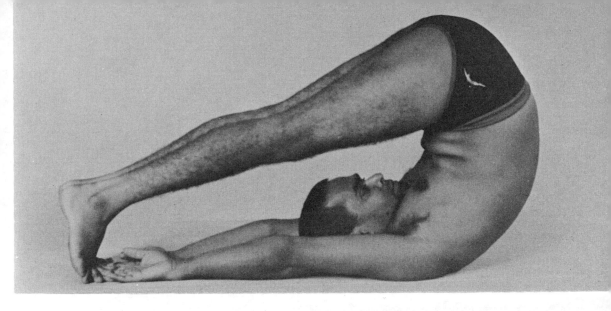

*plate 51*

## VARIATION 2

Lie down flat with the arms, palms up, over the head. Now slowly bring up the legs as in Variation 1, and touch the hands with the toes. This gives additional stretching to the lumbar and cervical regions of the spine.

## VARIATION 3

To come to this position, assume the original *halasan* position, then stretch the legs apart as far as possible, keeping the hands firmly on the floor. This stretches the muscles of the legs.

*plate 52*

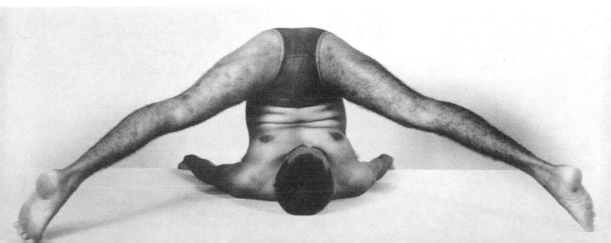

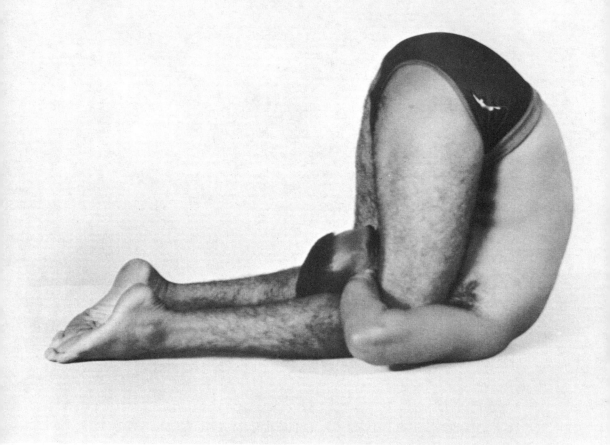

plate 53

Technique: **Karna Peedasan** [ear-knee pose]

In *karna peedasan,* the knees are bent toward the floor by each ear and pressed o the floor. This pulls the whole spine steadily, posteriorly. Every vertebra and ligament of the cervical region receives plenty of blood and becomes healthy.

All movements of the spine directly or indirectly give exercise to various internal organs and abdominal muscles. Any forward bending of the spine vigorously contracts the abdominal muscles and backward bending exercises and stretches the abdominal muscles.

Owing to accumulation of adipose tissue in the abdominal regions, more advanced exercises to the spine are found difficult to practice. But as you progress from the simple to the more complicated, you will find the difficult poses easier and there will be marked reduction of the extra fat of the abdominal muscles.

# YOGIC EXERCISES FOR LUMBAR REGION

### Technique: **Vatayanasan** [wind relieving pose]

This exercise is ideal for those suffering from excessive gas in the stomach and intestinal tract. People with indigestion and other abdominal ailments also find this very useful. Even very old people and obese people find this exercise easy and relief giving.

      Technique: Lie down flat. Now take a long, deep breath and hold it. During retention of the breath fold your right leg at the knee and press the folded leg with the abdomen. Use both hands in order to get the maximum pressure. Keep the left leg straight. Avoid bending the left knee. Repeat this exercise three times with each leg alternately. Now use both legs and press both the knees against the abdomen, three times, as before.

*plate 54*

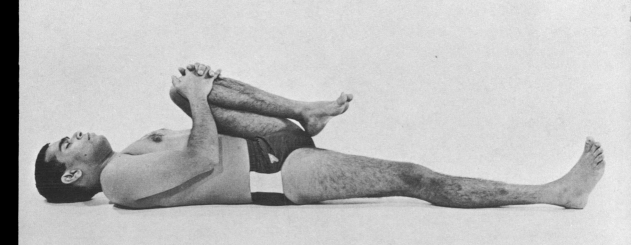

### Technique: **Paschimothan Asana** [head-knee pose]

Lie flat on your back on the blanket, with arms overhead on the floor. Keep the legs and thighs firmly on the floor. Stiffen your body. Slowly raise the head and chest and assume a sitting pose. Now exhale and bend yourself further until you are able to catch hold of your toes. You may even bury your face between the knees.

Remain thus for five seconds and then slowly raise the body and resume the supine position. You should now inhale.

Repeat this *asana* three to six times.

This is a powerful abdominal exercise. It stimulates such abdominal viscera as the kidneys, liver, and pancreas. This exercise is invaluable for diabetic patients. The hamstring muscles of the back of the knees are strengthened. The spine becomes elastic and thereby perennial youth is established.

*Paschimothan asana* can be practiced by balancing on the buttocks (see Plate No. 56, Variation 2). This gives more stretching to the leg muscles.

Advanced students practice this exercise without catching the toes, which gives them more flexibility of the spine (see Variation 3, Plate No. 57).

Immediately after this exercise, the spine should be stretched backward, resting on heels and hands and keeping the body straight. It can be repeated two or three times, each time remaining in the pose a few seconds, retaining the breath (see Plate No. 58).

*plate 55*

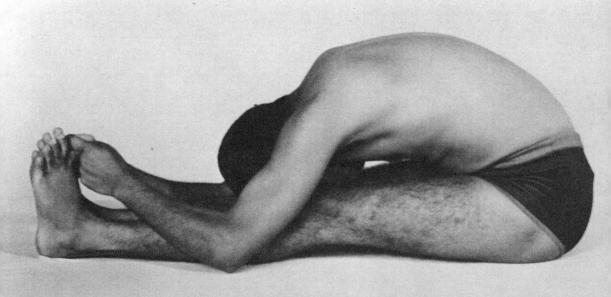

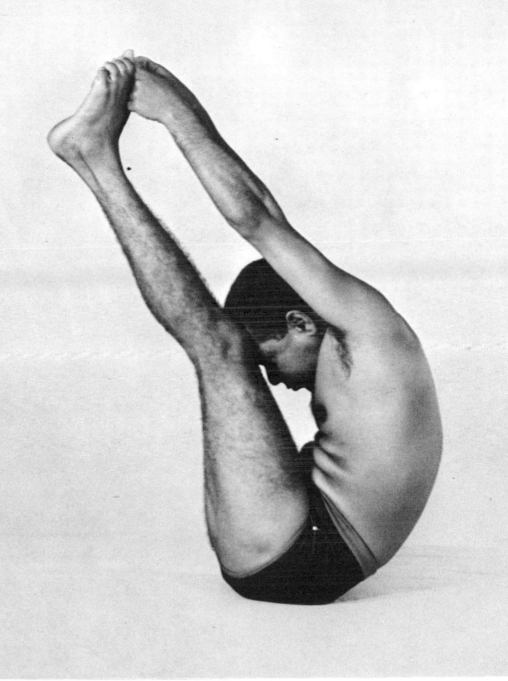

plate 56

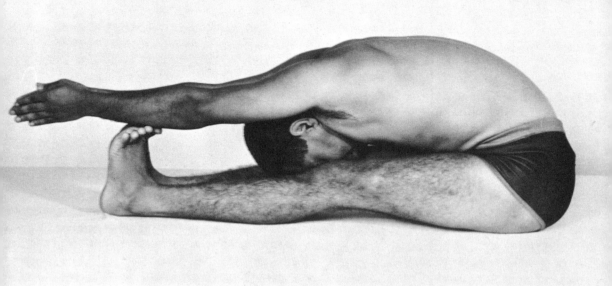

plate 57


plate 58

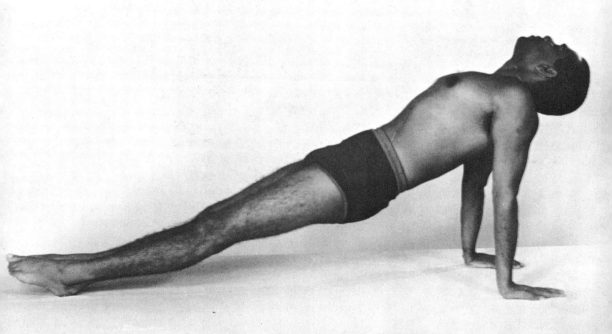

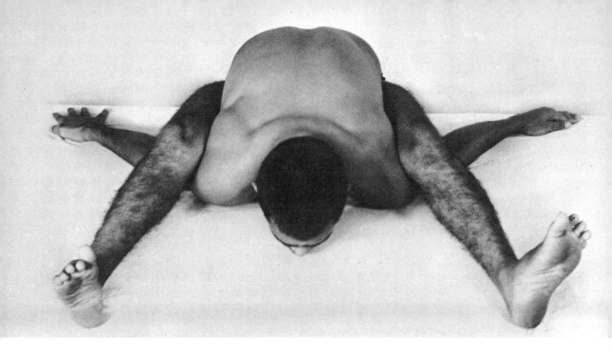

*plate 59*

## ADVANCED YOGIC EXERCISES FOR LUMBAR AND THORACIC REGION

### Technique: **Kurmasan** [tortoise pose]

Keep the legs apart. Bend the body forward and put the arms under the thighs. Keep the hands firmly on the floor. Stretch the legs.

### Technique: **Hastha Padasan** [leg and arm stretching exercise]

Sit, stretching the legs forward. Catch hold of the toes and draw the feet away from each other as much as possible. Bend forward and rest the chin on the floor. The knees and arms should not be bent.

Both *kurmasan* and *hastha padasan* are very good to bring maximum flexibility to the lumbar region and the ligaments.

*plate 60*

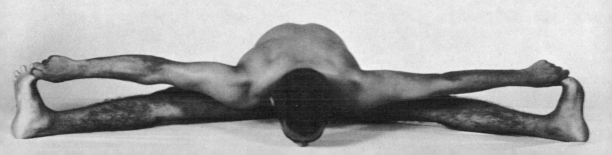

## Technique: **Janu Sirasan** [head-knee pose]

### VARIATION 1

Sit down. Press the perineal space with your left heel, stretching your right leg at full length. Keep it straight. Catch hold of the right foot with both hands. Exhale. Draw the belly inward. Slowly bend down and touch your right knee with the forehead. Keep this position for five to ten seconds and gradually increase the period. Then resume the normal position and repeat three to six times. Change the sides alternately.

### VARIATION 2

Instead of pressing the perineal space with the heel, keep the foot on the thigh. This will press the abdominal viscera when the spine is bent forward.

### VARIATION 3

This goes a little further, and here you must catch the toes of the foot kept on the thigh, and then bend forward. Along with the bending of the spine, the shoulder muscles and the thoracic region are pulled.

*plate 61*

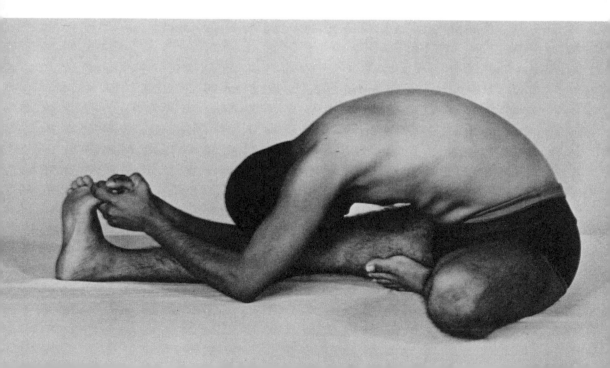

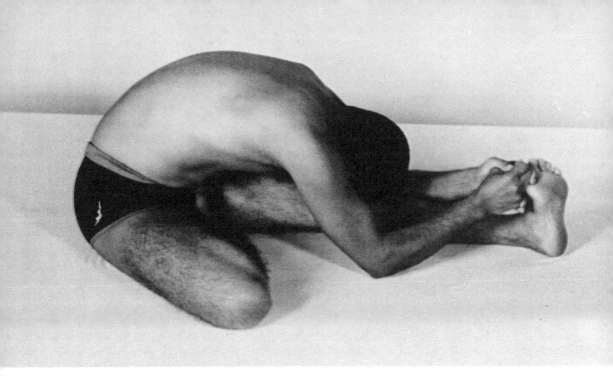

plate 62

plate 63

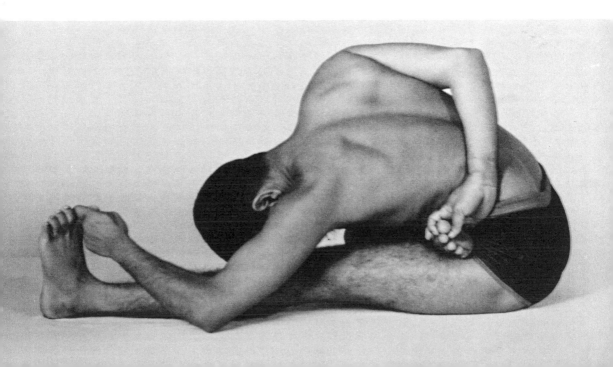

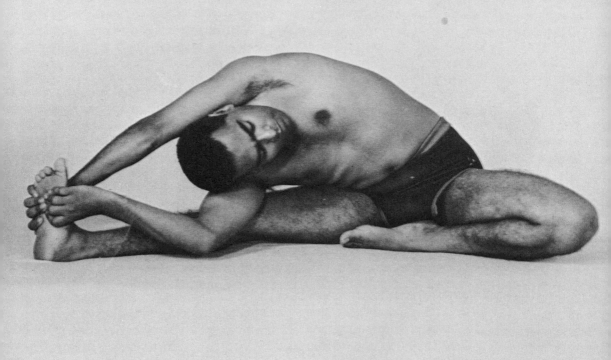

*plate 64*

### VARIATION 4, SIDEWAYS POSITION

Bend the right leg and stretch the left one sideways. Catch the left foot firmly and bend the trunk sideways.

### VARIATION 5

Stretch the legs, then bend the right knee. Keep the right foot close to the perineum. Now lift the left leg straight up and catch the foot. Bend the head and touch the knee.

Reverse the process and repeat several times.

*plate 65*

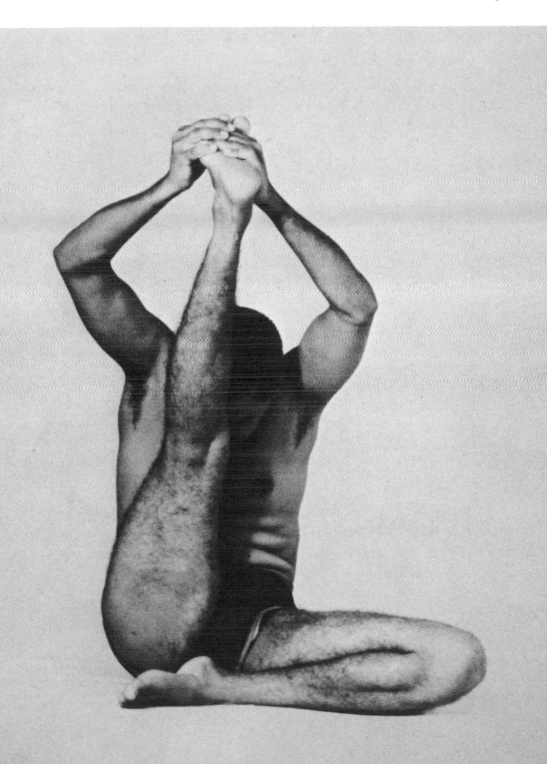

# STRETCHING THE LEG MUSCLES IN SITTING POSITION

## Technique: **Eka Pada Sirasan** [leg-head pose]

### VARIATION 1

Sit erect and stretch the legs. Now take the right foot with the hands and push it behind the head. Hold the leg firmly and keep the hands folded in front of the body for a few minutes. Reverse the pose.

*plate 66*

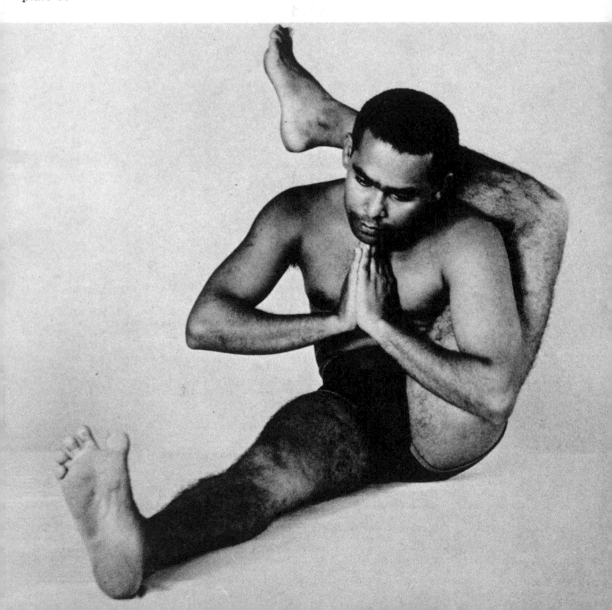

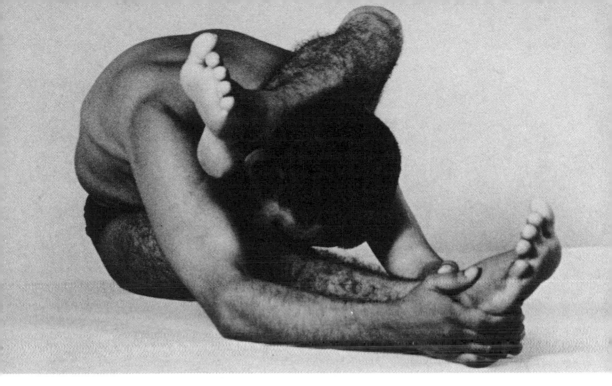

## Technique: **Eka Pada Sirasan** [bending in leg-head pose]

plate 67

### VARIATION 2

From the sitting position of *eka pada sirasan*, bend forward and catch the right foot. At the same time the left foot should be kept firmly behind the neck.

## Technique: **Eka Pada Sirasan** [leg-head pose while lying]

### VARIATION 3

From the sitting position of *eka pada sirasan*, slowly lie down while keeping the left foot straight and right foot behind the neck.

plate 68

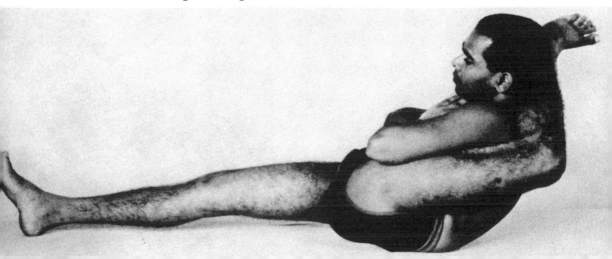

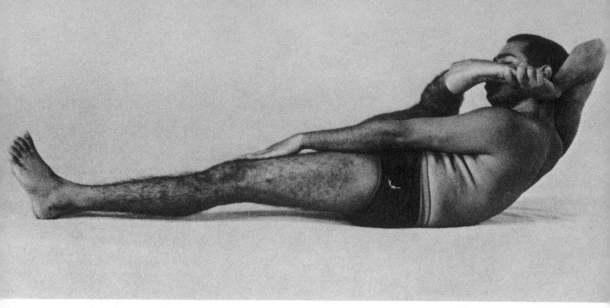

*plate 69*

## Technique: **Eka Pada Sirasan** [leg-head pose]

### VARIATION 4

Lie down flat. Bring the right foot to the left ear. Now with the right hand pull the right toes toward the left ear as much as possible.

## Technique: **Eka Pada Sirasan** [leg-head pose]

### VARIATION 5

*plate 70*

Lie flat on the back. Raise the head and thoracic portion of the spine. Now catch the right foot firmly, keeping the right knee straight. Bring the right knee to the forehead while keeping the left leg straight on the floor.

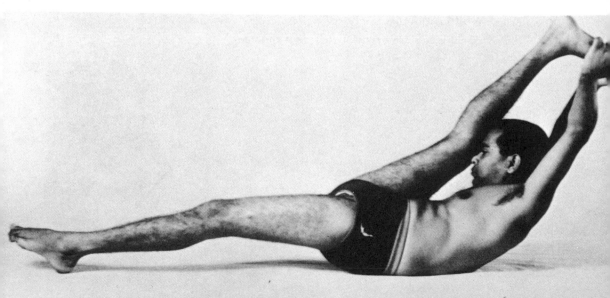

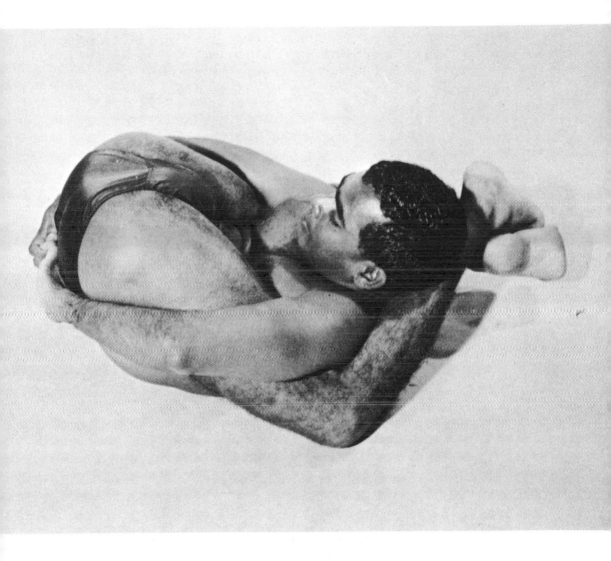

## Technique: **Dwipada Sirasan** [head-knee pose]

*plate 71*

Lie on the back and slowly pull the right leg over the head. Do not try to use too much force. Once the right foot is firm, pull the left foot over the head and the right foot. Interlock the fingers at the hipjoint.

This is one of the advanced exercises and should be practiced with caution. There is no other exercise in the forward-bending group that gives such a tremendous pressure on the abdominal muscles. Spine and neck get more exercise. The muscles of the legs and thighs are kept elastic and strong with this exercise.

## Technique: **Omkarasana, or Pranavasana** [OM pose]

This pose resembles the Sanskrit letter OM, as it is written; hence, it is named *omkarasan*.

Technique: Place the left foot over the right thigh. Now take the right foot and place it behind the head. This provides maximum stretching of the thigh muscles and puts tremendous pressure on the abdominal organs, as in the full spinal twist exercise.

*plate 72*

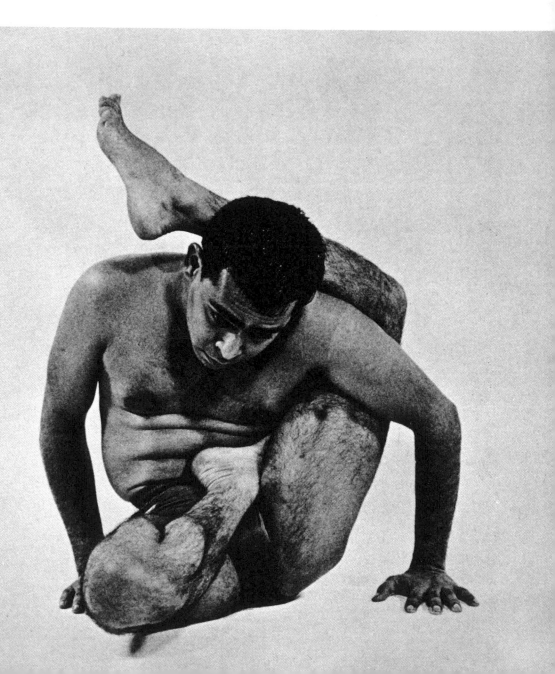

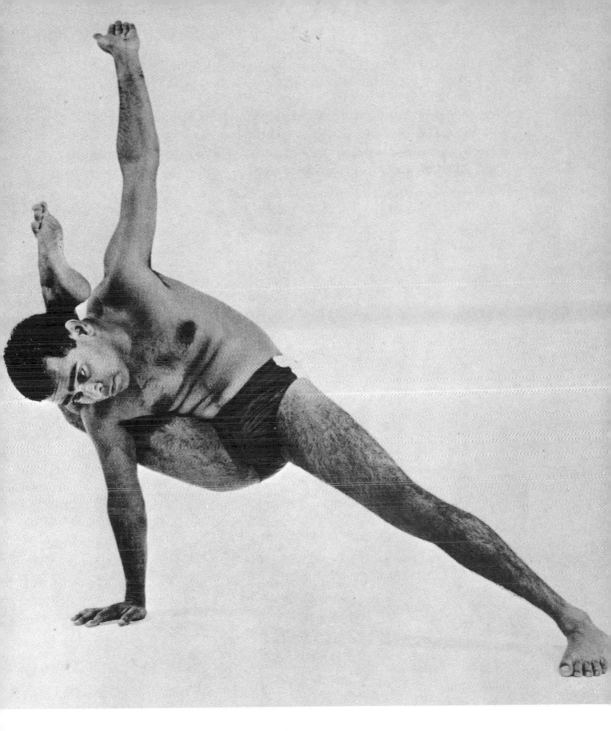

Technique: **Krishna Asana** [baby Krishna pose]

*plate 73*

One leg is passed over and behind the head and wedged against the nape of the neck; balance is kept on the other leg and opposite arm. This exercise offers a stretching and sideways motion simultaneously.

# Technique: **Uthitha Kurmasan** [tortoise pose, in balancing]

Place the right foot behind the head and wedged against the nape of the neck; then pass the left foot behind the right foot and form an ankle lock. Now balance on the hands. This is one of the more difficult poses and should therefore be done only by advanced students. This puts great pressure on the shoulder muscles and abdominal muscles.

*plate 74*

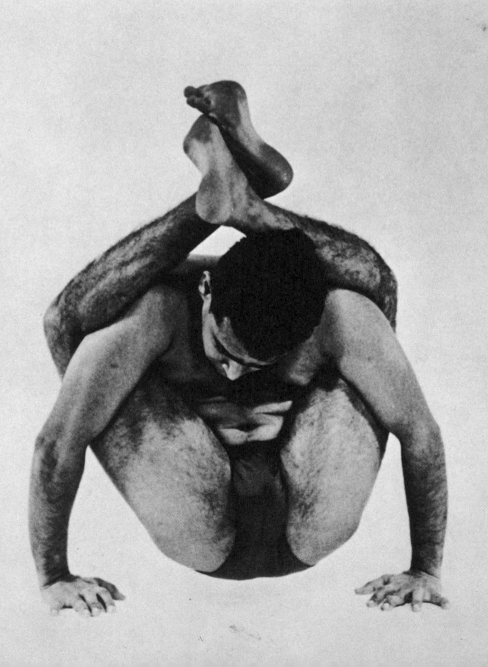

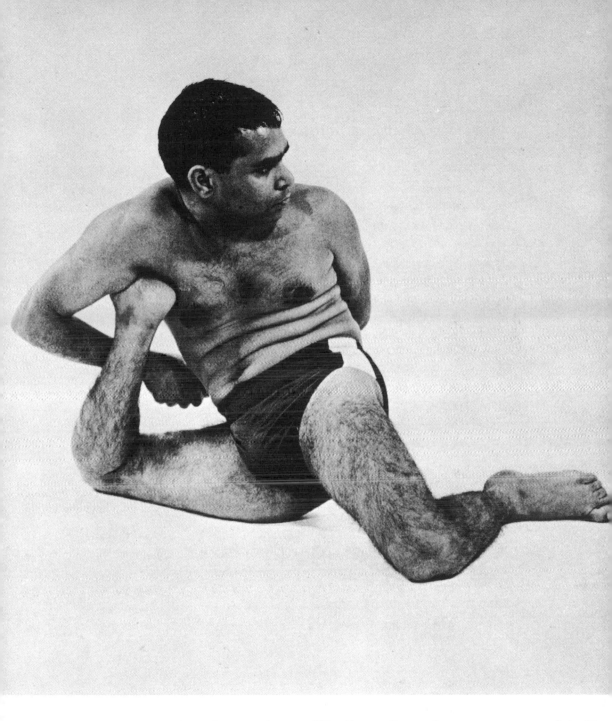

Technique: **Yoga Danta Asana** [Yogi's staff pose]     *plate 75*

In this exercise the knee joints are twisted and the foot is kept under the right armpit; the hands are locked behind the back. This increases the flexibility of the knee joints.

# BACKWARD BENDING EXERCISES

## YOGIC EXERCISES FOR SACRUM

## Technique: **Bhujangasan** [cobra pose]

### VARIATION 1

Lie face down on the blanket. Relax all the muscles completely. Place the palms on the blanket, below the corresponding shoulders. Raise the head and upper portion of the body slowly, just as the cobra raises its hood. Bend the spine well. Do not raise the body suddenly with a jerk. Roll back the spine slowly so that you can actually feel the bending of the vertebrae one by one and the pressure traveling downward from the cervical, dorsal, and lumbar regions and lastly to the sacral regions. Let the body from the navel downward to the toes touch the blanket.

Retain the pose for awhile and slowly bring down the head little by little. Breathe in while you bend backward, hold the breath while in the position, and exhale while coming down. Repeat the process six times.

There are many variations in this cobra pose in order to give a maximum bending to the spine.

The deep and superficial muscles of the back are well toned. This pose relieves the pain of the back that may have been caused by overwork. The abdominal muscles are pulled and thereby strengthened. It increases the intra-abdominal pressure. All the abdominal viscera are toned. Every vertebra and its ligaments are pulled backward and they get a rich blood supply. It increases bodily heat and destroys a host of ailments.

*Bhujangasan* is particularly useful for women for toning the ovaries and uterus. It is a powerful tonic. It will relieve amenorrhea, dysmenorrhea, leucorrhea, and various other utero-ovarine troubles.

*plate 76*

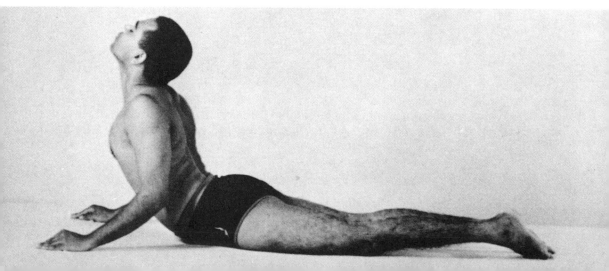

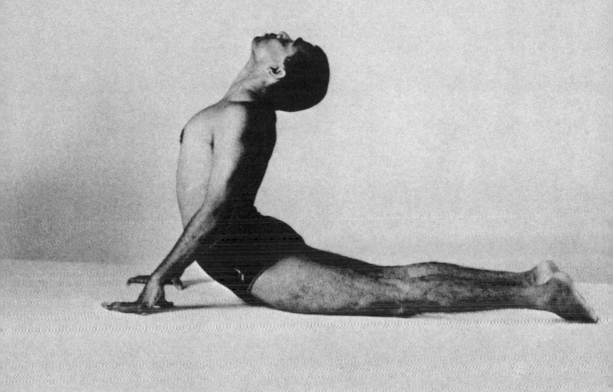

## Technique: **Bhujangasan** [cobra pose]

*plate 77*

### VARIATION 2

From the first position of cobra pose, rise further, keeping the elbows straight. In Variation 1, the elbows are not straightened and the sacral region of the spine is bent. In Variation 2, complete bending movement of the spine from sacral region to cervical region is done.

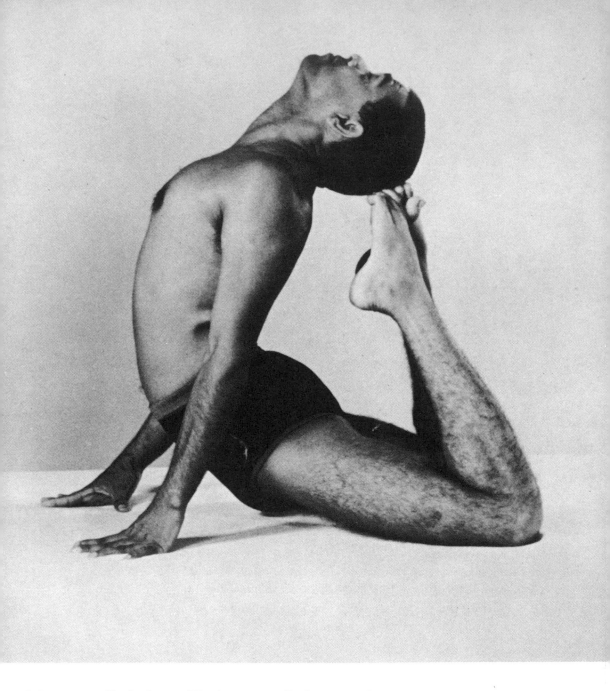

plate 78   Technique: **Bhujangasan** [cobra pose]

VARIATION 3

From Variation 2 of the cobra pose, bend the spine as much as possible.
Now fold the legs at the knees, bring the toes toward the head, and touch
the back of the head.

## Technique: **Salabhasan** [locust pose]

VARIATION 1

Lie prone (face down) on the blanket and keep the hands alongside the body, palms up. Rest the chin on the ground by raising the head a little. Now inhale slowly. Stiffen the whole body and raise the legs high. The knees should be kept straight. The sacrum too should be raised a little along with legs. Now the chest and the hands will feel the burden of the legs. Keep the thighs, legs, and toes in a straight line. Remain in the pose for twenty seconds and slowly come down. Repeat the process three or four times according to your capacity.

*plate 79*

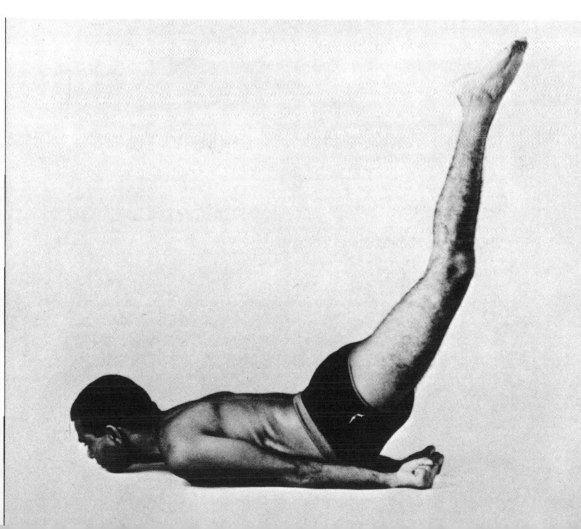

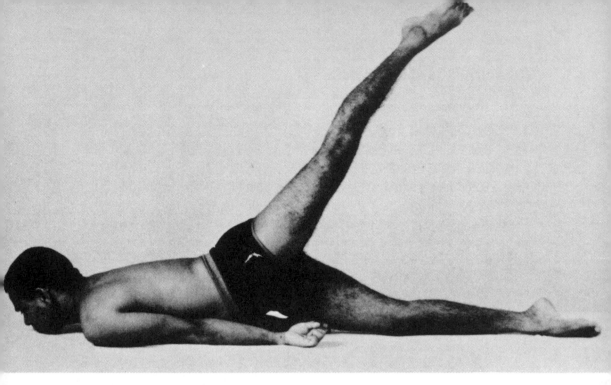

plate 80

## Technique: **Arhda-Salabhasan** [half locust pose]

### VARIATION 2

This is practiced by alternately lifting the legs. As you progress in this half pose, then you can start lifting both legs simultaneously. It is a preliminary to the complete *Salabhasan*.

## Technique: **Salabhasan** [locust pose]

### VARIATION 3

In this position, the cervical region and ligaments are used more. In the first variety, the sacrum and lumbar regions are used. The technique is the same except that more force must be used on the hands to raise the body till the whole body rests on the chin. This exerts tremendous pressure on the back muscles and shoulder muscles (platysma, trapezius, splenius capitis, sterno-cleidomastoid) and the biceps and deltoid of the upper arms and thereby stretches the muscles and tendons and increases the blood circulation. This exercise, when it is performed correctly, looks exactly opposite to the shoulderstand.

plate 81

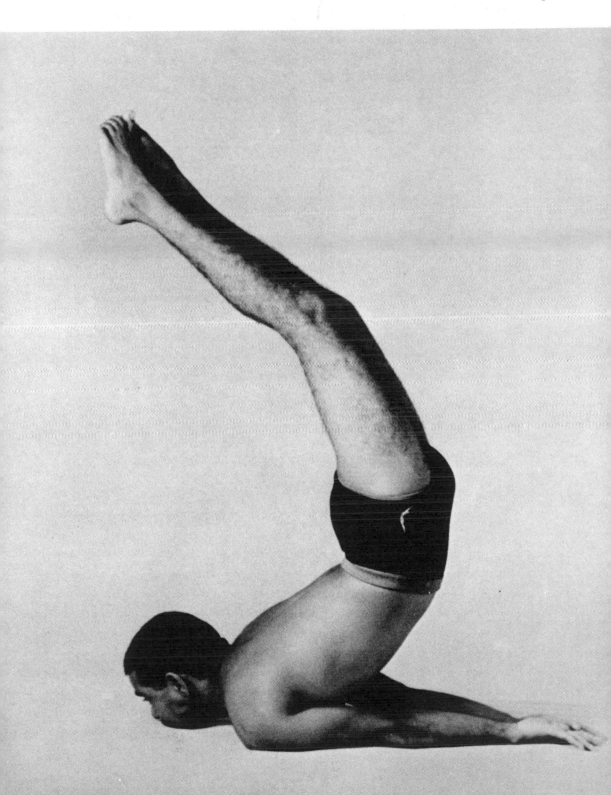

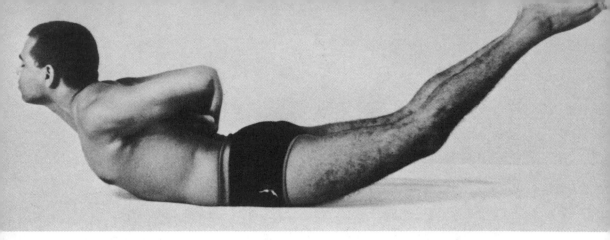

*plate 82*

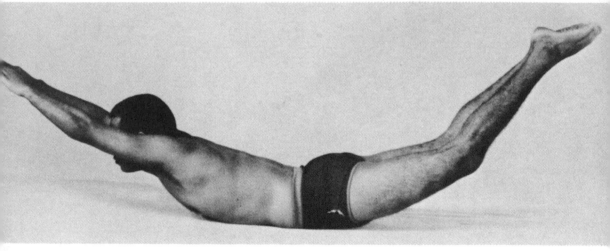

*plate 83*

## Technique: **Salabhasan** [locust pose]

### VARIATION 4

In the position of *salabhasan* (locust pose), keep the hands behind and raise the chin. Now without the help of the hands and chin, the legs and chest are raised, and one rests on the abdomen.

This pose puts more pressure on the lumbar region. It presses upon and tones the abdominal viscera.

## Technique: **Salabhasan** [locust pose]

### VARIATION 5

The technique here is the same as for Variation 4, except that the arms are stretched forward, bringing the fingertips and tip of the toes to the same level. This forms the shape of a boat.

## Technique: **Dhanurasan** [bow pose]

### VARIATION 1

When this *asana* is performed, it gives the appearance of a bow. The stretched hands and legs represent the string of a bow; and the body and thighs represent the bow proper.

Lie prone on the blanket. Relax the muscles. Now bend the legs over the thighs. Catch hold of the right ankle with the right hand and the left ankle with the left hand firmly. Raise the head, body, and knees by tugging at the legs with the hands so that the whole burden of the body rests on the abdomen and the spine is nicely arched backward like a bow. Maintain the pose for a few seconds and relax the body. Hold the breath while performing this pose. Do not permit jerks when you do this pose.

You can see by the illustration that the whole spine is bent like a bow. So this is the best exercise for cervical, thoracic, lumbar, or sacral region of the spine.

This pose gives the combined effect of the cobra and locust poses. The back muscles are well massaged. This removes constipation and cures dyspepsia, rheumatism, and gastrointestinal disorders. It reduces fat, energizes digestion, invigorates appetite, and relieves congestion of the blood in the abdominal viscera. This pose is recommended for women.

*plate 84*

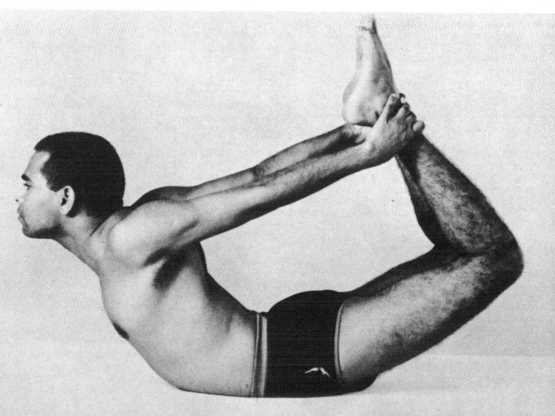

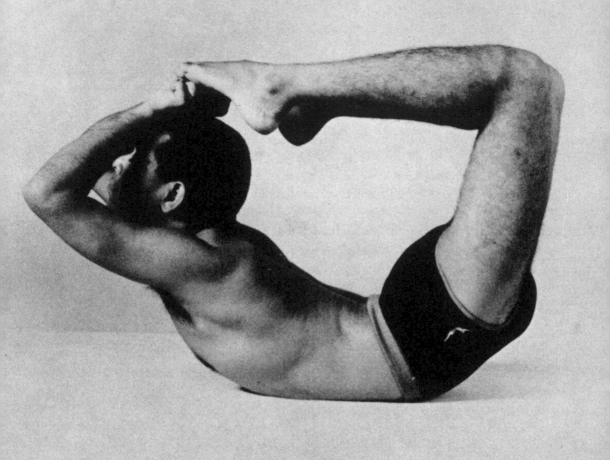

*plate 85*

## Technique: **Poorna Dhanurasan** [bow pose, full]

VARIATION 2

This is known as full *Dhanurasana* or *Poorna Dhanurasana*. To perform this, considerable flexibility of the spine is required.

Lie on the abdomen and fold the legs at the knees. Take hold of the big toes with the hands and slowly pull the feet toward the head.

This gives maximum exercise to the spine.

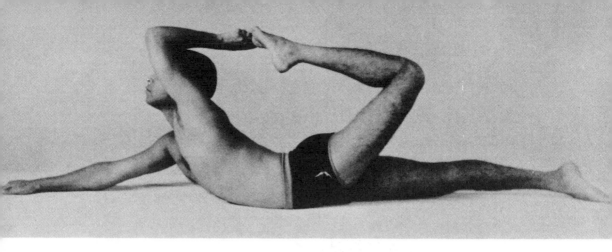

## Technique: **Dhanurasan** [bow pose]

*plate 86*

### VARIATION 3

In this pose, half of the body is bent and half is kept straight.

Lie down and fold the right knee. Catch the right toe with the right hand and slowly pull it toward the head, bending the right side of the back. Alternate the procedure for the left side. This can be done two times for each side.

## Technique: **Dhanurasan** [bow pose]

### VARIATION 4

This pose exercises more effectively the ankle, knee, and shoulder muscles.

Lie face down and fold the legs. Now press the feet with the hands until the heels touch the floor. Keep the head above the floor.

*plate 87*

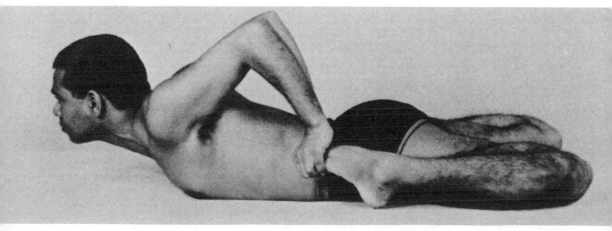

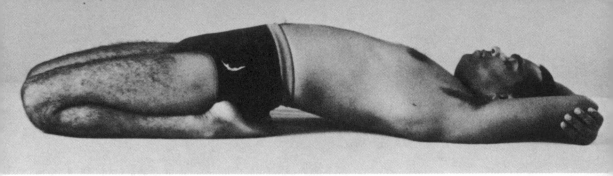

*plate 88*

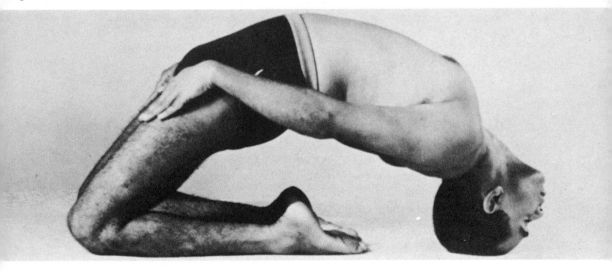

*plate 89*

## BACKWARD BENDING EXERCISES IN SITTING POSITION

### Technique: **Supta Vajrasan** [kneeling pose]

VARIATION 1

Sit on the heels. With the help of the elbows, slowly bend backward. Lie flat on the ground. Keep the arms folded behind the head.

This is very good for women. It stretches the muscles of the legs and muscles of the gluteal regions or buttocks.

### Technique: **Supta Vajrasan** [kneeling pose]

VARIATION 2

In this position, one must bend the spine as much as possible. Rest on the legs and head. Keep the hands on the thighs. This is a marvelous exercise for the spine. Cervical region and thyroid and parathyroid are exercised and get more blood supply.

Technique: **Poorna Supta Vajrasan** [diamond pose in full kneeling position]

Assume a kneeling position. Now slowly lie down on your back, keeping the knees together. As you touch the floor with your head, lift the buttocks and body from the floor, resting on the head and legs. Use the hands to push your head nearer to the heels. Through gradual practice you will be able to bring the head toward the heels. For beginners, this brings maximum flexibility to the back and develops the thoracic cage.

*plate 90*

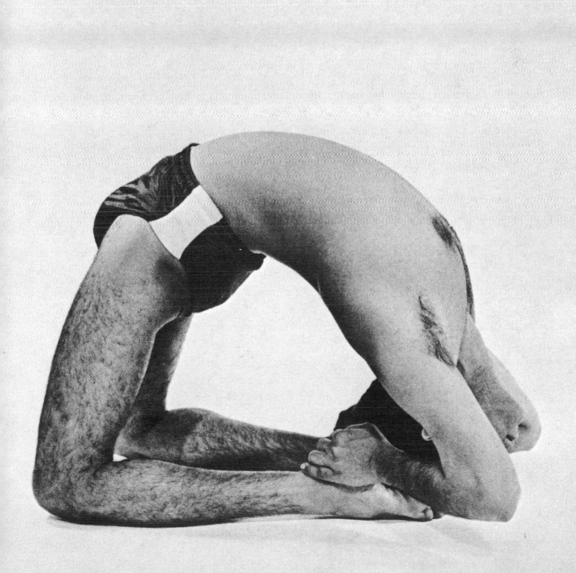

## Technique: **Kapotha Asan** [pigeon pose]

Bend the right leg at the knee and keep the right foot at the left thigh joint. Now stretch the left leg backward and bend the knee. With the hands, pull the left foot and touch the head. Bend the head and chest as much as possible. Practice this on alternate sides several times.

This is a very good exercise to stretch the muscles of the legs, thighs, and back.

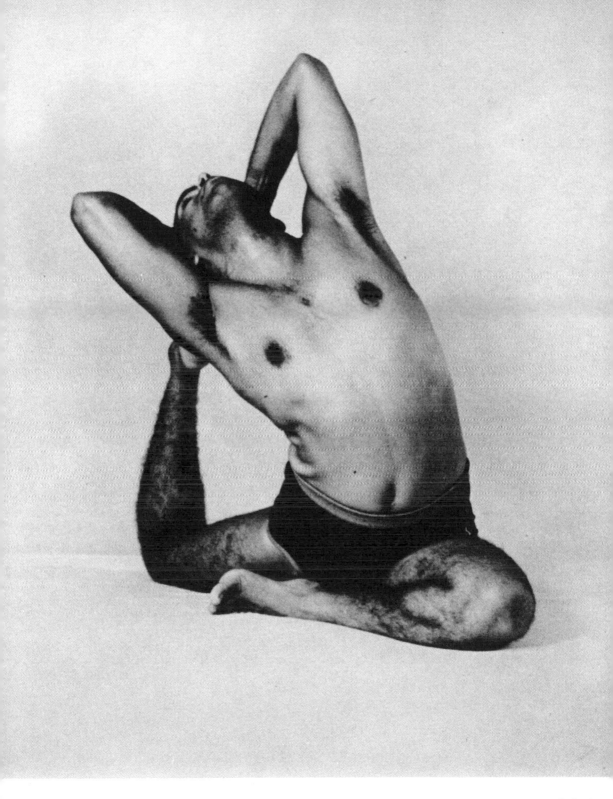

plate 91

# BACKWARD BENDING EXERCISES ON HAND

## Technique: **Vrischikasan** [scorpion pose]

First stage is to kneel on the floor, bend forward and place the forearms on the ground (palms down). Press the floor with the forearms and throw the legs up and straighten them. Keep the head above the floor and balance.

*plate 92*

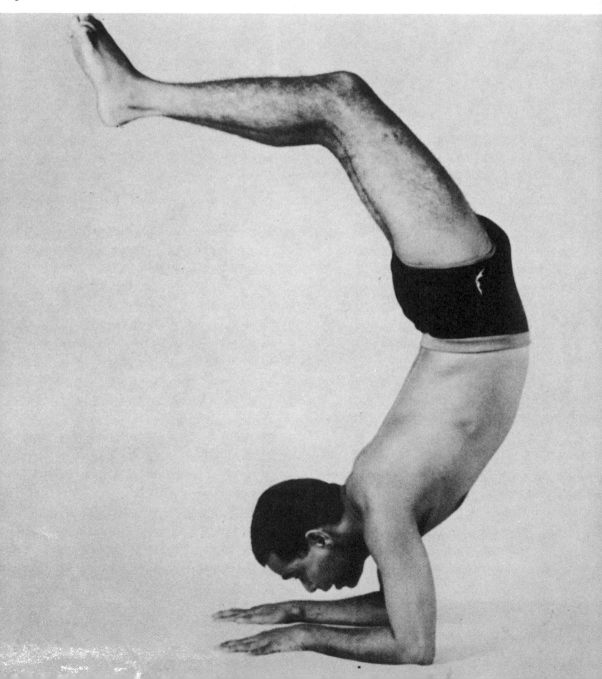

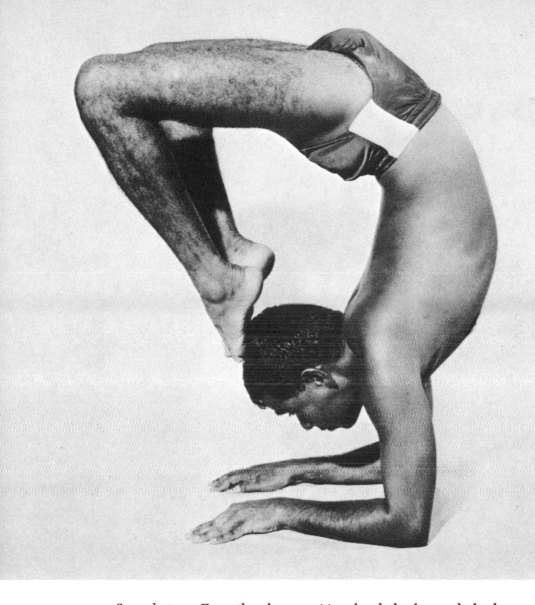

*Second stage*. From the above position, bend the legs and slowly bring them down over the head, which must all the time be above the floor, face parallel to the floor. Slowly touch the crown of the head with the soles of the feet.

*plate 93*

This *asana* gives maximum bending to the spine and imparts balance and harmony to the entire system. It should be practiced only after acquiring maximum proficiency in the headstand and *chakrasana*, the wheel pose.

Along with the spine and ligaments, this exercise stretches almost every muscle of the body and increases the circulation to every part, including the brain. As this pose is a difficult one, it takes a long time to achieve mastery over it.

## Technique: **Vrikshasana** [tree pose]

This is a hand-balancing exercise. One should be able to do a headstand properly and easily before attempting it. Beginners can use wall support until balance is secured. This strengthens the arms and shoulders. Because the head is not touching the floor (as in the headstand), there is no pressure on the vertebrae.

*plate 94*

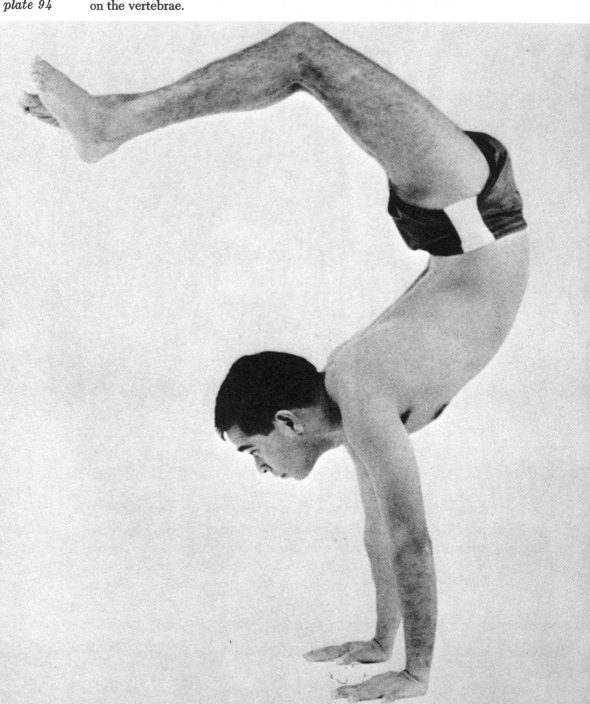

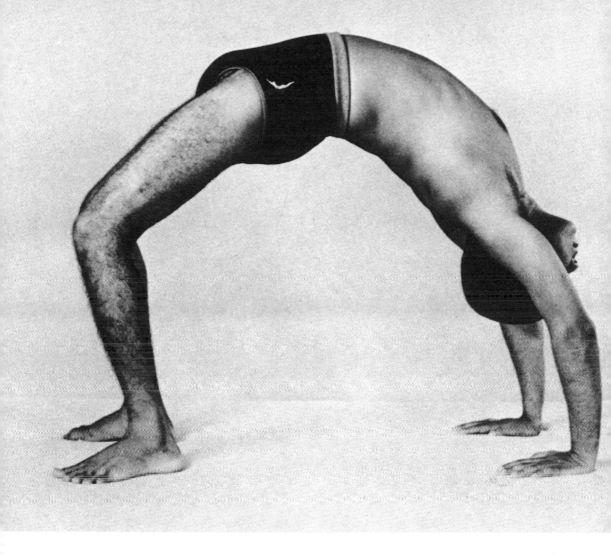

## Technique: **Chakrasana** [wheel pose]

VARIATION 1

This pose can be done in two ways.

Lie down. Bend the arms and legs. Raise the body and rest on the hands and feet. Bend the spine as much as possible by bringing the hands toward the feet.

In this pose the muscles of the legs, hips, shoulders, and arms along with the spine and its ligaments get complete bending and stretching. In this one pose, almost all the benefits of backward bending can be had. Advanced students take the variations to obtain more benefits.

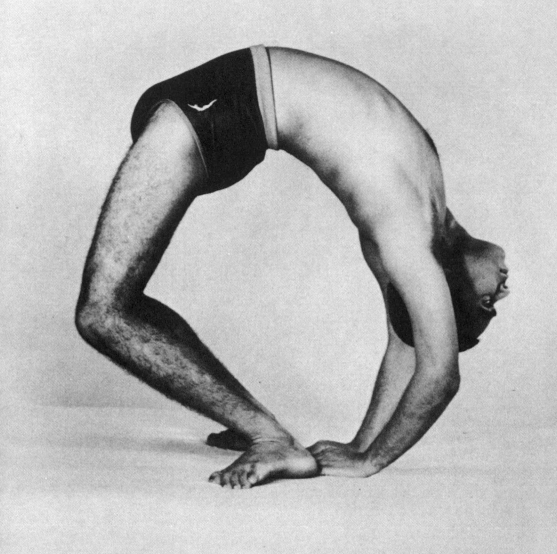

*plate 96*

Technique: **Chakrasana** [wheel pose]

## VARIATION 2

From the position of Variation 1, slowly bring the hands toward the heels and touch them. This is the final position and the whole body looks like a wheel.

## Technique: **Eka Pada Chakrasana** [wheel pose on one leg]

VARIATION 3

From Variation 1, raise the right leg and right arm and rest on the left foot and left hand. After relaxation, do the pose using the left hand and foot.

The second way of practicing the wheel pose is to stand erect and slowly bend backward until the hands touch the ground. Now rest on the arms and legs. Beginners should be careful when practicing this as they may fall backward and injure the head. This needs more balance and flexibility. To be on the safe side, first practice the first variation.

This pose may be done two to three times.

*plate 97*

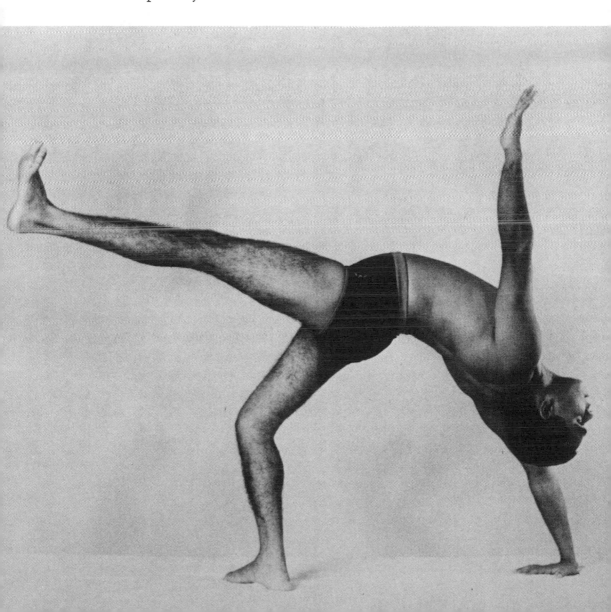

Technique: **Chakrasana** [wheel pose]

VARIATION 4

Stand erect with the hands along the thighs. Now bend backward, putting the weight on the heels and calf muscles. As you bend backward your hands will come nearer to the ankle. Now grab the ankle and pull your body downward as much as possible. (This exercise resembles the standing bow pose.)

*plate 98*

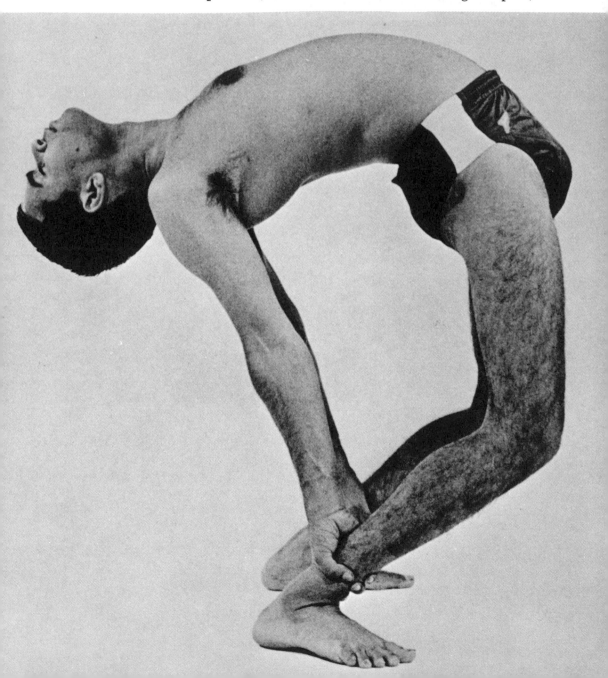

# Technique: **Chakrasana** [wheel pose]

VARIATION 5

Assume a kneeling position and bend backward, raising the buttocks. Now grasp the ankles. Breathe deeply and hold the breath for a few seconds and repeat the exercise three to four times. For beginners this pose is considerably easier than the two previous variations.

*plate 99*

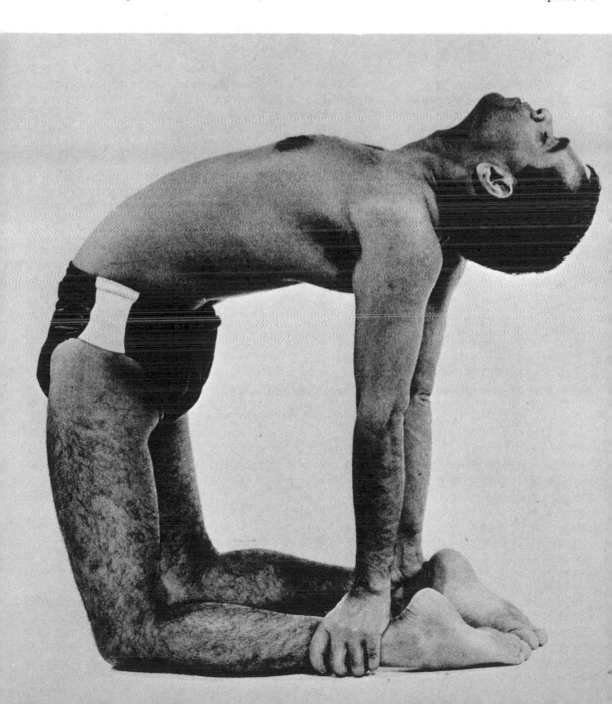

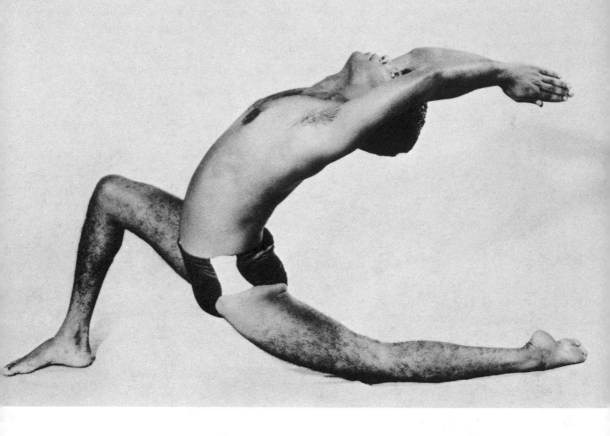

plate 100    Technique: **Anjaneyasana** [leg-split]

Stretch the right foot back as far as possible. Keep the left foot flat on the
floor with knees bending. Raise the hands above the head and slowly pull
the spine backward until the hands, spine, and legs have the appearance of
a semicircle.

# LATERAL MOVEMENTS OF THE SPINE

## Technique: **Ardha Matsendrasan** [spinal twist]

We have dealt with forward and backward bending of the spine. Now let us go to the lateral tilt in the dorsolumbar and lumbar spine and in the lumbo-sacral area, combined with extension of the pelvis at the hips.

Spread a blanket on the floor and sit on it with the knees close to the chest and resting on the feet. Bend the right leg at the knee and set the heel against the perineum. Do not allow the heel to move from this place. Now bend the left leg at the knee and with the hands arrange the foot to rest on the floor by the external side of the thigh. Then passing the right arm over the left knee, catch hold of the left foot firmly with the right hand. The left knee is now placed at the right axilla. In order to have more mechanical advantage for twisting the spine, the left hand is now swung back and the right thigh is caught. Now steadily pull and twist the spine. To help the spine to twist evenly all through, the neck too is turned toward the left shoulder. Keep the chest erect and forward.

Remain in this pose for five seconds. Then release the hands and legs. Repeat the same process, twisting the spine on the right side by changing the limbs, thus accomplishing the twist on both sides. This will complete the whole spinal twist.

This pose keeps the spine elastic and massages the abdominal organs well. Lumbago and all sorts of muscular rheumatism of the back muscles are helped. The spinal nerve roots and the sympathetic system are toned. They draw a good supply of blood. This is a very good *asana* for constipation and dyspepsia. In this pose every vertebra is rotated on both sides. The ligaments too that are attached to the vertebra get this movement and so receive a rich supply of blood. All the spinal nerves are toned.

On the following pages are shown the two variations of this pose (plates 101, 102).

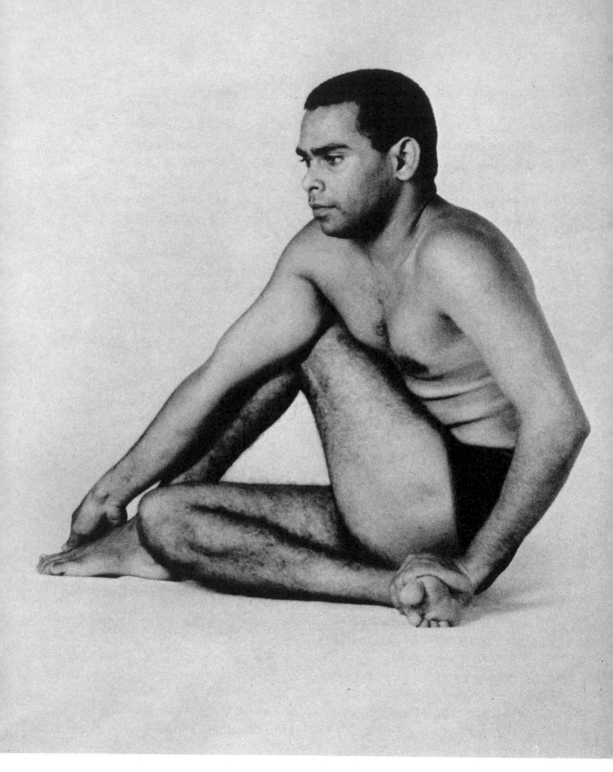

plate 101

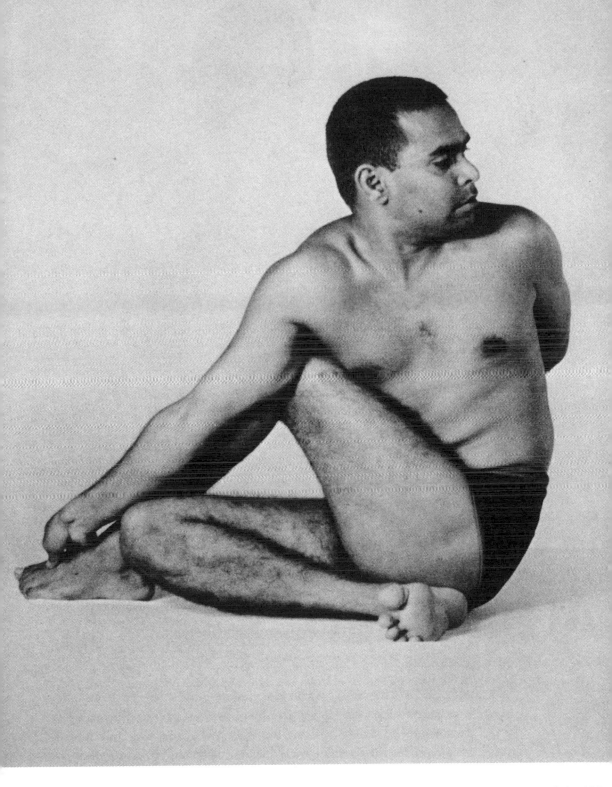

plate 102

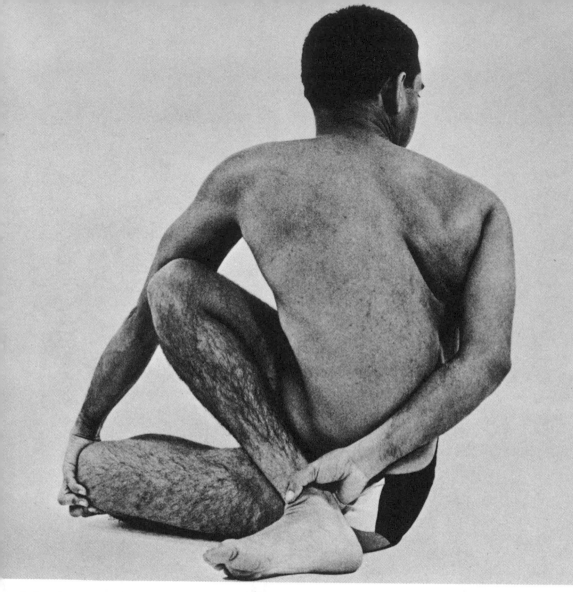

*plate 103*

## Technique: **Ardha Matsendrasan** [spinal twist]

### VARIATION 2

In Variation 1, twisting of the spine was almost even from top to bottom; in the second position, the upper shoulder muscles get additional twist.

    Technique: Sit down, bending the right leg so that the right heel is under the crotch. Pass the left leg over the right thigh and plant the foot flat on the floor. Pass the right arm behind the left knee and grasp the right knee. Now place the left arm behind the back and grasp the left ankle firmly. Keep this position for half a minute to one minute and then reverse the pose. By giving the body a side twist, the spinal column is made supple laterally, the tracts of the major sympathetic are toned up, and the muscles of the back are massaged.

# Technique: **Poorna Matsendriyasana** [full spinal twist]

### VARIATION 3

This pose is one of the most difficult to master. Before this exercise is practiced, you must be able to perform the lotus pose perfectly and with ease. The difference between variation 1 and the full position is only in placement of the foot. In the half position the right foot is under the thigh and the left foot is behind the right knee. In this position, the right foot is kept between the abdominal muscles and the thigh muscles and the left foot is in the same position as before (behind the right knee). When you bring the right arm behind the left knee to grasp the left foot, the right foot, which is between the abdomen and thigh, exerts tremendous pressure on the liver and stomach. In addition, the pressure is applied to the kidneys and intestines. In this way, all of the abdominal organs are massaged and circulation is increased, eliminating poisons produced in the digestive process.

*plate 104*

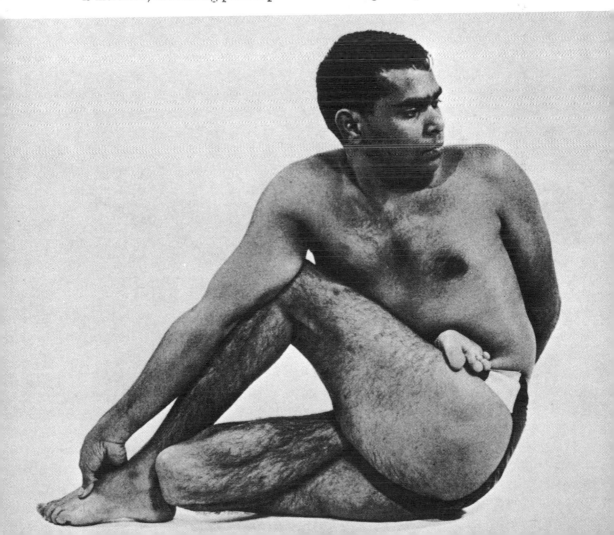

# BALANCING EXERCISES

## Technique: **Mayoorasan** [peacock pose]

### VARIATION 1

In Sanscrit, *mayur* means "peacock." When this *asana* is exhibited, the body resembles a peacock that has spread out its bundle of feathers at the back.

Kneel on a blanket. Join the two arms together and rest the hands on the floor, palms down with fingers pointing toward the toes. You may curve the fingers slightly. This facilitates balancing. Keep the hands firm. Now you have steady and firm forearms for supporting the whole body. Bring down the abdomen slowly against the conjoined elbows. Support your body on your elbows. Then stretch your legs. Inhale and raise the legs together from the floor. Raise the legs straight on a level with the head, parallel to the floor. Keep the posture steady for five seconds and then rest the toes on the floor and exhale. Rest for a few minutes. It can be performed two or three times.

*plate 105*

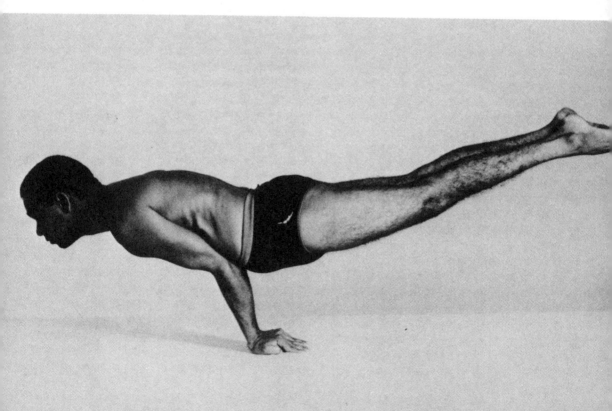

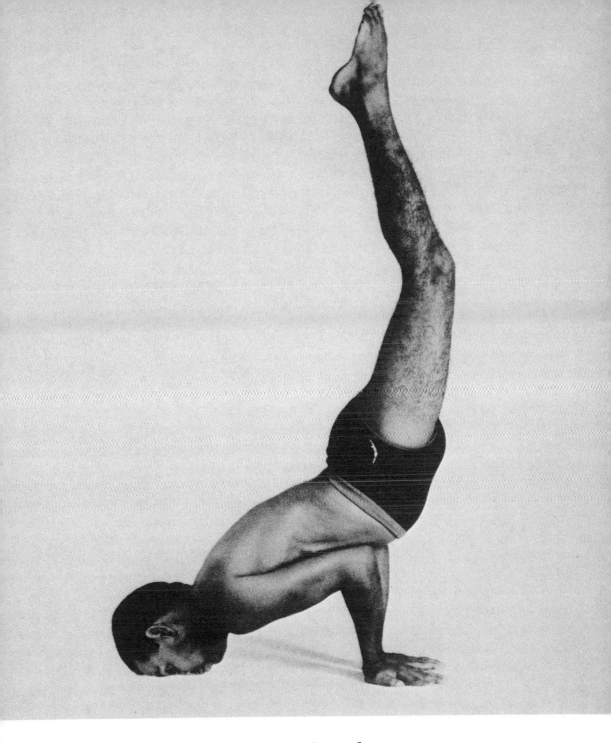

Technique: **Mayoorasan** [peacock pose]

plate 106

VARIATION 2

Assume Variation 1 of *mayoorasan,* then put the forehead down and raise
the legs as much as possible.

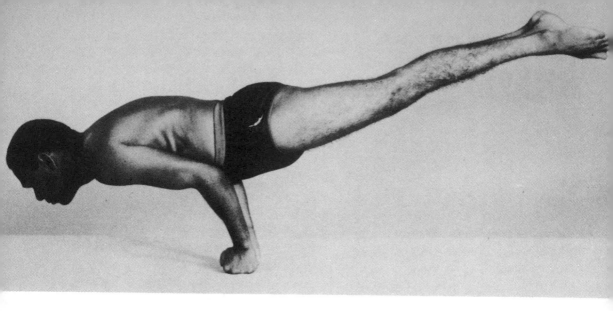

plate 107

Technique: **Mayoorasan** [peacock pose]

VARIATION 3

Perform *mayoorasan* by folding the fingers and balancing on the fists.

Technique: **Mayoorasan** [peacock pose]

VARIATION 4

*Mayoorasan* is done with the palms pointing toward the head. Now balance.
plate 108    In this, the wrist gets extra exercise.

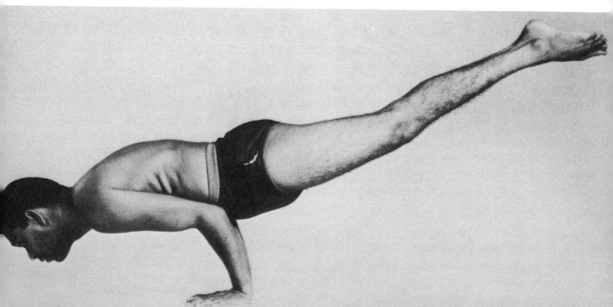

## Technique: **Mayoorasan** [peacock pose]

### VARIATION 5

Sit in the lotus pose. Keeping the thumb apart from the other fingers, balance in *mayoorasan*. This stretches the volar and dorsal carpal ligaments at the wrist, which are important.

All the balancing exercises strengthen the muscles of the arms and increase the breathing capacity.

Peacock pose especially is beneficial for all stomach disorders. Owing to the pressure of the elbows on the stomach below the navel, the abdominal aorta is partially compressed and the blood that is thus checked is directed toward the digestive organs. The liver, pancreas, stomach, and kidneys are toned. The intra-abdominal pressure is increased to a very high degree and the abdominal viscera are toned. *Mayoorasan* awakens *kundalini shakthi*, the spiritual power.

Sluggishness of the liver or hepatic torpidity disappears.

*plate 109*

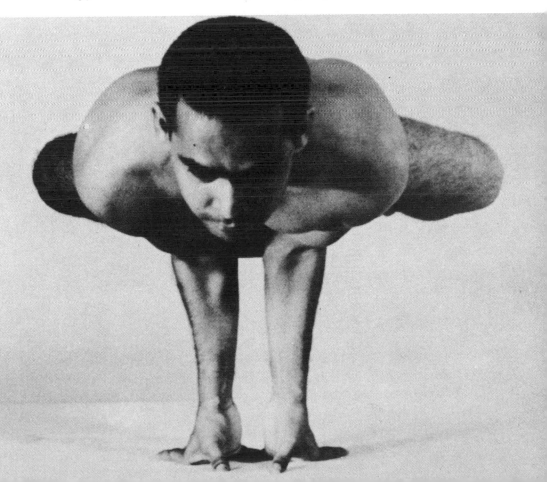

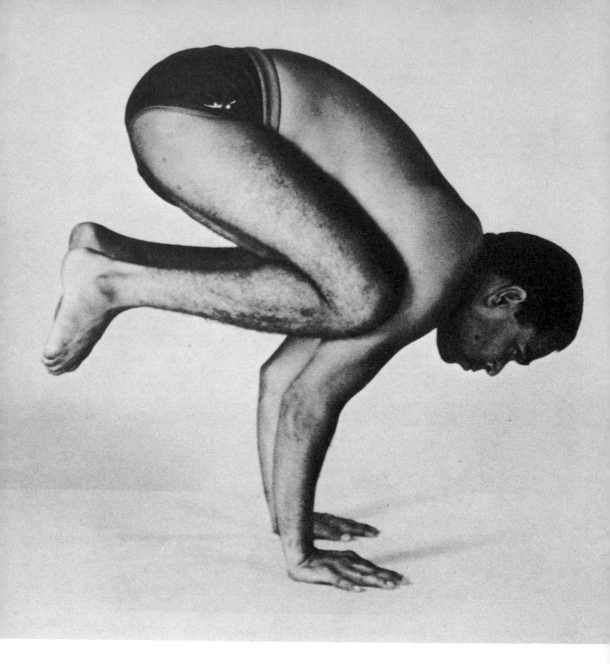

*plate 110*  **BALANCING POSE**

Technique: **Kakasana** [crow pose]

Sit on the toes keeping the knees apart. Now keep the hands firmly on the
floor. Rest the knees on the respective arms. Now raise the toes and slowly
balance yourself. Stand as long as possible.

Repeat three to four times.

# Technique: **Parswa Kakasana** [side crow pose]

Put the hands firmly on the floor. Now put both knees on the right thigh and balance. Repeat the same exercise on the other side.

*plate 111*

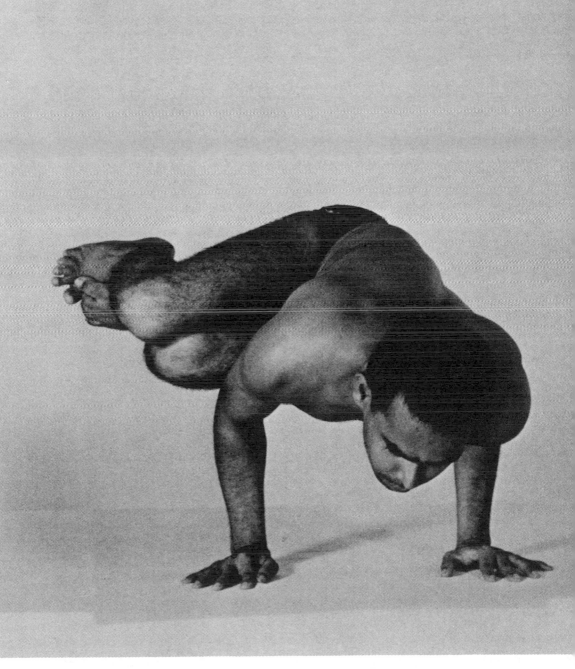

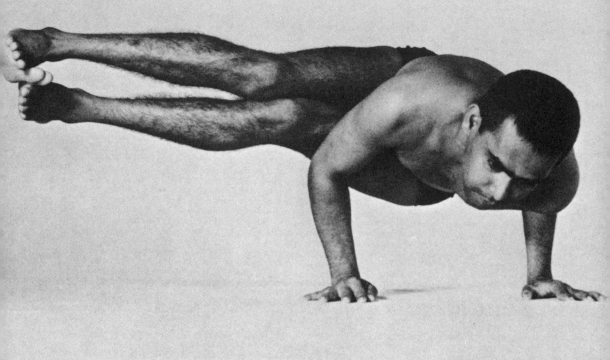

plate 112    Technique: **Vakrasana** [curved pose]

VARIATION 1

First of all, assume the *parswa kakasana* position. Then slowly straighten the legs.

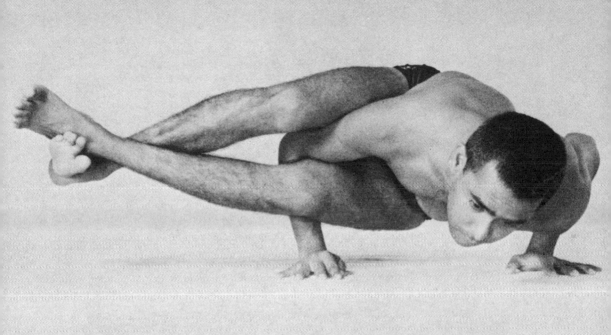

## Technique: **Vakrasana** [curved pose]

*plate 113*

### VARIATION 2

Stretch the legs and put the right hand in between the thighs. Now make an
ankle lock by placing left ankle over the right. Now slowly raise the body
and legs and balance on the hands.

This exercise is very good for muscles of arms and shoulders and can
be repeated several times.

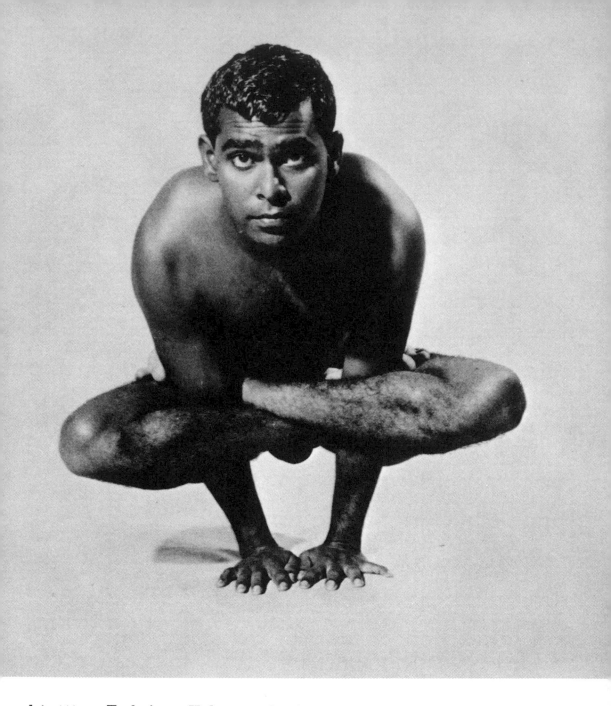

plate 114     Technique: **Kukutasan** [cock position]

Sit in lotus pose. Insert the hands in between thighs and calf muscles as far as the elbow. Now take a deep breath and raise the body above the ground, balancing on the palms.

Wrist and shoulder muscles are exercised in this position.

# Technique: **Parvatasana** [mount pose]

Sit in the lotus pose on a thick blanket. Slowly raise the body, and rest on the knees and hands. Now slowly raise both arms upward while balancing on the knees.

*plate 115*

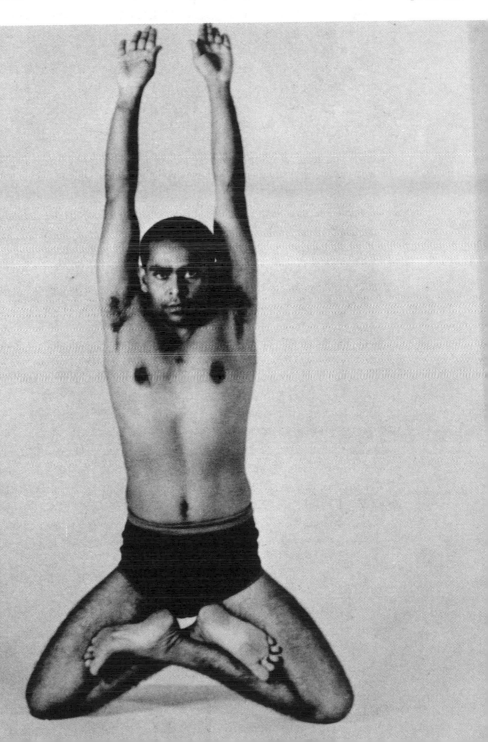

## YOGIC EXERCISES FOR THE LEGS

The movements of the feet and toes will be considered briefly. In the foot, upward movement is called flexion. Downward movement is called extension or plantar flexion.

In the toes, upward movements are called extension; downward movement is called flexion. Thus flexion and extension are movements opposite in direction at the ankle and metatarsophalangeal joints.

The muscles of the leg may be divided into the following groups: anterior, lateral, and posterior.

The foot is so associated with posture of the body generally and with the jarring of the tissues within the abdomen and skull that any interference with its function may affect the whole body. Many disturbances in the leg, the knee, the back, the hip, and disturbances of the health generally are associated primarily with deficiencies of action of the feet.

With the growth of civilization have come shoes and stockings, which affect the use of the feet and may be partially responsible for some of the difficulties commonly seen by the orthopedic surgeon and other specialists in diseases affecting locomotion.

It is now well established that the circulation to the feet must be well maintained if the toes are to be healthy. Such circulation is not maintained when the upper leg is too greatly constricted by tight garters or by rolling the stockings in a hard ridge or knot. Such constriction causes interference with the regular flow of blood and tends to break down the valves in the veins, resulting in varicosity.

Few persons understand how to take care of their feet with proper exercises. In many instances, feet are exceedingly painful because of a condition affecting a main bone of the foot, the astragalus. This is particularly the case in the condition commonly called fallen arch, a condition that occurs more often in women than in men.

Many of the foot ailments can be removed if one gives the feet simple exercises such as walking on the toes and heels alternately and avoiding shoes whenever possible.

The exercises suggested are very helpful in maintaining proper circulation and healthy muscles of the feet and legs.

The arches of the foot increase its strength and elasticity and provide protected places for the soft structures of the sole, such as the blood vessels and nerves. The foot constitutes a firm basis of support for the rest of the body.

The bones of the arch are arranged in longitudinal form, supported by a posterior and an anterior rest. There are two segments in the anterior portion of the arch. The medial segment is made up of the first three metatarsals, three cuneiforms, navicular, and talus. The medial division is especially important in the act of jumping; the lateral is more important as a basis of support in the upright posture. A transverse arch is formed by the metatarsal bones in front and distal row of the tarsus behind.

The ligaments that support the arch are:

1. Inferior calcaneonavicular (this fills the long gap left in the inner arch of the foot between the navicular and calcaneus); the tendon of the tibialis posterior runs under this ligament and supports it.

2. Long plantar, which makes a canal for the peroneus longus tendon, which runs beneath it.

There are numerous muscles deep in the sole of the foot; these act on the toes.

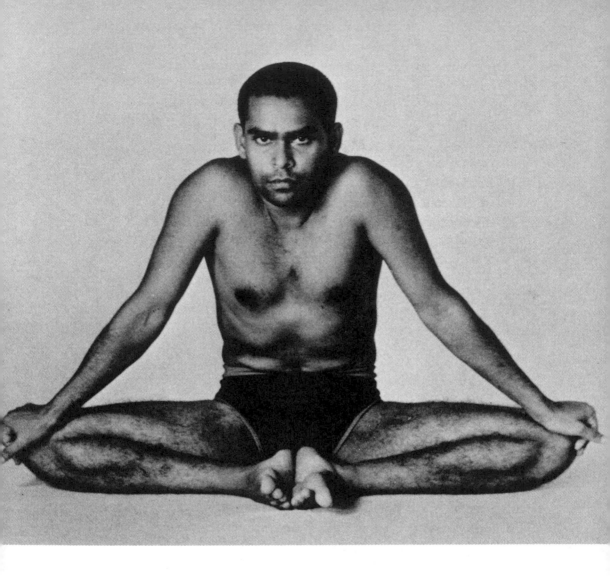

*plate 116*  **YOGIC EXERCISES FOR THE LEG MUSCLES AND FEET**

## Technique: **Bhadrasana** [ankle-knee pose]

Stretch the legs, the soles of the feet touching each other squarely. Fold the legs at the knees. Without letting the soles leave contact, draw them toward the body and place the heels close to the groin. Keep the hands on the knees and press the knees with respective hands to the floor.

This exercise stretches the muscles of the thighs and legs.

Do this pose once and hold from three to five minutes.

## Technique: **Goraksha Asana** [ankle-knee pose]

From *bhadrasana* position raise the body and bring the perineum over the heel. Sit for a minute and increase three to five minutes.

*plate 117*

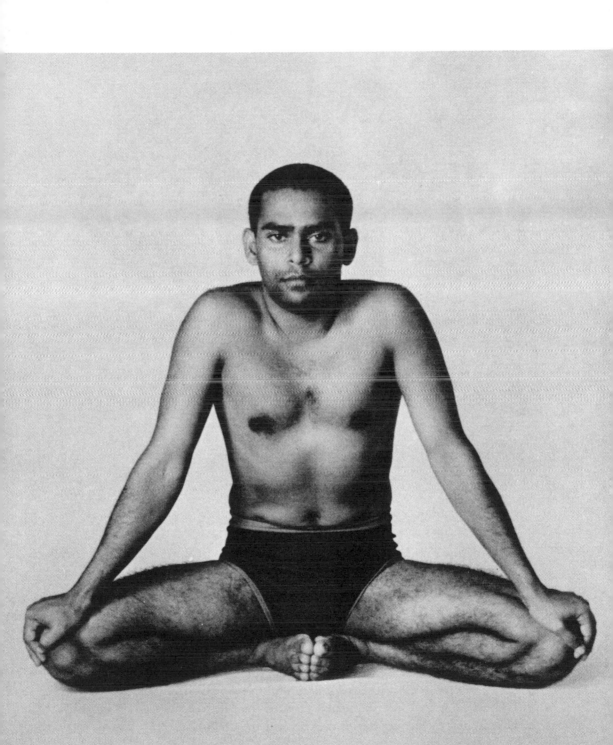

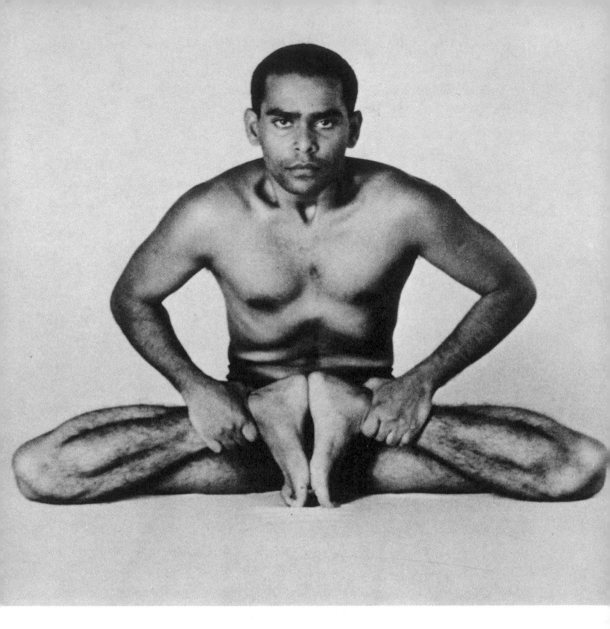

plate 118

## Technique: **Sakthi Chalini** [nerve power stimulation]

Before attempting the exercise, one should be able to do *bhadrasana* very well. Sit in *bhadrasana* pose, then insert the hands through the space between the calf muscles and the thighs. (If necessary, relax the *bhadrasan* a little, but keep the soles together.) Now catch hold of the toes firmly with both hands. Now draw the feet toward the body, at the same time twisting the feet at the ankles in such a way that the heels are above and the toes are touching the floor and the joined soles of the feet are perpendicular to the ground. Catch the ankles and pull toward the abdomen.

## Technique: **Khanda Peeda Asana** [ankle twist]

Perform the *sakthi chalini* pose first. Then take away the hands from the ankles. Raise yourself slightly from the floor and move forward with the toes in contact with the floor. Now sit over the feet. The toes are pointing backward now and the heels are in front. The feet joined together, soles facing each other, will now press against the *khanda*, i.e., the perineum or the space between the two legs.

This position is very difficult and, therefore, it should be practiced very carefully under the guidance of a teacher.

*plate 119*

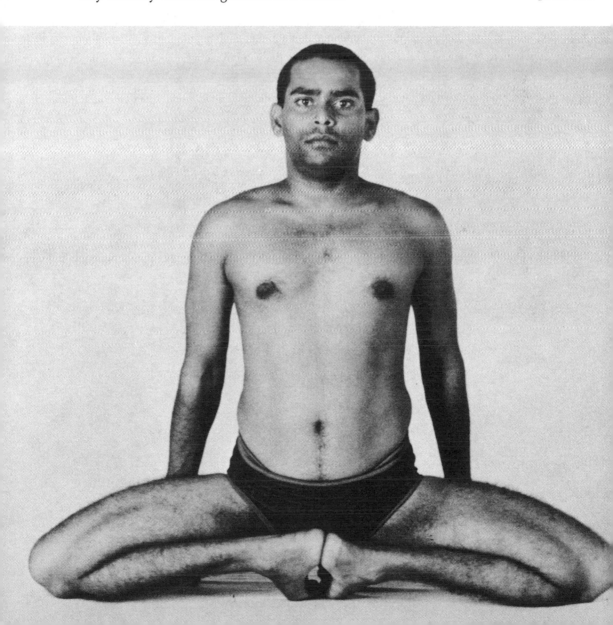

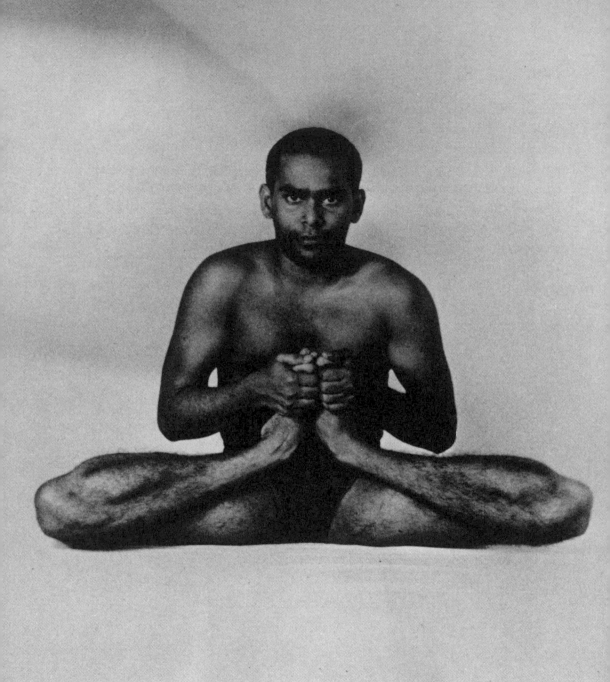

plate 120   Technique: **Nabhi Peeda Asana** [upward twist of ankle]

Keep the heels close together. Now with the help of the hands, bring the heels upward and toward the navel.

    This movement of the ankle is opposite to the *khanda peeda asana.*

## Technique: **Mandukasana** [frog pose]

Assume a kneeling position, keeping the feet together. Now separate the knees as far apart as possible. Sit firmly on the floor and keep the big toes of both feet touching. Place the hands on the knees. Sit in this pose for two to three minutes, gradually stretching the knees as far apart as possible. This exercise is very good for the ankle and knee joints.

*plate 121*

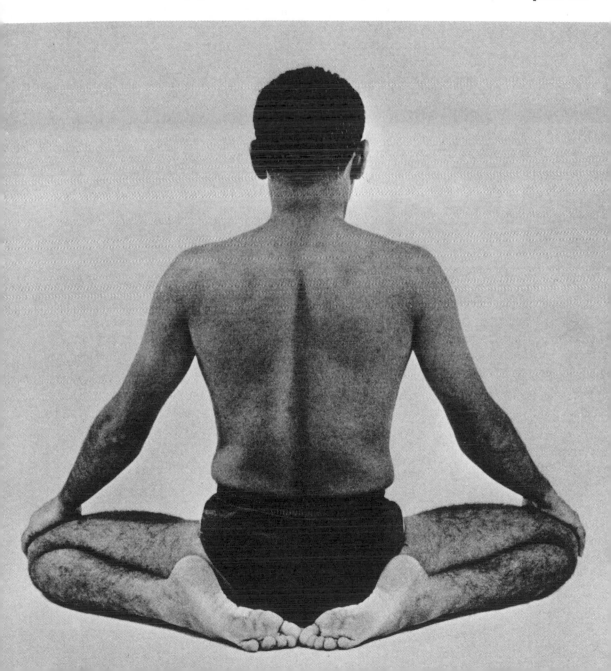

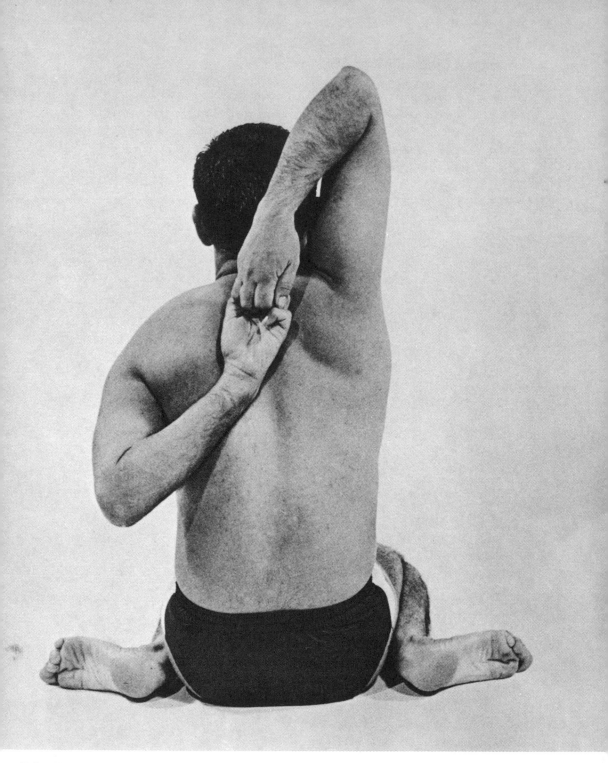

plate 122

## Technique: **Gomukhasana** [cow head pose]

In this exercise there is a peculiar ankle twist. (Look at the plate carefully.) It is the opposite of the frog position, in which the toes of each foot were pointing toward each other. In this position, the heels are kept sideways with the toes pointing away from the body, giving an extra twist to the knee joints. You will feel the pressure in two places when you do this exercise, one is at the knee joints and the other at the ankle joints. You should be very careful when performing this exercise, otherwise you might sprain your ankle and knee joints. Place the weight of the body on the hands by pressing against the floor and then slowly sit down until you are sitting firmly. It will take two to three weeks before you can sit comfortably. Once you master this position, you may go to the next stage, using the hands in order to exercise the shoulder muscles and arms. The next stage is performed by sitting firmly in the above described position. Now raise your right hand and bring it behind your shoulder. In the same way bend the left hand behind the back from the bottom and join the hands together. Do this exercise alternately. Proper execution develops the trapezoidal muscles and increases the capacity of the thoracic cage. This exercise also helps to prevent bursitis and the formation of calcium deposits at the shoulder joints.

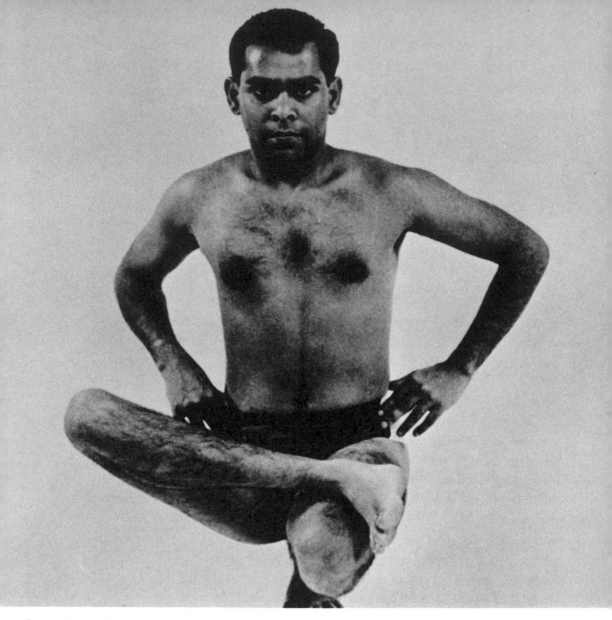

plate 123

## Technique: **Padandgushtasana** [tiptoe pose]

Assume a kneeling position. Now raise the knees slowly from the floor and come to rest on the toes. Use the hands to lift the knees. Now put the weight completely on the toes and balance yourself, without the help of the hands. Keep the hands either on the knees or on the hips. Sit in this position for two to three minutes at a time and gradually increase it to five minutes. After a few days of this practice, you should try to balance on one foot alone. When you balance with the right foot, put the left foot over the right thigh. Stay for half a minute to two minutes on each foot, alternately. This exercise is very good for the tired muscles of the ankle and toes, caused by feet squeezed into tight shoes. People with flat feet find this exercise useful.

## Technique: **Anjaneyasana** [split]

Stretch the legs. Now take the right leg backward by keeping the left one firm and straight. Now face toward the right foot while keeping both legs straight, opposite to the body.

*plate 124*

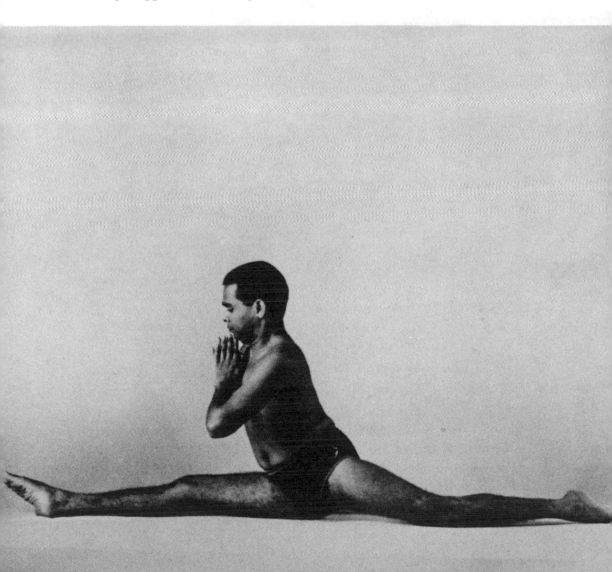

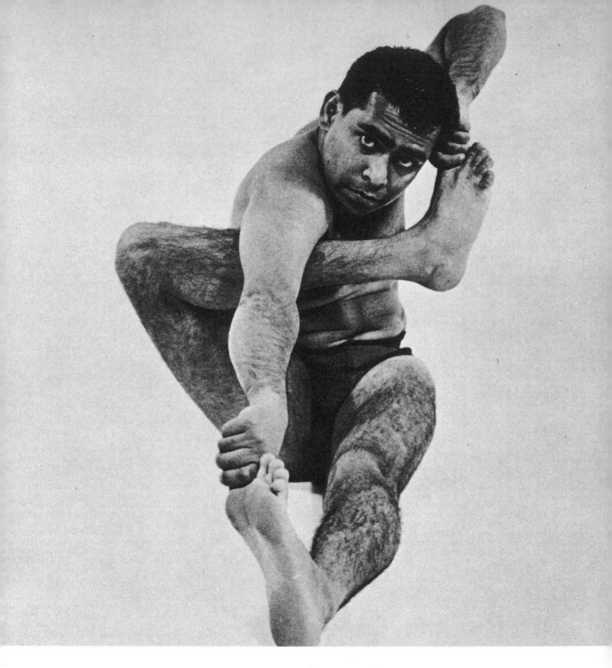

plate 125  Technique: **Akarna Dhanurasan** [shooting bow pose]

VARIATION 1

Stretch the legs and bend your right foot and keep it over the right thigh. Now extend the left leg and grasp the left foot with the right hand. When the left foot is firmly grasped, pull the right foot with the left hand until you touch the left ear with it. Repeat this three times, alternately. This exercise brings flexibility to the lower joints and strengthens the abdominal muscles.

Technique: **Akarna Dhanurasan** [shooting bow pose]

VARIATION 2

Stretch the legs and catch the right foot with the right hand and the left foot with the left hand. Then pull the right foot to the right of the right ear. This exercise stretches the leg muscles and the thigh joints become flexible.     *plate 126*

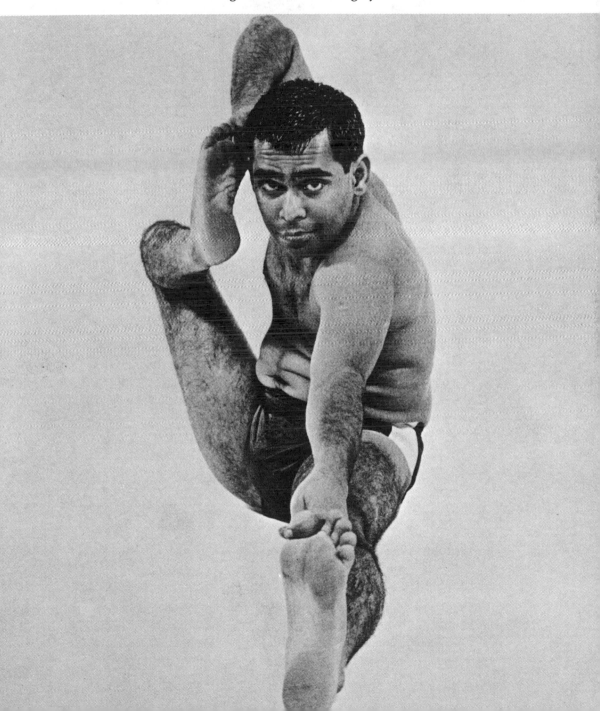

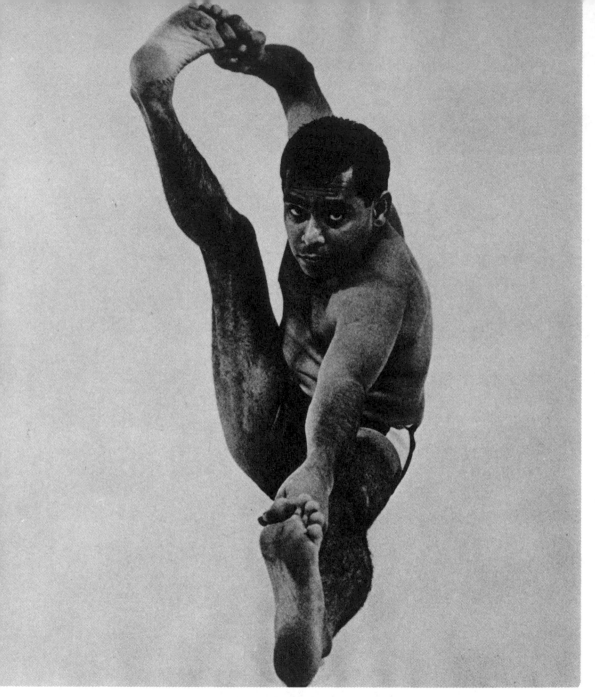

*plate 127*   Technique: **Akarna Dhanurasan** [shooting bow pose]

### VARIATION 3

There is only a slight difference between Variation 2 and Variation 3. In this position, instead of pulling the foot to the right ear or the left ear, the foot is pulled directly above the head in order to get maximum stretching of the thigh muscles. Repeat this exercise three to four times, alternately.

# YOGIC EXERCISES IN SITTING POSITION

## Technique: **Yoga Mudra** [lotus position with forward bending]

### VARIATION 1

Sit on a blanket. Form a foot lock as in lotus position. Fold the palms and place them in between the heels and abdomen. Now exhale and slowly bend forward, bringing the forehead to the floor. Remain in this pose for ten seconds and then assume the original sitting posture and inhale slowly. Repeat this pose six times.

*plate 128*

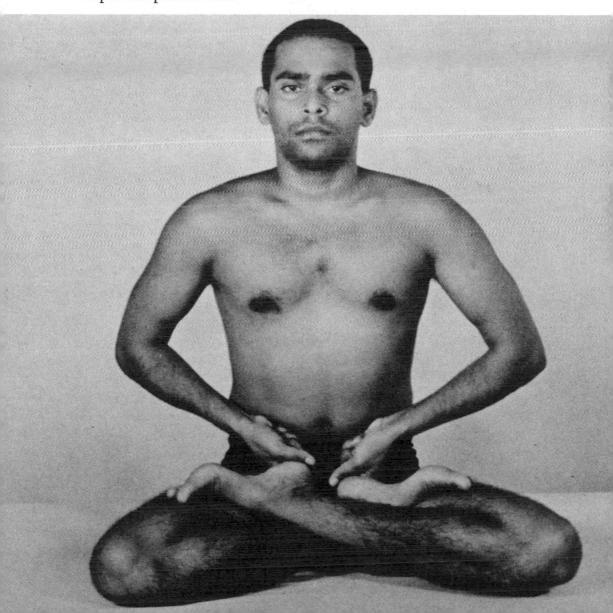

## Technique: **Yoga Mudra** [bound lotus pose, with forward bending]

### VARIATION 2

In this advanced exercise every muscle of the back and abdomen is exercised.

The muscles of the back, trapezius, infraspinatus, deltoid, and rhomboideus major and muscles of the abdomen, obliquus abdominis externus, rectus abdominus, obliquus abdominis internus, are the important ones toned during this pose. The pressure by the folded hands exerts more stimulation for pancreas, liver, and spleen in the first variety of *yoga mudra;* see the position of the first during the practice.

*plate 129*

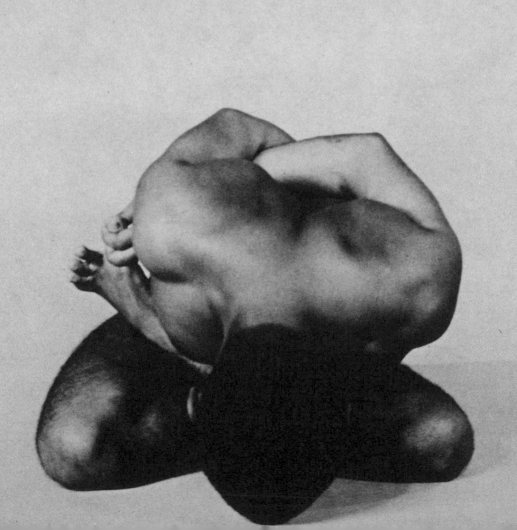

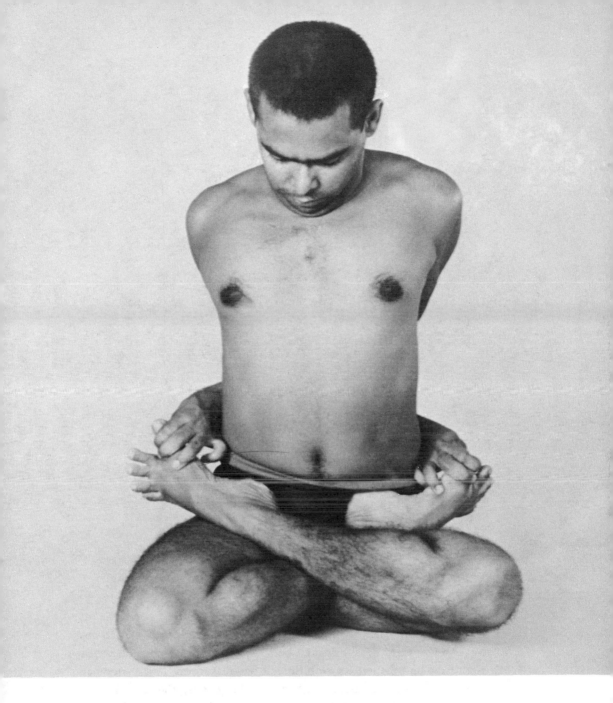

Technique: **Bandha Padmasan** [bound lotus pose]        *plate 130*

Assume the lotus position. Now bring your right arm around your back and catch the right foot. In the same way, catch the left foot with the left hand.

This pose is a little difficult for beginners. It expands the chest and pulls the ribs and intercostal muscles and the shoulder muscles.

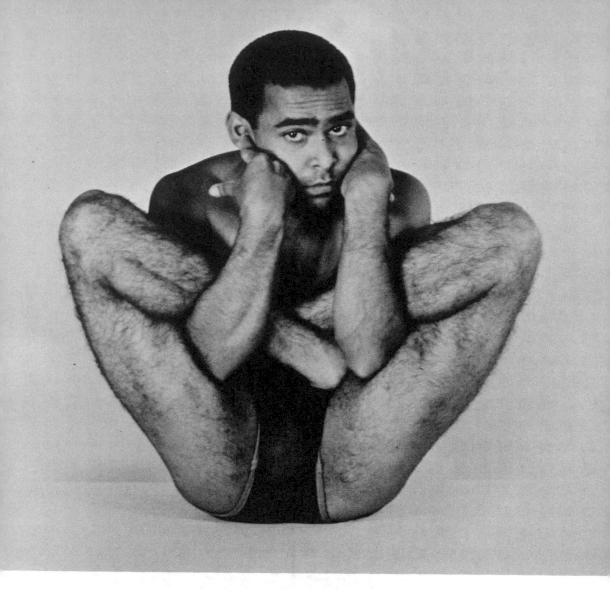

plate 131

## Technique: **Garbhasana** [foetus pose, bending]

As described in *kukutasana* or cock pose, insert both hands in the space between the thighs and calves. Bring out both elbows. Grasp the right ear with the right hand and the left ear with the left hand. Perform the last stage of this *asana* with great care, because when one tries to grasp the ears with the hands, one may fall backward. By practice, one can slowly balance the body on the buttocks and be able to remain steady.

The digestive power is augmented. Appetite increases. Bowel movements become freer. Many intestinal diseases are removed. Hands and legs will become strong. Hip joints will get sufficient movement and blood circulation will increase in the lower part of the body.

## Technique: **Veerasana** [warrior pose]

Stretch the legs. Now bend the right leg under the left thigh and keep the right foot close to the left thigh. Now take the left leg over the right thigh and keep the left foot close to the right thigh. Bring the left hand behind the back and the right hand above the shoulder toward the back. Now interlock the fingers of the left and right hands. This pulls the shoulder and arm muscles.

This resembles *Gomukhasana* [cow head pose], except for the position of the legs.

*plate 132*

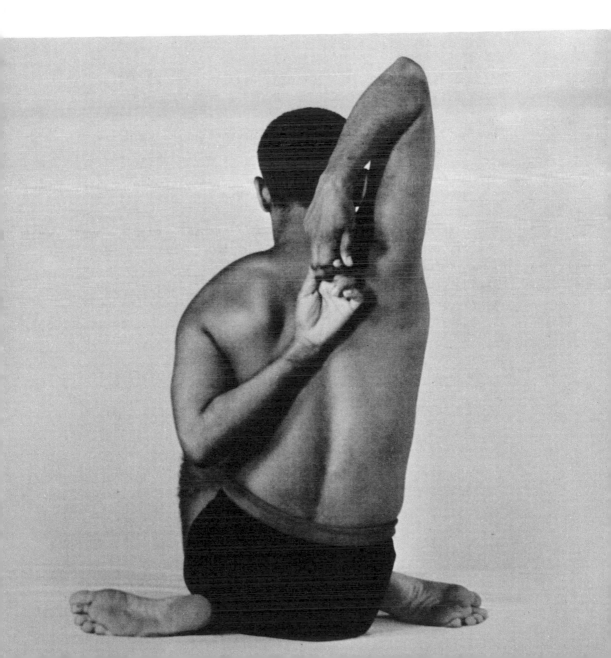

# YOGIC EXERCISES IN STANDING POSITION FOR THE BACKBONE AND LEG MUSCLES

## Technique: **Pada Hasthasan** [hands to feet pose]

### VARIATION 1

Stand erect. Raise arms overhead and inhale deeply. Then exhale slowly and while exhaling, bend the body until the hands reach the toes and the nose touches the knees. The raised arms should be in contact with the ears throughout, even while bending the body. After a little practice, one will be able to bury the face between the knees and keep the palms firmly on the floor. Remain in this pose for five seconds and slowly assume the standing position. When the body is raised, inhale slowly. Repeat this pose four times.

The spine becomes supple and is lengthened. The adipose tissue on the abdomen will disappear. This *asana* is very suitable for women who wish to reduce excess fat and for developing a graceful figure.

plate 133

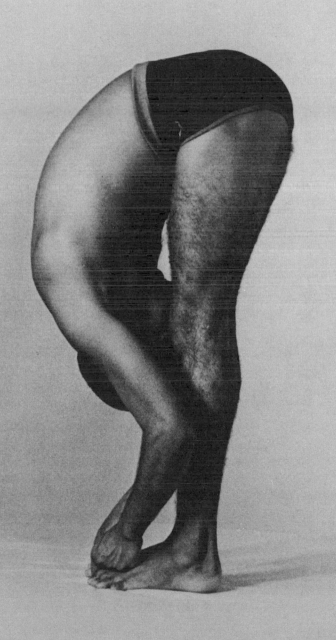

# Technique: **Pada Hasthasan** [hands to feet pose]

VARIATION 2

Keep the legs a little apart. Put the hands back and catch hold of the right hand with the left. Now bend toward the right leg. Slightly turn the body toward the right leg. Repeat this same process with the left leg by bending to the left side.

*plate 134*

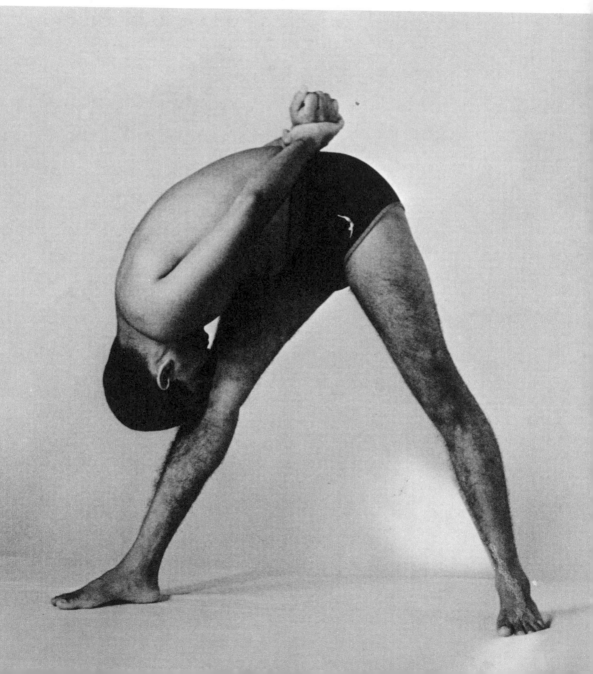

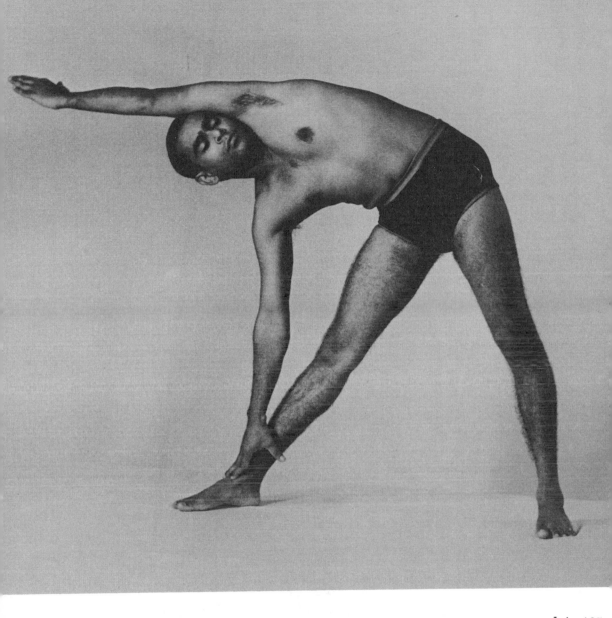

## Technique: **Trikonasan** [triangle pose]

*plate 135*

### VARIATION 1

Stand erect keeping the feet two or three feet apart. Now bring the arms shoulder height, the palms down. Bend to the left slowly and touch the left toes with the left hand. Remain thus for five seconds and slowly return to the standing position. Do not bend the legs or arms when bending down or when getting up. From the standing position, bend to the right and touch the right toes with the right hand. Remain for five seconds in this position and then come back to the original standing position. Repeat four times.

plate 136

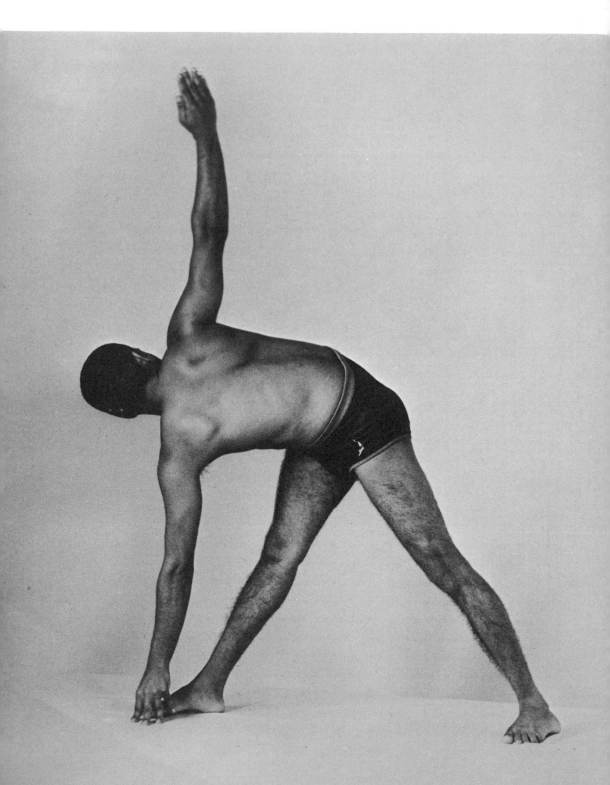

Technique: **Trikonasan** [triangle pose]

Keep the legs apart. Now twist the body and look back. Slowly bend and touch the right foot with the left hand. The right hand should be kept straight, making a straight line from the left hand to the right.

Triangle pose tones the spinal nerves and the abdominal organs, increases peristalsis of the bowels and invigorates the appetite. The body becomes light. The trunk muscles are contracted, relaxed, and stretched. The spine is bent laterally on both sides and the muscles are fully stretched. This keeps the spine elastic.

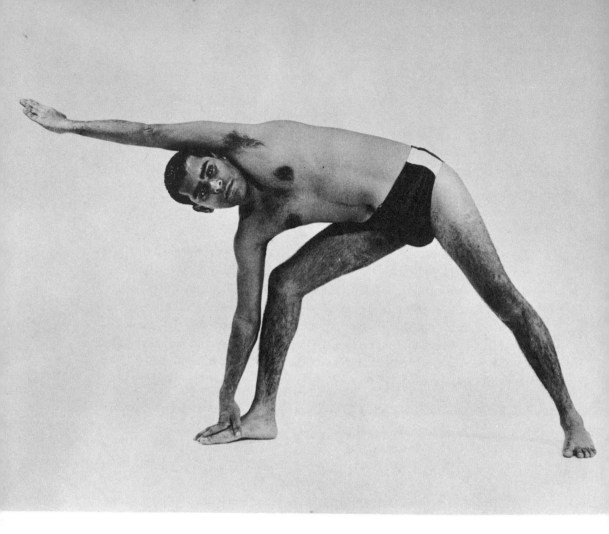

*plate 137*

Technique: **Trikonasan** [triangle pose]

### VARIATION 3

Place the feet three to four feet apart while standing. Now bend your right knee slightly and bend the whole body sideways until you touch the right foot with the right hand. This exercise is easier than the first one. Beginners and old people should start with this exercise before they attempt Variations 1 and 2.

# Technique: **Trikonasan** [triangle pose]

## VARIATION 4

The technique is the same as in Variation 3, except that you twist the spine and touch the right foot with the left hand. Back muscles will get a twist along with bending.

*plate 138*

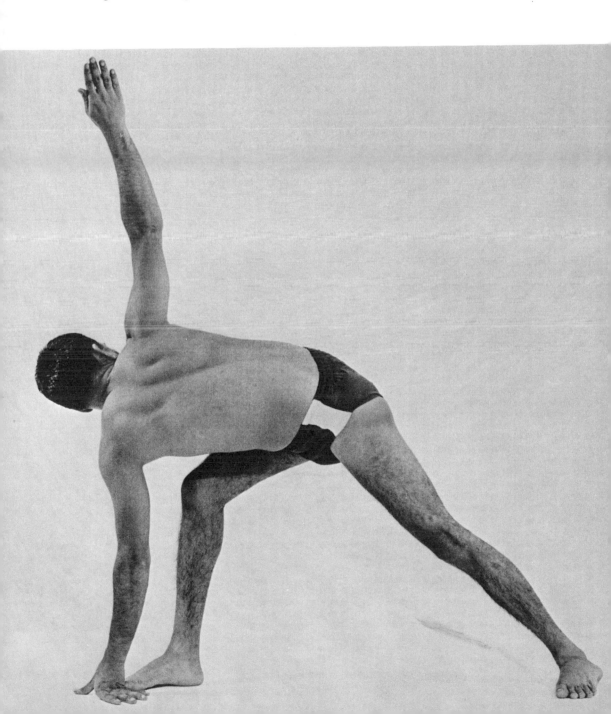

## Technique: **Sirangushtasana** [head-toe pose]

This is also a variation of the triangle pose. Keep the legs as far apart as possible while standing. Now fold your hands behind the back and bend toward the right foot until the nose comes in contact with the foot. This is a stretching exercise for the thigh and calf muscles.

*plate 139*

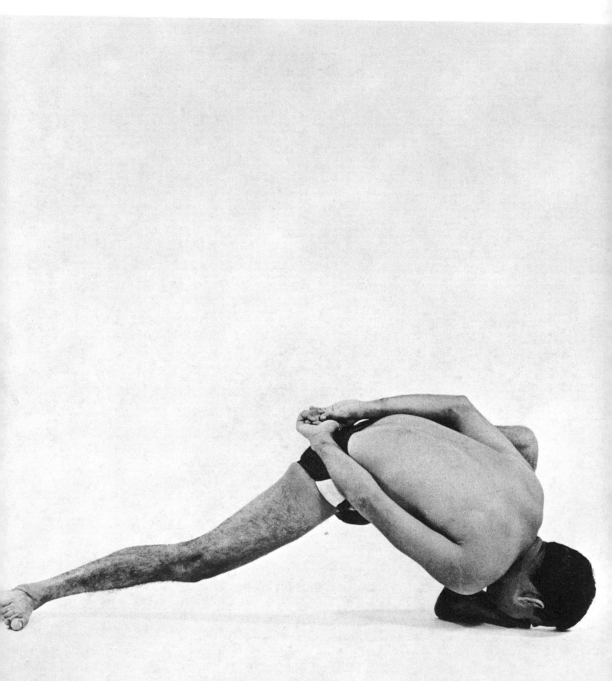

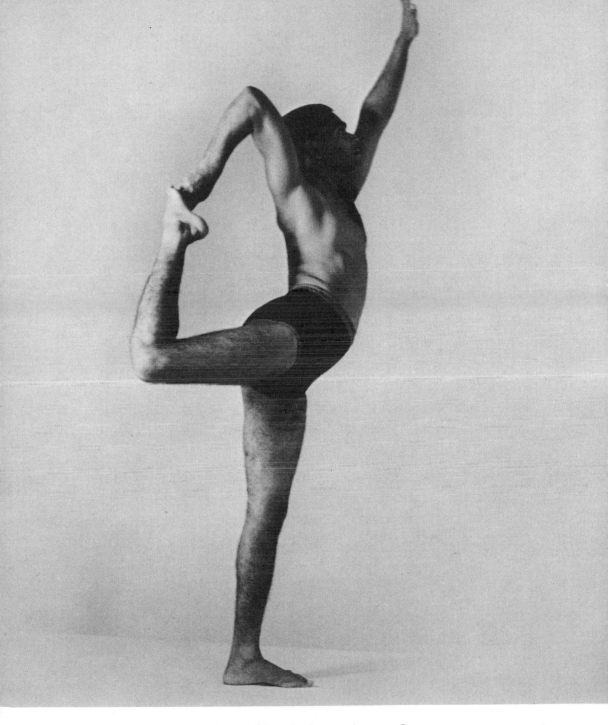

### Technique: **Natarajasan** [Lord Nataraja pose]

*plate 140*

Stand erect. Now bend the right leg at the knee, grasp the big toe, and pull toward the head.

This gives wonderful exercise to the leg muscles and spine. It stretches various ligaments.

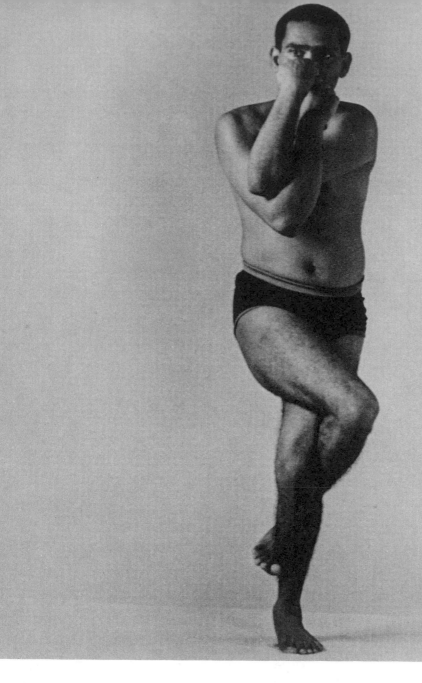

plate 141

## Technique: **Garuda Asana** [eagle pose]

Stand erect. Lift the right leg and twist it over the left leg. Cross the elbows in front with the left elbow on top, and press the arms together. Reverse the position and stand on the right leg.

  This strengthens the calf muscles and reduces the extra fat from the thighs.

## Technique: **Vatyanasana** [one knee and foot pose]

Stand erect. Bend the right leg and put the foot on the left thigh joint. Now slowly bend the left leg and bring the right knee toward the floor, resting on the knee and the foot.

This is a very good exercise to bring flexibility to the lower part of the body.

*plate 142*

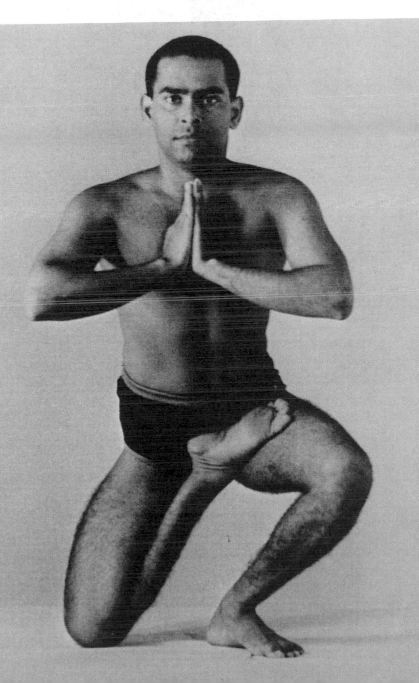

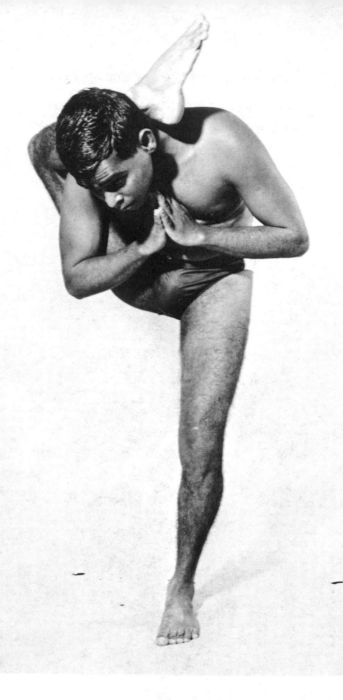

*plate 143*  **Technique: Beka Asana** [crane pose]

Stand erect. With the help of the hands slowly lift the right foot over the head. Now straighten the left knee and pull the body as straight as possible.

Fold the hands and balance on one foot. One may use the help of the wall in the beginning.

## Technique: **Eka Pada Hasthasan** [leg hands pose]

Assume the crane pose. Now slowly bend forward, keeping the right foot firmly over the back of the head until the head touches the left knee.

*plate 144*

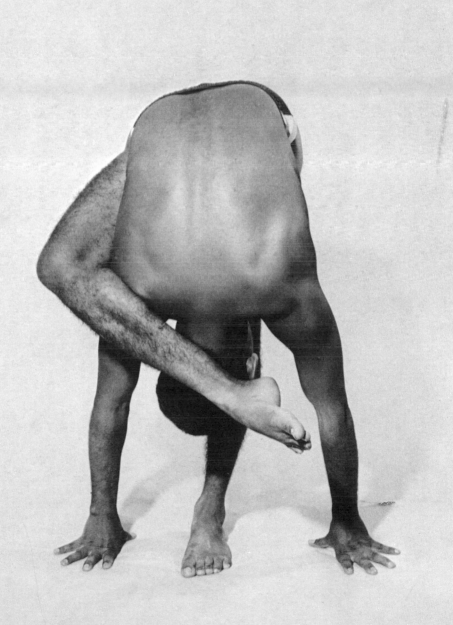

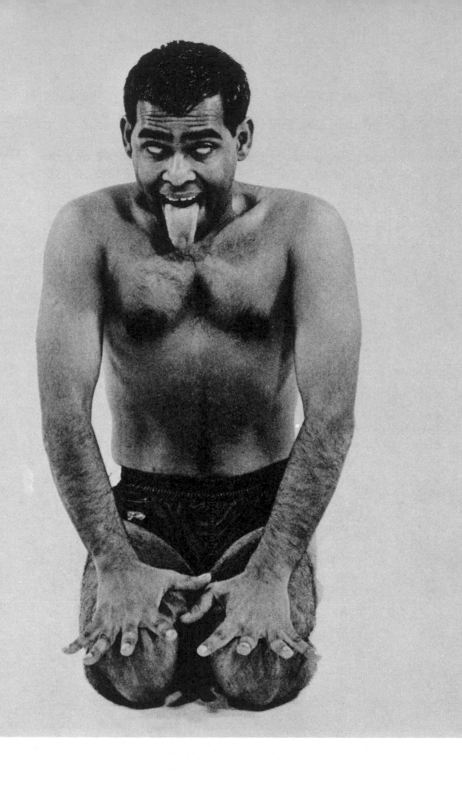

plate 145

## Technique: **Simhasan** [lion pose]

This pose resembles a lion in action and is therefore called the lion pose. This is practiced specifically for the throat and tongue. The tongue must be stretched out as far as possible, in order to increase the circulation to the root of the tongue and to the throat. The eyeballs are turned upward and the whole body is stiffened as though the lion is about to spring upon its prey.

Technique: Assume a kneeling position (or *japrasan*) and keep your palms over the knees and gently lean over the hands. Now protrude the tongue as far as possible by contracting the throat muscles, meanwhile rolling your eyeballs upward. During this position exhale the breath as much as possible. Repeat this exercise four to six times.

**Caution.** All the difficult postures should be practiced under the guidance of a teacher. Any twisting of the muscles and joints without proper guidance may bring agonizing pain and the student may stop the practice of even simple exercises altogether, because of pain.

Another important point is never to do any exercise beyond your capacity.

At the end of the exercise relax for ten to fifteen minutes.

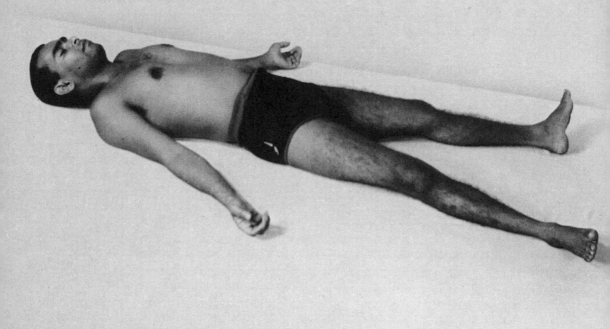

plate 146

# SAVASAN—CORPSE POSE; AND RELAXATION

Elsewhere in this book we mentioned that one of the five things necessary to keep an automobile in good condition is cooling the engine when it gets hot; the same principle applies to the human body also. When the body and mind are constantly overworked, their efficiency in performing their natural work diminishes. Modern social life, food, work, and even the so-called entertainments, such as boxing and wrestling, make it difficult for the civilized man of today to relax. Not only is it difficult for him to relax, but he has even forgotten nature's way of recharging the body during relaxation and rest. Even while resting, the average person spends a great deal of physical and mental energy.

Most of the energy produced by the body is wasted uselessly. For one thing enormous amounts of energy are wasted on unnecessary muscular tension.

There is no use in increasing energy if we are going to waste it unnecessarily, because if production of energy is increased while the useless waste remains unchecked, the new energy produced will merely increase this useless waste. Therefore, before learning any physical or mental exercise one should first learn to observe and be aware of muscular tension and be able to relax unnecessary tension of the muscles. The whole of the Yogic exercises is based upon this principle.

Every physical action puts tension in the muscles. Sometimes you can observe the tension of your muscles, without any reason, when you are resting. When you learn to drive a car, tremendous physical

and mental tension go into the driving. Even fifteen minutes will make
a new driver tired and his muscles ache. On the other hand, when an
experienced driver drives for a hundred miles he feels no fatigue, because in this case the muscles are relaxed during driving. Though most
of us drive, only a few know how to drive with perfect relaxation. This
does not mean the relaxed driver is careless. On the contrary, his reflexes respond more readily than do the reflexes of those who are always
tense to meet an emergency; at the same time he uses a lesser amount
of energy. The same applies in the fields of the arts, painting, music,
and so forth. Every genius consciously or unconsciously relaxes during
his particular job; that is why he is efficient in his art.

Before we can study relaxation we must first understand the
opposite contraction. When we wish to perform an action, four things
happen one after another to complete the action. First of all a thought
arises in the mind, say, to take a book from the table. This thought wave
is transmitted to the brain, and the brain sends an impulse to the muscles needed for the particular job, along with an extra supply of pranic
energy for those muscles. The *prana* travels over the motor nerves,
reaches the muscles, and causes them to draw the ends together—and
finally the book is in the hands. Every action, conscious or unconscious,
uses up a certain amount of pranic energy. In the conscious action, the
conscious mind sends a message to the subconscious mind, which immediately obeys the order by sending the *prana* to the desired part.
When an action is automatic, that is, when the conscious mind plays
no role, the subconscious mind takes up the whole work itself, both
ordering and finishing the job. When the amount of pranic energy spent
is more than the body can restore, the body feels weak. This is one way
of spending energy.

Another way of spending energy without any muscular movement is through the emotions, such as worries, sorrow, anxieties, anger,
and greed. No one is without emotions, and only a few can keep them
under control or at least within limit. Uncontrolled emotions can very
quickly use up the *prana* that is stored in the body. A few minutes of
anger can cost more energy than a day of physical labor. Look at a person in anger; see how all muscles are tensed; watch his irregular breathing, clenched fists, and bloodshot eyes. Is any part of the body inactive
during that moment? His heart beats fast; blood pressure increases; his
digestive system is disturbed. The sudden outburst of anger produces
a shock wave in the nervous system. Imagine how much energy is
necessary to restore order to the various muscles and organs that were
co-operating with the emotions! This phenomenon is not limited to

anger; every emotion takes its toll on the body. No amount of tonics, injections, vitamins, or balanced diet for a person who is suffering from worries and anxieties will provide an ultimate solution to his problems.

After the anger, worries, and sorrows have disappeared, there is still another demon waiting to swallow the energy, which is called mental fatigue or tension. We can compare the waste of pranic energy as the result of tension to the waste of water as the result of not turning off a faucet and allowing the water to trickle away hour after hour. So we allow our *prana* to trickle away in a constant stream of tension, which in turn results in wear and tear on our muscles and internal organs.

When man is inflamed with anger, there is a desire to strike the person who caused the anger, and all the muscles are ready so to act. But our higher faculties, the reasoning power by which man controls his fighting instinct, send out a repressing impulse that in turn holds back the action. This double action of ordering and withdrawing is done so quickly that there is no time for the mind to decide and the muscles begin to quiver from two opposite thought currents. When the anger has subsided, there is still no definite command for the muscles to relax and they remain activated. When we are excited by lower emotions, the mind constantly keeps the nerves in action and our muscles tense by unrestrained and uncontrolled mental states. An enormous amount of energy is wasted, in the first place, owing to unnecessary activities that we tend neither to stop nor to control and, secondly, there is the unnecessary constant tension of the muscles of our organism. Even at rest, muscles are under tension and as soon as we start to do even a small amount of work, a whole system of muscles is put into action just as if we were to do the hardest and most strenuous work. Under such conditions even to lift a book may require as much energy as should be required to lift a big man, or to type a few pages may use up as much energy as should be necessary to type a whole volume, because we continuously spend muscular energy. Observe how some persons walk. Their shoulder muscles are tensed. Even when they sit or write, the muscles of their shoulders, arms, legs, and stomach are tensed unnecessarily. During sleep, too, muscles are tensed and continue to spend energy, though we are unaware of it.

More of our energy is spent in keeping the muscles in continual readiness for work than in actual useful work done during our lifetime.

In order to regulate and balance the work of the body and mind, it is necessary to learn to economize the energy produced by our body, which is the main purpose of learning how to relax.

It is to be remembered here that our body usually produces in the course of one day all the substances and energy necessary for the next day. But it often happens that all these substances and energy are consumed within a few minutes by bad moods, anger, injury, or irritation, when they reach a certain degree of intensity. At times a single violent flash of anger can destroy practically all man's energy.

This process of eruption and repression of violent emotions often grows into a regular habit, and the result is very disastrous, not only for the body, but also for the mind.

During relaxation there is practically no energy or *prana* consumed, although a little is kept in circulation to keep the body in normal condition, and the remaining portion is being stored up and conserved.

We should not confuse relaxation with laziness. In infancy the child relaxes naturally; some adults possess this power of relaxation. Such persons are noted for their endurance, strength, vigor, and vitality. It was stated that Napoleon could relax and sleep on horseback during continuous fighting. Many great statesmen and sages depend upon their power of relaxation to enable them to carry out the tremendous amount of work they have shouldered. Mahatma Gandhi and Swami Sivananda are the best examples of our times.

Observe a cat crouched before a mouse hole, in an easy, graceful attitude without any muscular contraction or tension, but ready for action. Though devoid of any tension in the muscles, the repose of the cat is a live repose that very seldom fails at the time of action.

In order to achieve perfect relaxation, three methods are used by the Yogis. The three methods are known as physical, mental, and spiritual. No relaxation is complete until man reaches the stage of spiritual relaxation, which only Yogis know.

1. *Physical Relaxation.* We all know that every action is the result of thought originated in the mind consciously or subconsciously. Thoughts take form in action and the body reacts to it. When we want to perform an act, the thought is generated in the mind, is transmitted to the brain and, simultaneously, the brain telegraphs the message through the nerves, and the muscles contract. Just as behind the muscular contraction or tension there is thought, so also behind the relaxation there is again thought vibration. Just as we send a message to contract the muscles, so also another message will bring relaxation to the tired muscles. This relaxation message is known as autosuggestion or suggesting one's own muscles and internal organs relax. But as we have no control over such involuntary organs as the heart, lungs, liver, brain, etc., we cannot directly send the thoughts for relaxing to these

organs. Yet they, too, need rest and relaxation to increase their efficiency to do their work. Here the Yogis use the subconscious mind,
which controls all the automatic functions of these involuntary organs
for relaxation. Elsewhere in this book we have dealt with the subconscious mind and how suggestions consciously given are promptly carried out by it. During relaxation, the conscious mind sends a message
to a particular organ, such as the heart or liver. This message is received by the instinctive mind and the order is immediately carried out.
Thus one could relax all the involuntary organs too. First, physical
relaxation starts from the toes upward and the autosuggestion passes
through the muscles and reaches up to the eyes and ears at the top.
Then, slowly, messages are sent to the kidneys, liver, and so on,
internally.

2. *Mental Relaxation.* The constant tension put on the mind
owing to unnecessary worries and anxieties takes away more energy
than physical tension. During mental tension one should breathe slowly
and rythmically for a few minutes and concentrate on breathing. Slowly
the mind will become calm and one is able to feel a kind of floating
sensation, as if one were as light as a feather; one feels peace and joy.

3. *Spiritual Relaxation.* However one tries to relax the mind,
one cannot completely remove all tensions and worries from the mind
unless one goes to spiritual relaxation. As long as man identifies himself with the body and mind there will be worries, sorrows, anxieties,
fear, and anger which, in turn, bring tension. Yogis know that unless
man can withdraw himself from the body idea and separate himself
from the ego consciousness, there is no way of obtaining complete
relaxation. So, from the mental relaxation, he withdraws himself and
identifies himself with the all-pervading, all-powerful, all-peaceful and
joyful self, or pure consciousness within himself, because all the source
of power, knowledge, peace, and strength are in the soul and not in
the body. Man has become prey to all evil emotions of the mind by
identifying himself with the body and mind, and the only sure way to
free himself from its clutches is by asserting his real nature, that is,
"I am that pure consciousness or self." This identification with the self
completes the process of relaxation. This relaxation position is known
as *savasan,* or dead body pose. Plate No. 146.

# 7

# NATURAL DIET OF MAN

We have considered the body as a motor car. To run it we need gas. The energy for the physical body is obtained through food, water, and air. In this chapter, we will explain man's need for a natural diet.

The body needs food for two purposes: as fuel to supply energy, and to repair body tissues. If fuel in the form of food were not available to the body, it would consume itself. A loss of body tissue then means a loss of weight, as excessive weight is reduced in proportion to the food intake withheld from the body.

The following four elements are needed for the body's repair and upbuilding: (1) protein or nitrogenous food; (2) carbohydrates; (3) hydrocarbons or fat; (4) minerals.

These elements are found in larger proportions in vegetable than in animal tissues. Nuts, peas, beans, milk, and cheese contain a large percentage of nitrogenous matter (protein), whereas wheat, oats, rice, and other grains, potatoes, etc., are mainly carbohydrates (starches and sugar).

Nearly all the protein foods and vegetable oils furnish hydrocarbons or fats, while the valuable organic mineral elements of iron, potassium, lime, soda, etc., which serve as eliminators, antiseptics, blood purifiers, and producers of electromagnetic energy are mostly found in the plant kingdom. The main supply of organic minerals comes from fruits and vegetables.

Fruits and vegetables also aid in keeping an alkaline reserve in the blood. This is essential in maintaining its capacity for carrying carbon dioxide to the lungs for elimination.

The most important sources of vitamins in a diet are vegetables. Those which can be eaten raw, such as lettuce, spinach, cabbage, and tomatoes contain the three main types of vitamins: A, B, and C. Vitamins A and B are not appreciably affected by boiling, but frying may destroy them. Vitamin C, which is necessary for sound bone formation and healthy teeth, is found only in fruits, green-leaved vegetables, and to some extent in fresh milk. It is rapidly destroyed in heating, drying, dehydrating, preserving, canning, and washing.

Milk is a complete protein food. Thus, a diet containing milk and dairy products, fresh fruits, oranges, lemons, and pineapples, leafy vegetables (salads), and whole grains should be man's ideal vitamin-rich diet.

Fruits and raw vegetables contain antiscorbutic substances that prevent various diseases. Meat, on the other hand, may be affected to a high degree with such dreaded diseases as trichinosis, intestinal worms, etc., which are readily transmitted to those who eat it.

A large number of medical men and dieticians today forbid their patients to eat meat, not only as a means of eliminating such ailments as gout, rheumatism, etc., but also as a preventive against uric acid diseases. It has been found that injuries suffered by vegetarians heal more quickly, and the danger of contracting fever and high temperatures is considerably minimized.

Eminent French and English physicians have proved that a large number of ailments suffered by the civilized race are caused by uric acid deposits in the muscle fibers of the meats consumed. When extra uric acid is introduced into the system, the body must eliminate its own manufactured supply, plus the extra supply taken in the form of meat.

For example, a pound of liver contains 19 grains of uric acid and a pound of beefsteak 14 grains, whereas the daily amount of uric acid the body produces and eliminates through the kidneys is only about six grains. As a person's liver and kidneys are not able to deal with the extra intake, the uneliminated uric acid becomes the seedbed of gout, rheumatism, headaches, epilepsy, convulsions, nervousness, etc. From this it is evident that cures cannot be effected while a person continues to eat meat.

Though the eater of meat shows bodily vigor, he does not possess the vegetarian's endurance. A vegetarian can work for long periods under the most trying conditions and not tire, while the meat-eater can do a large amount of work for a short time only, but soon will get weak and hungry.

Natural diet gives more disease resistance and prolongs life.

The oldest man in English history, Thomas Parr, who died in 1635 at 152 years and 9 months, did not die of old age. He had lived on an exclusive diet of milk, cheese, and hard bread, remarried at the age of 120, and finally died after moving to London where for the first time he ate rich food and drank wine. After performing a post-mortem on Parr, Dr. William Harney found his body in excellent condition and gave as cause of death "mere plethora brought on by luxurious living."

A noted geologist, Professor H. M. Ami, of Montreal, has reported in his *Geography of North America* that the diet of the human race in prehistoric times did not include flesh in any form. According to the professor, man did not become a flesh-eater until he was forced into it by the destruction of the great forests of nut trees and wild fruits by the great ice cap that crept down over the northern hemisphere during the glacial period.

All food is originally produced by the vegetable kingdom, which absorbs and stores the sun's energy. The energy found in flesh is the balance stock that has not been used by the animal. When one animal eats the flesh of another, it is taking vegetable food at secondhand from the unused portion of the flesh, as vegetable food is the original source of all animal energy.

An interesting point to be noted here is that man utilizes mainly the flesh of those animals which live on plant life: cows, pigs, sheep, goats, horses, poultry, etc.; even in wild animals, man prefers the flesh of such as deer, rabbits, boar, and not the flesh of tigers, lions, or leopards, which are carnivorous. This in itself shows that man draws secondhand vegetable energy from the flesh of animals that live on vegetables.

All flesh foods, as commonly consumed by man, are highly unbalanced, containing a great excess of protein, while almost completely lacking in calcium and growth-promoting vitamins, which are originally derived from the vegetable kingdom. Gathered from the soil, calcium is changed by the vegetables into organic or food calcium and, with the help of the sun's rays, vitamins are manufactured by the green leaves.

Another case of drawing secondhand food energy is noted in the Eskimos, who eat the raw and frozen stomachs of the reindeer in order to get the vitamins contained there as grass and other vegetables. But the Eskimo diet is one of necessity and not of choice.

Another important objection to eating meat is that, of all the foodstuffs, it most readily putrefies. Even eggs undergo putrefaction, but not so milk or vegetables, which decay or ferment, a process not as harmful as is the putrefaction of flesh. During putrefaction, a poisonous toxin is released. It has been proved that animal protein putrefies twice as fast as vegetable protein.

Several types of animal parasites can be found in the human intestine, the more common being the beef, pork, and fish tapeworm, roundworm, pinworm, hookworm, and liver fluke. These parasites usually enter the body by way of the mouth through food contaminated with eggs or adult parasites. Later the eggs hatch into adult worms and continue to live and reproduce in the intestines. With certain species the embryonic forms are absorbed into the blood stream and travel through the body, at times lodging in the liver, brain, lungs, and muscles, to return to the intestines.

The common sources of these worms are infected beef, pork, fish and, of course, contaminated waters. Worms do not always produce absolutely typical symptoms, and many cases show no symptoms at all over long periods. Some of the main symptoms from which people suffer are abdominal pains, irregular evacuation of the bowels, itching of the rectum, vomiting, headaches, mental depression, and loss of appetite.

In some cases there may even be severe anemia, and the bowel contents may at times contain blood and mucus, plus the parasites and eggs.

Ordinary cooking as a rule does not destroy these worms, as they are able to withstand very high temperatures.

When alive, animal muscle tissue is tender, but after death, stiffening from the coagulation of the muscular tissues sets in. The meat toughens and never becomes tender again until it putrefies. This is why meat is kept for some time to "ripen" or, in other words, to decay.

Experiments reported by Farger and Walepole in the *Journal of Physiology and Pathology* show that putrefied meat contains many poisonous substances, some of which cause the blood pressure to rise. This is why some physicians forbid meat to patients suffering from arteriosclerosis or from high blood pressure. This restriction is a protection, not only against putrefaction in meat, but also against further putrefaction of the undigested remnants of meat that takes place in the patient's intestines.

The following report of experimentation with rabbits indicates that one of the causes for the hardening of arteries is an excessive meat diet.

The first group were fed bread and meat. The second group were fed no meat at all. Both groups were kept in the laboratory under the same conditions. After several weeks all the rabbits in the first group, which had been fed on a 36 per cent protein (mostly meat) diet, developed extensively hardened chalky deposits in their blood vessels, while none of the rabbits in the second group showed any arterial diseases. Upon examining the hardened arteries of the animals, experts found them to be identical to those of humans with arteriosclerosis.

Another important point to be noted here is that the dreaded disease of cancer is practically unknown in vegetarian countries. But cancer is rapidly increasing in the countries whose meat consumption is on the increase because of economic prosperity.

Aside from the harmful effects of meat on the human body, we must consider the ethical objections to killing innocent animals.

Horses, dogs, and cows can learn, remember, love, hate, mourn, rejoice, and suffer just as humans can, though the animals' sphere of life is more limited. Every creature is endowed by nature with an instinct, and knows how to protect its life. When animals learn that human beings are harmless, they forget this natural instinct.

In the Ganges River, in Hardwar, pilgrims can see hundreds of big fish waiting to be fed by the visitors. Those fish have learned by instinct that humans are harmless, as fishing is forbidden in this pilgrim center. One cannot wade into the water without pushing the begging fish away. But in other parts of the same river a fish can hardly ever be seen, not to mention caught.

The amazing tricks displaying the intelligence of porpoises and seals of the Los Angeles Marine Land have to be seen to be believed. They play basketball, blow horns, put out fires, and obey the commands of the trainer as if they could understand the human language.

Animals know instinctively when they are destined for the slaughterhouse; though they are dumb, their watery eyes appeal for mercy from man's cruelty. The bleating of the calf, the bellowing of the bull, the cackling of frightened geese, and the cries of hundreds of other animals are protests against the wrongful and merciless destruction of the lives of innocent and helpless animals by so-called civilized and superior beings.

As we do not have the power to restore life, we certainly do not have the right to kill. Every action has its reaction and every good or bad action brings forth good or evil fruit. This is a Divine law and no law of man can void it. When man was given permission to kill animals and eat their flesh, according to the Bible, animals were also given permission to slay and eat humans: "And your life will I seek; at the hand of every beast will I seek it."

Many religious devotees and monks abstain from eating meat. A sect of Catholic monks in Iowa even abstains from eating fish and eggs. Today science has verified the accuracy of the Biblical accounts of the dietetic habits of the first men on earth, as recorded in Genesis, 1:29: "Every herb bearing seed, . . . and every tree, in which is the fruit of a tree yielding seed; to you they shall be for meat."

If meat is not man's food, then what are the foods he can eat for his physical and mental devlopment? Every diet has its effect on the human mind.

According to the *Bhagavad Gita*, there are three types of food: namely, *sattvic* food (pure food), *rajasic* food (stimulating food), and *tamasic* (impure and rotten food).

Milk, butter, fruits, vegetables, and grains come under the category of good or *sattvic* foods. Spices, hot substances, meat, alcohol, fish, and eggs, which stimulate the nervous system, come under the heading of stimulating or *rajasic* foods, while food that is rotten, putrefied, and overripe comes under the *tamasic* or impure food category.

Man's preference for one of the above-mentioned food types is in accordance with the evolution of his mind. Spiritually and mentally advanced people prefer the pure type of food. Average worldly people prefer the *rajasic* or stimulating food, and the *tamasic* or impure type of low, undeveloped man prefers the last type of rotten and putrefied foodstuffs.

Pure food brings purity and calmness to the mind and is soothing and nourishing to the body. Rajasic food arouses animal passion in man and brings a restless state of mind. It also causes nervous and circulatory disorders such as high blood pressure, hardening of the arteries, and uric acid diseases mentioned previously.

The third type, *tamasic* or impure food, makes a person dull and lazy. His thinking capacity diminishes and he sinks almost to the level of animals or bushmen. He has no high ideals or purpose in life; on the physical side, he suffers from chronic ailments of the body. Thus, according to man's degree of mental purity, he instinctively chooses certain types of food.

In every country we can see people suddenly change from impure and stimulating foods to the pure type as they progress in mental purity. Foods that once pleased their palates and minds now disgust them and leave a bad feeling. It is interesting to note that seldom do vegetarians change to the lower types of food, but nonvegetarians change increasingly to the pure type of food. Man ceases to desire meat as he grows spiritually.

It is not necessary nor is it desirable for Yoga students to become food cranks who weigh, measure, and analyze every mouthful of food. It is far better to keep as close as possible to natural foods. Always remember that nature is marvelously wise, since it represents the infinite wisdom of all creation.

This is the general rule of the Yoga student's diet: By the combination of nuts, cereals, and plenty of fresh fruits and vegetables, he can get all the important vitamins, minerals, proteins, and carbohydrates.

Yogis not only advocate a nonanimal diet, consisting of fruits, nuts, and bread made of whole wheat, but insist on masticating their food slowly. It is interesting to note that once students return to the natural habit of proper mastication, the sensation of abnormal appetite that compels a person to eat more will decrease and he will have only natural hunger. The natural appetite is nature's instinct in the animal kingdom to protect its life upon the earth, and the instinct very seldom fails. But man, as he developed his reasoning power, confused nature's instinct. Moreover, though he is a rational being, he seldom uses his reasoning power to substitute for his lost instinct. Hence, he suffers from various ailments and makes others suffer too. When we go back to nature, our instinct once more will guide us, provided we are not again spoiled by indulgence in absurd and palatable dishes and drinks common in these days, which are the cause of abnormal appetite and diseases.

Yogis advocate occasional fasts, especially during sickness, in order to give the stomach a rest. The recuperative energy may thereby be directed toward the casting out of the toxins and poisonous matter that have been causing the trouble. Nature's precaution of fasting to restore health is to be noted even in animals. They stop eating while they are sick, and lie around until they are normal once again, when they return to their food.

Raw, freshly made vegetable and fruit juices are very good for those who suffer from chronic ailments. Do not think that raw vegetable juices are like drugs to cure ailments. They are rather the most vital rebuilding and regenerating foods that the body can use for construction. These raw fruits and vegetables are the storehouses of nature's energy to nourish the starved cells of the body. When one intends to fast for a week or two on only freshly made juice, one can drink several pints of juices a day. At times one can feel discomfort from fasting on raw juices, usually because of the stirring up of poisons accumulated in the system, which nature is anxious to eliminate, but soon energy and vigor return when the toxin is eliminated.

Here I want to mention a very interesting experience, how I once felt aches and pains when my system was loaded with poisons. When I first arrived in the United States, I was the guest of a devoted couple in Oakland, California. They were so eager to show their American hospitality to a foreigner that they gave the best of everything they could afford, such as fruits, juices, whole wheat bread, etc., which a Yogi prefers. After a few days I developed a pain in the muscles of my thighs and knee joints. I did not remember having had such pain in my life but now it was a reality, even though I was living in the same way and was very careful about my diet. According to the Yogic theory, pain is nature's warning of accumulation of poison through food, so I watched my diet carefully to see if anything was wrong with it; I noticed a small change—that I was taking a glass of canned pineapple juice with my lunch. I wanted to know whether the pineapple juice was the cause of the pain, so I avoided taking it for two days. Miraculously the pain disappeared. To complete my test, once again I added the canned juice to my lunch and the next day the pain returned to warn me that I was taking wrong foods into my system. Does this not prove that nature is wise and pain is a blessing in disguise? But modern, civilized man never heeds nature's warning. He uses modern pain-killing drugs to suppress pain and, thus, merely adds more poison through the drugs themselves. Of course, even the perfect system cannot carry out its functions if we do not stop eating unnatural foods and drinks and using modern man's daily companion, the pills.

To achieve rapid results, serious students who practice Yoga are advised not to use the following while they are practicing Yoga: acids, pungent substances, salts, mustards, bitter foods, and articles roasted in oil, long walks, early morning bathing in cold water, slaughter of animals and eating their flesh. Cruelty toward animals and human beings, pride, and enmity are also forbidden. Long walks will bring fatigue and consume large amounts of energy that the Yoga student uses for concentration and serving humanity. Early morning bathing is forbidden to full-time Yoga students who practice *asanas* and breathing three times daily, so as not to chill the body after the heat of the exercises.

*Prevention is better than cure.*    Use food as medicine chiefly by eating foods in their natural state as much as possible. Fresh fruits and vegetables, nuts, whole wheat, and milk and its products should be taken in the natural state for nourishment of the body as well as prevention of diseases.

Avoid the processed, refined, and packaged foods. Use real stone-ground whole grain bread made without synthetic ingredients. For prevention of disease omit all white sugar and white flour products from your daily meals, including soft drinks, desserts, and bakery products. This is not difficult even if you eat all your meals in restaurants.

Eat organically grown food if you possibly can. Yogis live a natural life, including natural food. Prevention of disease is not merely a factor of food alone. Even after following a natural diet you may not achieve perfect health because you are subjected to many poisons and unhealthful influences every day with pollution of the air you breathe, insecticides, chemicals in drinking water, dry heat in winter, air conditioning in summer, the use of such household supplies as soaps, detergents, cleaning fluids, and so forth. Within the last fifty or sixty years since chemistry began to make our lives more convenient by surrounding us with all kinds of chemical preparations, our state of nutrition has been degenerating—partly because our food is refined and processed, partly also because most of these chemicals use up some of the body's vitamins. Inhaling tobacco smoke, for instance, uses up vitamin C, and use of soaps and detergents often makes the skin alkaline rather than acid and results in "dish-pan hands."

Prevention of disease is possible only if we follow the five important Yogic rules for health: (1) proper exercise to stimulate circulation, (2) proper breathing exercise, to absorb more oxygen, (3) proper relaxation of the body and mind, (4) natural wholesome food, and (5) proper thinking and concentration of the mind.

VITAMINS

The vitamins are substances of a highly complex nature and each one of them has a special work to perform in connection with the proper functioning of some particular organ or group of organs in the human body. Vitamins control the body's use of minerals. If the mineral supply is deficient there is less for vitamins to do. Without vitamins the body can appropriate and use minerals to some extent, but without minerals the vitamins are less useful. Therefore a proper balance of vitamins and minerals is necessary for the functioning of the endocrine glands and the formation of hormones.

### Vitamin A

It is soluble in fats and oils and insoluble in water, not affected by dilute alkalies and acids, stable to heat with no loss of activity even at 200° F. if air is kept away but unstable in presence of air, even at room temperature. It is stored to some extent in the subcutaneous fatty tissues, the kidney, and liver; however, the supply should be augmented by definite daily amounts. The body uses vitamin A best in conjunction with vitamin D in the proportion 7 to 1.

Vitamin A helps to maintain the skin in a moist condition, increasing the resistance of the body to infection of the urinary and respiratory tracts, is essential for proper growth and vision, and also increases resistance to coughs and colds.

Lack of vitamin A brings dry, horny, or scaly skin, low resistance to infection, formation of gall and kidney stones, poor tooth formation, poor digestion, sinus troubles, catarrh, ear abscesses and night blindness.

Apricot, asparagus, cabbage, carrot, celery, dandelion, endive, lettuce, orange, parsley, prune, spinach, tomato, turnip leaf and watercress are all good sources of vitamin A.

### Vitamin B1

This vitamin is not affected by dilute acids but destroyed by alkalies and sulphites. It is soluble in water and not in oil. Crystalline vitamin B1 is obtained from rice polishings.

It is unstable to ultraviolet irradiation; boiling in slightly acid solution results in partial destruction while heating in an alkaline solution results in complete loss. Pasteurization brings partial destruction and the usual cooking processes may entirely destroy vitamin B. It is stored in small amounts in the liver and must be taken daily. Vitamin B1 intake must be increased when the carbohydrates in the diet are increased.

It has a marked stimulating effect upon the appetite. It also aids digestion and absorption of foods, promotes growth, increases resistance to infection, and is essential for the proper functioning of nerve tissue. Age, exercise, fevers, and weight increase the body's need for vitamin B1.

The lack of vitamin B may result in slow heartbeat, poor appetite, nervousness, intestinal and gastric disorders, poor lactation, diminished peristalsis, nerve degeneration, enlargement of adrenals and pancreas, and beriberi (a disease of the peripheral nerves).

Asparagus, cabbage, carrot, celery, coconut, dandelion, grapefruit, lemon, parsley, pineapple, pomegranate, radish, turnip leaf, and watercress are good sources of Vitamin B1.

### Vitamin B2

Soluble in water, and acting as an oxidizing agent, this vitamin is not affected by dilute acid or air but alkalies bring almost complete destruction. It is stable to heat except in alkaline solution.

It is readily stored in the body and in greater amount than B1. The supply of vitamin B2, however, is depleted when the consumption of minerals and fats is increased. The fibrous foods tend to conserve the supply. It is necessary for healthy skin, good vision, and for the healthy functioning of the entire gastrointestinal tract. This vitamin also aids the body to assimilate iron and aids protein metabolism.

Lack of vitamin B2 brings retarded growth, lack of stamina and vigor, digestive disturbances, reduced tissue respiration or exchange of gases between the tissues and the blood, loss of hair, cataract, tongue ulceration, etc.

Apple, apricot, cabbage, carrot, coconut, dandelion, grapefruit, prune, spinach, turnip leaf, and watercress are good sources of vitamin B2.

### Vitamin C

Vitamin C is insoluble in oils, soluble in water. It is less affected by dilute acids than alkalies. It is stable to heat but not in the presence of oxygen. Steam cooking causes little loss but ordinary cooking methods destroy it; pasteurization causes considerable loss. It is not affected by cold storage if air is absent. Copper cooking vessels cause serious loss. Dried fruits lack vitamin C unless dried in vacuum.

Though it is stored in small amount in the liver, intestinal walls, and adrenal cortex, it must be replenished daily.

It promotes fine bone and tooth formation, helps to increase resistance to infection and bacterial toxin, and keeps the blood vessels in a healthy condition. Vitamin C is a distributor and diffuser of calcium to the tissues from the blood.

Lack of vitamin C may result in shortness of breath, physical weakness, rapid heart action, rapid respiration, tendency to disease of heart and blood vessels, headache, defective teeth, tender joints, peptic and duodenal ulcers, impaired adrenal function, and scurvy. Lack of this vitamin also makes difficult the knitting of broken bones.

Cucumber, grape fruit, orange, papaya, parsley, pineapple, radish, rhubarb, spinach, tomato, turnip, watercress, cabbage, carrot, and asparagus are good sources of vitamin C.

*Vitamin D*

This is insoluble in water but soluble in fats and oils and not affected by dilute acids, alkalies, or air.

Vitamin D2 is stored in the skin as ergosterol, which is converted to vitamin D2 by sunshine or ultraviolet irradiation. An excessive amount of vitamin D results in general depression, diarrhea, severe toxic effects, and abnormal calcium deposits in blood vessel walls, liver, lungs, kidneys, and stomach.

Vitamin D controls the calcium content in the blood and so governs muscular action and regulates the absorption and metabolism of calcium and phosphorus, the bone-forming elements.

Lack of vitamin D may result in soft and fragile bones, rickets, bowed legs, enlargement of elbows and wrists, malformation of pelvis and chest, poor retention and deposition of calcium and phosphorus, and tetany, a condition manifested by flexion of the ankle and wrist joints, muscle twitchings and cramps resulting from abnormal calcium metabolism.

Vitamin D is not found in vegetables, fruits, and cereals. For vegetarians butter gives the supply of vitamin D though there are a number of concentrates and artificial sources of vitamin D, among them irradiated ergosterol and many irradiated foods. Viosterol is activated ergosterol, and it is a source of vitamin D without vitamin A, as is cod liver oil.

*Vitamin E*

Soluble in oils but insoluble in water, this vitamin is not affected by alkalies or acids, though ozone or chlorine destroys it. It is also not affected by sterilizing, drying, or cooking. Though stable to ordinary light, ultraviolet light gradually destroys it. It is stored in the muscles and fat, rapidly depleted, and therefore must be renewed regularly.

According to investigators, lack of vitamin E may produce sterility in both sexes, loss of hair, miscarriage, etc.

Celery, lettuce, parsley, spinach, turnip leaf and watercress contain food amounts of vitamin E. The most important source is wheat germ.

MINERALS

It has been recognized by most authorities that the elementary composition of the human body is as follows, hundred pounds body weight, in pounds: oxygen, 65; carbon, 18; hydrogen, 10; nitrogen, 3; calcium, 1.5; phosphorus, 1; potassium, 0.35; sulphur, 0.25; sodium, 0.15; chlorine, 0.15; magnesium, 0.05; iron, 0.004; manganese, 0.003; iodine, 0.00004; and aluminum, copper, fluorine, silicon and zinc in very minute amounts.

Research authorities have determined that of the above elements calcium, chlorine, copper, iodine, iron, magnesium, manganese, phosphorus, potassium, sodium, and sulphur are absolutely essential. The body must have a proper amount of these minerals in addition to the vitamins.

### Calcium (Alkaline)

Calcium builds strong bones and teeth, aids in the clotting of the blood, aids in the metabolism of vitamin D, and regulates the proper performance of the heart muscles. It aids in regulating general mineral metabolism and helps greatly in correcting disturbance of the acid-alkaline equilibrium. It is also necessary for reducing fatigue and increasing mental alertness and resistance. Calcium in the average meal of the person who lives on a bread, meat, and potato diet is usually deficient. According to the nutrition experts, all the body calcium is completely replaced in about six years; to maintain the proper balance in the body an adequate supply should be added daily in the diet. Calcium is withdrawn from bones and teeth if the food intake is deficient in calcium. About 90 per cent of the calcium in the body is in the bony structure.

Important sources of calcium are cheese, milk, blackberry, cabbage, carrot, celery, cranberry, endive, fig, grapefruit, lettuce, lemon, orange, rhubarb, parsley, spinach, turnip and watercress.

Daily requirements: adults, 10 grains, children, 15 grains.

*Phosphorus (Acid-forming)*

Phosphorus is necessary to every living cell in the body and helps maintain the slight alkalinity of the blood stream by means of the phosphates it forms. Along with calcium, phosphates help in building sound bones and teeth. Phosphorus also keeps the hair, skin, and nails in healthy condition. An adequate supply of vitamins A, C, and D is necessary.

The lecithins (phosphorus compounds) are widely distributed in the tissues and liquids of the body and white matter of the nervous system. Lecithin is found in the gray matter of the brain to the extent of about 17 per cent and seems to be related to the higher intellectual activities. About 90 per cent of the phosphorus is found in the skeletal structure of the body and it takes about three years to replace all the body phosphorus.

Important sources of phosphorus are almonds, Brussels sprouts, chickpeas, corn, dandelion greens, grapes, lentils, peas, pecans, brown rice, rye flour, soybeans, spinach, walnuts, whole wheat, wheat germ, and apple, apricot, blackberry, coconut, cranberry, cucumber, orange, prune, tomato, watermelon.

Daily requirements for adults, 20 grains; for children, 15 grains.

*Iron (Alkaline)*

Iron builds red corpuscles and plays an important part in absorbing and carrying oxygen in the blood stream to various organs of the body. Iron deficiency results in anemia. For the proper assimilation of iron there must be an adequate supply of chlorophyll and some copper in the diet. Nutrition experts are of the opinion that for a given body weight a woman requires three to four times more iron than a man, this because of her special biological functions of menstruation, pregnancy, and lactation. Iron also is necessary for making the respiratory enzymes, such as peroxidase, catalase, etc., these enzymes being necessary for the health of every cell in the body.

Dried beans, dried peas, whole wheat, oatmeal, dried prunes, spinach, cheese, lima beans, watercress, dates, raisin, figs, oranges, turnips, tomatoes, bananas, carrots, cabbage, fresh string beans are common sources of iron for our daily requirements.

Daily requirements for adults, 12 to 15 milligrams; for children, 5 to 8 milligrams per 1,000 calories.

### Copper (Acid-forming)

Some amount of copper is necessary for assimilation of iron in the diet, though the exact amount of the daily requirement is not established yet.

Dried fruits, leafy vegetables, and fresh fruits are the common sources of copper.

### Iodine (Acid-forming)

Iodine is very essential for the proper functioning of the thyroid gland and deficiency results in goiter. It also helps to balance the development of the general glandular system. Kelp and sea lettuce are excellent sources of iodine. Asparagus, cabbage, carrot, cranberry, cucumber, lettuce, pineapple, prune, radish, spinach, tomato, and watercress contain a fair amount of iodine.

### Potassium (Alkaline)

Potassium is the mineral basis of all muscular tissue, giving muscles their pliancy. In the constructive and synthetic processes of the body, potassium plays an important part in the formation of glycogen. The liver, which is principally concerned with glycogen formation, contains twice as much potassium as sodium. Potassium is necessary for every cell in the body and for the life of every living thing. Practically all fruits and vegetables are good sources of potassium.

### Sodium (Alkaline)

Sodium plays an important part in the formation of the digestive juices, the saliva, bile, and pancreatic juices, and is necessary for the elimination of carbon dioxide. According to some authorities, deficiency of sodium in the blood is one of the causes of diabetes.

Though sodium chloride is important to the body, it is better to obtain it in natural form rather than by the use of much table salt. Whole wheat bread, rye bread, buttermilk, cream cheese, banana, and celery, beet, dandelion, lettuce, spinach, and watercress are rich in natural sodium chloride.

*Magnesium (Alkaline)*

Magnesium makes teeth and bone harder and gives strength and firmness to the bone tissue. Approximately 70 per cent of the magnesium in the body is found in the bones and it is an important constituent of muscle. It aids in building cells, particularly of lung tissue and the nervous system, and helps in the formation of the albumin of the blood. Adequate intake of magnesium helps to avoid constipation, excess acidity, poor circulation. It is also necessary for cell growth and reproduction. Magnesium is well distributed in most foodstuffs. The common sources of magnesium are almonds, cashew nuts, peanuts, lima beans, whole wheat, brown rice, oatmeal, dates, raisins, spinach, and most of the fruits and vegetables.

*Sulphur (Acid-forming)*

Sulphur is found in all body tissues; it is a constituent of the hemoglobin of the blood, keeps up body resistance, and has an antiseptic and cleansing effect on the alimentary canal. It also tends to stimulate the bile secretion, purify the blood, improve the hair, and prevent accumulation of toxic impurities. Most foodstuffs that contain sulphur also contain phosphorus, although in widely different proportions. According to nutrition experts, many disease conditions usually ascribed to the accumulation of uric acid in the system are frequently caused by the use of foods too high in phosphorus and deficient in sulphur. Foods typical of the group are cereals, milk, nuts, cheese, and eggs. These items of diet should always be well balanced with vegetables and fruits rich in sulphur to offset the phosphoric acid salts. Practically all fruits and vegetables are good sources of sulphur.

*Chlorine*

Chlorine is a general body cleanser, expels waste, helps clean the blood, tends to reduce excess fat, and keeps joints supple. It is also important in the formation of the digestive juices, particularly the gastic juice.

Most of the fruits and vegetables are fair sources of chlorine.

Though the above minerals and vitamins are also found in animal food and other foodstuffs, they are omitted here, particularly because the Yogic student needs a pure, nontoxic balanced diet for the development of the body and mind in order to reach the highest spiritual perfection.

8

# PRANAYAMA OR YOGIC BREATHING

Yoga has been broadly divided into four forms: Karma Yoga (path of action), Bhakthi Yoga (path of devotion), Raja Yoga (the science of mental control), and Gyana Yoga (the path of knowledge). The aim of these Yogas is realization of the *brahman* or the absolute even though they differ as to the means employed.

Karma Yoga (the path of action) removes *mala* or gross impurities of the mind, such as selfishness and egoism, and develops the giving hand of generosity. Bhakthi Yoga or path of devotion destroys *vikshepa* or tossing of the mind and develops the heart. Raja Yoga steadies the mind and makes it one-pointed and Gyana Yoga removes the veil of ignorance (*avarana*), develops will and reason, and brings in knowledge of self. Though it appears that these various Yogas are separate from one another, in reality they are not antagonistic to each other. Just as one and the same suit will not suit Mr. Smith and Mr. Shyam, so also one path will not suit all people. But students are advised by such great teachers as Sri Swami Sivananda to take up one of the Yogas as the main path and the other Yogas as auxiliary to the main one in order to achieve quick progress.

Again, Raja Yoga has been divided into three more subdivisions known as Mantra Yoga, Kundalini Yoga, and Hatha Yoga. These are all various modes of practice whereby the *chitha vrithi* or mental modifications are brought into control and the absolute is in various ways realized. Each of these branches of Raja Yoga has the same eight limbs (*ashtanga*):

1. *Yama* (internal purification through moral training preparatory to Yoga)
2. *Niyama* (cleanliness, contentment, mortification, study, and worship of God)
3. *Asanas* (postures)
4. *Pranayama* (breath control)
5. *Prathyahara* (making the mind introspective)
6. *Dharana* (concentration)
7. *Dhyana* (meditation)
8. *Samadhi* (the highest superconscious state)

These eight accessories may be divided into five exterior methods chiefly concerned with the body and *prana* (vital air) and three inner methods affecting the development of the mind.

Hatha Yoga gives first attention to the physical body, which is the vehicle of the soul's existence and activity. Purity of the mind is not possible without purity of the body in which it functions and by which it is affected. Through the practice of *asanas* and *pranayama*, the mind becomes one-pointed and thus one can progress quickly in concentration and meditation.

For the mind is by nature unsteady and it is at every moment being affected by sight, sound, and other factors of external objects, which mind perceives through the agency of the senses. In order to get control over the mind, Hatha Yoga prescribes various *pranayama* or breathing exercises. Before we proceed into the details of *pranayama*, the reader may do this simple experiment. It will convince everybody why Hatha Yoga emphasizes *pranayama* or breath control.

Place an alarm clock approximately twelve to fifteen feet away from you. Now concentrate on the ticks, keeping all other thoughts from the mind. You may find it hard to keep all other thoughts from the mind but apply a little more effort and you will succeed, at least for a few seconds. Repeat this experiment until you are successful in keeping the mind for a few seconds completely without distraction. After doing this experiment read the following explanation.

Now let us see what happened while hearing the ticking sound of the clock. The majority must have completely suspended the breath; the others, who have less concentration, must have had very slow breathing. Thus it proves that where there is concentration of the mind, the breathing becomes very slow or even suspension may take place temporarily.

The Sage Patanjali, in his *Yoga Aphorisms*, defines Yoga as the suspension of the modification of the thinking principle, which is not practicable without controlling the *prana* or breath, which is intimately connected with the mind.

This connection is proved by our daily experience of life. When we are absorbed in deep thinking or meditation, the process of breathing becomes slow. The suspension of mental activity increases in proportion to the slowness of breath. In cases of asphyxia, mental activity ceases altogether until respiration is revived. Again, when the mind is afflicted by sorrow or anger, the breath becomes irregular and broken, the opposite of the slow, smooth flow of the breath when the mind is calm.

These considerations prove that the mind and *prana* or vital breath are interdependent, each unable to act independently of the other.

It has been said in the *Siva Gita* that the vehicle of mind is *prana* and therefore mind functions where *prana* moves.

The great Sage Vasishta, in his *Yoga Vasishta*, has thus described the relation between the mind and the *prana*:

> O Rama! For the motion of the chariot, which is the physical body, the God has created the mind and *prana* (vital breath), without which the body cannot function. When the *prana* departs, the mechanism of the body ceases and when the mind works *prana* or vital breath moves. The relation between the mind and *prana* is like that between the driver and the chariot. Both exert motion one upon the other. Therefore, the wise should study regulation of *prana* or vital breath if they desire to suspend the restless activity of the mind and concentrate. The regulation of breath brings all happiness, material and spiritual, from the acquisition of Kingdoms to Supreme Bliss. Therefore, O Rama! Study the Science of Breath.

The word *hatha* is composed of the syllables *ha* and *tha*, which mean sun and moon: that is, *prana vayu* (the positive vital air) and *apana vayu* (the negative vital air). *Prana* (vital air) in the body of the individual is a part of the universal breath. The regulation of the harmonized breath helps the Yogi to the regulation and steadiness of mind. Similarly, by controlling the mind *prana* is also controlled. *Prana* is not something related to breath alone. Breathing is only one of the many exercises through which we get to the real *pranayama*. The breathing is a manifestation of a vitalizing force called *prana*. By regulating the physical breathing, the *prana* is controlled and this process of controlling the subtle *prana* is called *pranayama*.

This vital energy is found in all forms of life from mineral to man. *Prana* is found in all things having life. This *prana* is not the consciousness or spirit but is merely a form of energy used by the soul in its material and astral manifestations. The whole body is controlled and regulated by the force of *prana*. Every cell in the body is controlled by it. *Prana* is in all forms of matter and yet it is not matter. It is the energy or force that animates matter.

*Prana* is in the air, but is not the oxygen, nor any of its chemical constituents. It is in food, water, and in the sunlight, yet it is not vitamin, heat, or light-rays. Food, water, air, etc., are only the media through which the *prana* is carried. We absorb this *prana* through the food we eat, the water we drink, and the air we breathe. Animal and plant life breathe this energy with the air and it also penetrates where the air cannot reach.

*Prana* is also known as universal energy. It is the *prana* that is manifesting itself as gravitation, electricity, as the actions of the body, and as the nerve currents and thought force. From thought down to the lowest physical force, everything is thus the manifestation of *prana*.

Knowledge and control of *prana* manifested in individuals is called *pranayama*, which opens to us the door to almost unlimited power. The control of *prana* being the one idea of *pranayama*, all the training and Yogic exercises advocated in Hatha Yoga are for that one end. This little wave of *prana*, which represents all mental and physical energies, is the easiest to control through the regulation of physical breathing.

There are people in every country who consciously or unconsciously have control over the *prana*. In the West there are spiritualists, mind healers, faith healers, the Christian Scientists, and the hypnotists who have some control over *prana* whether they know it or not. These healers of various sects have stumbled on the discovery of pranic energy and of manipulating it without knowing its nature. Yogis use this *prana* consciously for awakening the dormant spiritual force in man.

The finest and highest manifestation of all *prana*'s action in the human being is thought. By the trained manipulation of this subtle force of *prana*, the Yogi is able to give a push to the mind to go higher up into the superconscious plane and to act from that plane.

The grossest manifestation of *prana* in the human body is in the motion of the lungs. If the motion of the lungs is stopped, all other manifestation of energy and movements of the body will stop automatically. In order to reach and control the subtle *prana*, the Yogi uses various breathing exercises. The motion of the lungs acts like the flywheel that sets the other forces of the body in motion. So *pranayama* means the controlling of this motion of the lungs, by which the subtle *prana* is controlled. When the subtle *prana* is controlled, then all other gross manifestations of *prana* in the body will slowly come under control. Every part of the body can be filled up with *prana* and when we are able to do this, the whole body will be under our control. All diseases of the body can be destroyed from the root by controlling and regulating the *prana* and it brings the secret knowledge of healing. If our body is strong and healthy with much pranic energy, we will have the natural tendency to produce health and vitality in those who live near us because the pranic energy of our body will be, as it were, conveyed to other bodies just as the water flows from the higher level to the lower.

Thus in the case of one man trying to heal another, a sick person, it can be done by transferring his own *prana* to the sick person. This can be successful only when one is able to recharge his body consciously with pranic energy through *pranayama*. This healing process can also be carried on at a distance. The *prana* can really be transmitted to a great distance, though such genuine healers are rare. *Prana* can be stored up in the body, especially in the solar plexus, as in a storage battery. This *prana* we constantly inhale through the air we breathe. Though *prana* is found in all elements, most of the *prana* we extract for our body is found in its freest state in the atmosphere.

In ordinary breathing we extract this *prana* only very little, but when we concentrate and consciously regulate our breathing, we are able to store up in our various nerve centers and brain a greater amount of *prana*.

Various powers of the advanced Yogis are due to the control of this stored-up *prana*. The main storage battery of the *prana* is the solar plexus, in the navel, and even the brain receives its energy for its function from this source.

He who has abundant pranic energy radiates vitality and strength, which can be felt by those coming in contact with him. Many psychic powers come to a Yogi through the practice of *pranayama*, though a real Yogi never demonstrates those powers. By demonstrating such powers, one not only loses the powers, but also one gets terrible reactions.

The pure man who has controlled the pranic energy has the

power of bringing it into a certain state of vibration that can be conveyed to others, bringing in them a similar vibration. These kinds of powers are used purely for good purpose by the real Yogis. Magnetic healing, faith healing, are performed in this way without any selfish motive. Such great people will not even accept thanks in return for their service.

We knowingly or unknowingly use the power of *prana* in our various daily activities. When you visit a sick friend who is having pain all over his body and head, you often unconsciously put the palm of your hand on his forehead or stroke gently over his body. You are at this moment unconsciously trying to transfer your pranic energy through your palm to your sick friend. Just see what happens to you when you fall down and knock your knee accidentally. The first thing you do is to hold the breath and then you hold the knee tightly with your palms. This is an instinctive act. But the real fact behind this is that by holding the breath you are able to get an extra supply of pranic energy, which you unconsciously transmit to that knee through your hands. When you want to lift a heavy object you again hold the breath automatically, because lifting needs more energy, which you get by holding the breath. Thus it proves that breathing plays a great part in controlling and regulating the pranic movements in the body.

All of us know the fact that the speech of some persons penetrates to the heart of the hearers while the speech of another will bring no effect on the mind, though he speaks beautifully. In the former, the speech is charged with *prana* and in the latter it is merely intellectual. The great prophets and saints had the most wonderful control of *prana,* which gave them that sort of tremendous will power that brought thousands toward them and made them think as the prophets. They could produce a tremendous amount of *prana* and their thought vibrations were charged with the pranic energy that gave them the power to sway the world. All will power arises from the control of *prana.*

All the functions of *prana* will have to be learned and mastered slowly and gradually under the guidance of a truly unselfish teacher. By proper training one can find out the fact that there is more or less supply of *prana* in one part of the body than in another part. The feeling will become so subtle that mind can feel where there is less supply of *prana* and also possess the power to supply it. This is one among the various functions of *pranayama* or Yogic breathing.

Sometimes the supply of *prana* in our body moves to one part, leaving the other parts partially empty. This brings various mental and physical illnesses. Through regulated breathing, the superfluous *prana* that is accumulated in one part is transferred toward other parts as well and thus brings energy and strength.

If we look at the vast ocean, we see big and small waves arise and dissolve with innumerable small bubbles. But the background of all these waves and bubbles is the same vast ocean. Everything from the smallest bubble to the biggest waves is connected with the ocean though in appearance they differ. Similarly every human being or animal or plant is connected with the infinite ocean of energy or *prana*. In reality, wherever there is motion and life, behind there is the storehouse of pranic energy.

The Yogi, using the method of *pranayama*, is able to absorb the energy from the infinite mass that exists behind, uses this energy for his quick spiritual growth, and within a short time is able to reach the highest perfection.

*Pranayama* teaches men how to intensify the power of assimilation of this great energy and thereby reach perfection quickly instead of progressing slowly with the retarded of the human race.

All the great saints, prophets, and Yogis, in one life span of time, lived the entire life of race, bridging the great length of time that it takes for a whole race to reach perfection. Through the power of concentration they are able to absorb and assimilate a tremendous amount of energy from the infinite storehouse, by which they are able to intensify the process of evolution in a short time. For ordinary people such power of concentration is not possible and therefore the science of Yoga teaches the science of *pranayama* in order to gain the power of concentration and energy.

Yogic breathing is that part of *pranayama* which attempts to control the physical manifestation of *prana* in the physical body. As the student progresses in the spiritual side, he is taught to control the *prana* manifested as mental power, which can be controlled only by mental means. This process of controlling the *prana* through mental concentration is called Raja Yoga. Therefore, Hatha Yoga and Raja Yoga are like the obverse and reverse of the same coin.

For the vast majority of the people to attain perfection through Raja Yoga alone is very difficult. For such people the Hatha Yogic breathing brings quick results and they are able to understand the law of *prana* upon the mind and establish themselves quickly in the path of Raja Yoga or the process of controlling the mind.

Many people think Hatha Yoga is merely physical exercises. But in reality there is no difference between Hatha Yoga and Raja Yoga.

In the *Hatha Yoga Predeepika,* the well-known, authoritative treatise on Yoga, the great author Swatma Rama emphasizes the necessity of Hatha Yoga "to those who wander in the darkness of the conflicting sects unable to obtain Raja Yoga, the most merciful Swatma Rama Yogin offers the light of Hatha Yoga" (Chap. I, Stanza 3). Here the author says that it is impossible to obtain Raja Yoga by any other means than the *hatha vidya.*

The way to higher paths is now smooth and easy after mastering body and mind through *asana* and *pranayama* prescribed in Hatha Yoga. But the ground is hard to tread and very few have the patience to persevere after repeated failures. They read of the magnificent and stupendous results laid down as following the easiest physical processes alone for a short time and take to it with avidity for some months. But finding they do not see even a shadow of the glorious powers prophesied, they give up Yogic practices in disgust and perhaps become the bitterest enemies of Yoga. They do not realize the important fact (nor do their selfish pseudo-teachers who come to the public platforms showing some magic stunts, such as eating glass and lying on a bed of nails) that these tremendous powers are promised as a result of a course of *pranayama* only when it is practiced by one who has perfected himself in the moral and spiritual qualities prescribed in the Yogic lessons. In the following story from the *Yoga Vasishta* this point is brought out very beautifully.

A Yogi retired into the jungle and practiced *pranayama* (Yogic breathing) for many years but without realizing any of the powers foretold. He then went to a teacher and asked him to teach him the Yoga. The sage told him to remain with him. For the first two years the sage met all his pupil's eager solicitation for instructions with "Wait." Gradually the Yogi pupil got accustomed to the situation and forgot to trouble his master any more for instructions. At the end of twelve years the sage called his pupil and asked him to repeat mentally the sacred syllable *Aum* (*Om*). When the pupil came to the first syllable *A*, the process by which the air in the lungs is pumped out set in naturally. When he finished the second syllable, *U* (*oo*) the process of inhalation set in naturally. At the end of the third syllable (*M*) the process of retention set in.

As a spark of fire ignites a whole field of sun-dried grass and the whole is in flame in a few minutes, so the pronunciation of the sacred word *OM* roused into activity the spiritual faculties that lay dormant hitherto in the pupil and in a short time he had passed the initial stages of *pranayama,* concentration and meditation and settled into the superconscious state.

This story illustrates the fact that the sage patiently waited for the natural unfoldment of the pupil's spiritual tendencies and the purifying of his nature through his association and surroundings. He chose the right time to initiate him only after many years, when the pupil was purified through preliminary exercises, *pranayama,* prayer, and the long association with the sage.

If purification of the mind as an essential part in the process of Yoga is understood and tried, through the prescribed method, then there would be fewer victims of failure.

### IMPORTANCE OF PRANAYAMA AND RULES

*Pranayama* is one of the most important practices in all forms of Yoga. By practicing *pranayama,* the Yogi is able to control the nervous system and thereby obtains gradual control over *prana* or vital energy and the mind.

To breathe means to live and to live means to breathe. Every living thing depends upon breathing and cessation of breathing is cessation of life itself. From the first cry of the infant to the last gasp of a dying man there is nothing but a series of breaths. Yogis count life not by number of years but number of breaths. We constantly drain our life force or pranic energy by our thinking, willing, acting, etc. Every thought, every act of will, or motion of muscles uses up this life force and in consequence constant replenishing is necessary, which is possible mainly through breathing alone.

Just as oxygen is carried through the blood stream to all parts of the body, building up and replenishing, so is the *prana* carried to all parts of the nervous system. If we know that Yogis get most of their energy from the air, then the importance of proper breathing is readily understood. Whoever practices breathing regularly and systematically can feel in his own body this great effect of absorption of *prana.*

When one inhales, he is taking in *prana* and storing it in various nerve centers, especially in the solar plexus. The more *prana* one can take in, the more vitality he will possess. In the practice of *pranayama,* mind plays a great part and it is important to observe consciously everything that takes place in the phenomenon of breathing.

In the West there are numerous schools where correct breathing is taught for the sake of physical health. Even pregnant women are taught certain types of breathing exercises that resemble Yogic breathing for natural painless childbirth. During the birth of the child, with each contraction the expectant mother breathes rapidly in quick succession and holds the breath. This act of breathing relieves the pain and the child is born in a natural way while the mother is conscious of every process of nature's act of bringing her child into the world.

Yogis declare that the correct habit of breathing, with natural diet, would regenerate the race and the modern diseases of civilized man, such as blood pressure, heart diseases, asthma, tuberculosis, etc., would be only medical names in the dictionary. In addition to the physical benefits derived through breathing, Yogic teachings further show that through *pranayama* man's will power, self-control, concentration power, moral qualifications, and even his spiritual evolution can be increased.

## EFFECT OF PRANA ON THE NERVOUS SYSTEM

There are two nerve currents on either side of the spinal column and there is a hollow canal named *sushumna* running through the spinal cord. At the base of this hollow canal is the seat of the *kundalini* or the serpent power.

When the coiled power of *kundalini* awakes through various *pranayama* and concentration, it tries to force a passage through this hollow canal and as it rises from lower nerve plexuses to the higher ones, layer after layer of mind opens and many powers and visions come to the Yogi. And when the *kundalini* reaches the last and highest center, *sahasrara chakra* (thousand-petaled lotus) in the brain, he becomes perfectly detached from his body and mind and his soul is freed from all limitations caused by time and space. Here the Yogi realizes his eternal existence and enjoys the bliss of the superconscious state.

Yogis, through the *pranayama*, open the canal of *sushumna* in the spinal column, which is closed at the lower end, situated near what is called the sacral plexus. The six plexuses that have their centers in the spinal cord can very well stand for the six *chakras* in the *sushumna*.

We shall have to remember here from physiology that there are two kinds of action of the nerve currents—one afferent or sensory, which carries the sensations inward to the brain, and the other efferent or motor, from the brain outward to the body. Another point to be remembered here is that the center that regulates the respiratory system has a sort of controlling action over the nerve currents.

There are ten *nadis* (subtle nerve tubes) through which the nerve currents or *prana* moves. Out of these ten *nadis,* the principal *nadis* are three: *ida, pingala,* and *sushumna.* Again, among these three *nadis* the *sushumna* located in the spinal column is the most important for Yogis. *Sushumna* plays a great part in *pranayama.* Through certain *pranayama* and concentration, Yogis withdraw *prana* from the *ida* and *pingala* consciously and take it to *sushumna,* which will become active. When the *ida* and *pingala nadis* are devitalized by the operation of *sushumna nadi,* there is no night or day for the Yogi. When the *sushumna* is in operation, the Yogi can transcend the limitation of time and space.

We shall see now why *pranayama* has been taught in order to make the *sushumna nadi* function. The brain receives all sensations through nerve fibers; similarly all the messages are telegraphed from the brain through the nervous system only. The *ida* and *pingala nadis* of the Yogins correspond to the column of sensory and motor fibers in the spinal cord through which the afferent and efferent currents are traveling. Now according to the Yogic system, the mind can send nerve currents without the use of *ida* and *pingala.* If we take the analogy of the telegraph system and wireless system, we can easily understand how the mind can send and receive nerve currents without the help of *ida* and *pingala.* For the telegraphic system the message is sent through the wires but in the wireless system there is no need of any wires. Yogis use the wireless method to send the nerve currents. Now the question arises, what is this use of it and how is it done? The answer is that, by doing so, we will be able to get rid of the bondage of matter.

When the *sushumna nadi* in the spinal column is made active by *pranayama* and by certain other processes prescribed in Hatha Yoga, then alone can we get rid of the bondage of matter. By such practices, a Yogi makes his *sushumna nadi* active. By this the knowledge of his relations with the objective world is held in abeyance and he sees his self pervading the whole universe and becoming one with it.

In ordinary persons, the *sushumna* is closed up at the lower extremity and no nerve current passes through it. This canal of *sushumna* can be opened through *pranayama.* When the *sushumna* canal is open and active, the *prana* acts upon the coiled power *kundalini* at the *muladhara* and then the *kundalini* is consciously made to travel up the *sushumna nadi.* When the entire coiled power travels from center to center, layer after layer of the mind, as it were, will be perceived by the Yogi in its fine or coarse form. And when this tremendous mass of energy is made to move along the *sushumna* by the power of intense meditation and *pranayama* and strike on the last center *sahasrara chakra* in the brain, the knowledge and sensation are superior to the knowledge that comes through the ordinary senses. This direct perception of the self without the help of ordinary senses is called illumination or superconscious perception wherein there is no limitation of self caused by mind or matter.

Thus the rousing of the *kundalini* through *pranayama* and other Hatha Yogic methods is one of the ways to the realization of the self or pure consciousness. This *kundalini shakthi* can be aroused through other methods also, such as through devotion and love for God, through intense meditation on the *kundalini shakthi*, through the power of the analytic will of the *Gyana* Yogis or Vedanta philosophers, etc.

Wherever there is supernatural power of wisdom or knowledge, there must have been at least a partial manifestation of *kundalini*. All kinds of worship,. from the primitive man to the civilized man, lead to this one end of rousing this power and many of such worshipers had ignorantly stumbled onto some practice that set in motion a portion of this *kundalini shakthi* for a very short time.

Thus that supreme, universal mother nature whom men worship under various names and faiths, through fear and tribulations, the Yogi declares unto the world to be the living power that is lying coiled up in every being as *kundalini shakthi*, the giver of immortality and eternal happiness.

## FIVE PRINCIPAL PRANAS OR FIVE TYPES OF VITAL FORCE

Before the student takes up *pranayama* for awakening *kundalini*, he should have a proper understanding of the five major *pranas* or five types of vital forces and their functions. Though *prana* is one, it assumes five forms: (1) *prana*, (2) *apana*, (3) *samana*, (4) *udana*, and (5) *vyana*, according to the different functions it performs.

The seat of *prana* is the heart; of *apana*, the anus; of *samana*, the region of the navel; of *udana*, the throat; while *vyana* is all-pervading and moves all over the body.

The function of *prana* is respiration and its color is that of a red gem; *apana* does excretion and its color is a mixture of white and red; *samana* performs digestion and its color is between that of pure milk and crystal; *udana* does deglutation (swallowing of the food) and is plain white color. *Udana prana* also assumes the function that takes the individual to sleep. *Vyana* performs circulation of blood and it resembles the color of archil (or that of a ray of light).

Thus, according to the Yoga philosophy, all visible and invisible happenings in the universe and in the body are the functions of one *prana*, which manifests in various forms. The activities of the human body automatically come under the control of *prana* and this cosmic *prana* as it functions in the body is named *pancha pranas* or five vital forces, according to the nature and function it performs.

These five *pranas* function through the five subsidiary nerve centers in the brain and spinal cord.

*Prana* through the cervical portion of the autonomic nervous system governs the verbal mechanism and the vocal apparatus, the respiratory muscles, and the movements of the gullet.

*Apana Prana* controls mostly the autonomic action of the excretory apparatus of the body such as kidney, bladder, genitals, colon, and rectum through the lumbar portion of the autonomic system.

*Samana Prana* controls such secretions of the digestive system as that of the stomach, liver, pancreas, and intestine through the sympathetic portion of the autonomic system in the thoracic region.

*Udana Prana* functions above the larynx and controls all the automatic functions that come under the cephalic divisions of the autonomic nervous system. It also functions as a psychic force that separates the astral body from the physical body at the time of death.

*Vyana Prana* pervades all the body. This *prana* controls the voluntary and involuntary movements of the muscles of the whole body and the movements of the joints and structures around them. It also helps to keep the whole body in erect position by generating unconscious reflexes along the spinal cord.

In addition to the five principal *pranas,* there are five more *upa pranas* or five minor vital forces: *naga, kurma, krikkara, devadatha,* and *dhananjaya.* The *naga vayu* performs the function of belching and gives rise to consciousness; *kurma* opens the eyelids (drooping of eyelids before sleep) and causes vision; the *krikkara* causes sneezing and causes hunger and thirst; the *devadatha* produces yawning, and *dha-*

*nanjaya* pervades the whole gross body and does not leave the physical body even after death.

Every one of these five *pranas* is governed by five *vayus* or nerve impulses. These five *vayus* are also named in the same way as the five *pranas*: (1) *prana vayu*, (2) *apana vayu*, (3) *udana vayu*, (4) *vyana vayu*, (5) *samana vayu*.

The word *vayu* in the Yogic literature is used to describe a particular nerve current or impulse, which is one of the properties of a nerve. These *vayus* or nerve currents are either received or generated by *pranas* located in different plexuses of the sympathetic portion of the autonomic system. Each plexus is an independent nerve center, which can receive and generate a nerve impulse.

During *pranayama* exercises, *prana vayu* is generated by the intaking of breath and *apana vayu* is generated by the exhaling process. The *prana vayu* is an afferent impulse going to the brain or nerve centers and *apana vayu* is an efferent impulse that moves away from the brain and nerve centers. During retention time in *pranayama*, the Yogi unites these *prana vayu* and *apana vayu* (afferent and efferent nerve impulses) at the *muladhara chakra* (pelvic plexus). When the two impulses are united at this basic nerve center (pelvic plexus), then this center will act like a dynamo, sending tremendous amounts of pranic energy to stimulate the coiled power *kundalini* lying dormant at this center.

When the *kundalini* becomes active it will try to move upward through the canal in the *sushumna*. This is the first awakening of the *kundalini shakthi*. When *kundalini* is awakened, various reactions can take place in the body. At first the canal of the *sushumna* in the spinal column is not well opened and there will be a great struggle to raise the *kundalini* upward.

Here I would like to add some of the initial reactions I had during my *pranayama* exercise, which will be helpful for advanced students in breathing exercises.

The first reaction, especially during the *bhastrika pranayama*, is a feeling of a pleasant warmth at the pelvic plexus (*muladhara*). This is due to the initial vibration caused by the partially united *prana* and *apana* nerve impulses. This feeling of heat is felt for several days during the *pranayama* exercise. Then one day the heat at the lower spine became very intense but very pleasant throughout the period of retention: This experience continued for some days. As the heat increased at the lower spine, a peculiar sensation is felt like a whirlpool in a river. This churning sensation is due to the reaction of the *kundalini shakthi*. Slowly and gradually this sensation of the coiled power of *kundalini* moving upward became intense. At first when the power started rising upward through the *sushumna* in the spinal column, it became active as though it were a high tension wire sending pranic current to every cell of the body throughout the nervous system. At first the body started trembling and quivering when the *sushumna* was active. At times the reaction was so intense that the body was thrown out of its seat. But all the time during the period of retention there was a peculiar joy that cannot be expressed in words.

As the *pranayama* exercises continued with proper diet for some months the *prana* started moving steadily in the *sushumna*, which can be felt with various kinds of sensations and joy while the trembling and quivering sensation of the body became less and less and finally stopped. The trembling of the body was due to the sudden striking of *prana* on the *sushumna nadi* and to forcing a way through it while still not completely purified. It took long practice of purificatory breathing exercises before the *sushumna* became fully opened and active. At first the control of the body when it started trembling was not possible consciously. This was due partially to impurities in the *sushumna* and partially to not using the locks or *bandhas* properly (*moola bandha* or the anus contraction and the *jalandhara bandha* or the chin lock), which will be described at the end of this chapter.

When these locks are done properly during the retention time and when the *sushumna* is free of impurities, then at will the *prana* could be taken to *sushumna*, which was not possible previously. It took several months before this control was possible. Purification of the *nadis* (physical and astral nerve tubes) is essential to get psychic experience, which may take several years of practice. This purification exercise for *nadis* is known as *anuloma viloma pranayama* or alternate nostril breathing.

These experiences are convincing and can be achieved by anyone who sincerely practices *pranayama* with proper diet and under direction of a teacher. *Pranayama* is important in the control of the body and mind.

PRACTICAL LESSONS ON YOGIC BREATHING
OR PRANAYAMA

We have now to deal with the exercises in *pranayama*. The first lesson in *pranayama* is to learn to control the motion of the lungs. The reason for doing so is to feel the finer motions that are going on within the body, which the Yogi says can be learned by controlling the motion of *prana* manifested in the lungs.

Before we go to breathing exercises, let us take a hasty glance over the mechanical arrangements whereby the respiratory movements are affected. The respiration takes place through elastic movements of the lungs and the activities of the side and bottom of the thoracic cavity. The trunk is divided into two portions, the thoracic cavity and abdominal cavity. The thoracic cavity is occupied mainly by the lungs and the heart and is bounded by the spinal column, the ribs, the breast bone, and at the bottom of the lungs by the diaphragm. There are twenty-four ribs, which emerge twelve from each side of the spinal column. There are two types of ribs, true ribs and false or floating ribs.

The upper seven pairs are the true ribs, which are fastened directly to the breast bone and the lower five pairs are floating ribs. The thoracic cavity is separated from the abdominal cavity by the muscular partition known as the diaphragm, which plays an important part in respiration.

In the process of inhalation, the ribs are moved by the intercostal muscles and the diaphragm descends toward the abdominal cavity. The movement of the ribs and the intercostal muscles and the pull of the diaphragm downward expand the two elastic lungs. When the lungs are expanded by these respiratory muscles, a vacuum is created in the lungs and the air from outside rushes in.

The science of *pranayama* starts with the proper control of the diaphragm and the respiratory muscles, which will bring the maximum degree of lung expansion in order to absorb the greatest amount of the life-giving energy from the air.

In order to secure the greatest amount of air through minimum effort, you may do the following tests. These tests of your respiratory system will bring the knowledge that certain types of breathing bring a maximum amount of air into the lungs with less effort.

*Test No. 1.* Sit erect by keeping the spine, neck, and head in a straight line. Now relax the abdominal muscles. Do not raise your chest and do not bend forward. If you have a watch with a second hand, count the number of seconds while you inhale. Now take a long breath while allowing the diaphragm to descend without raising the chest and shoulders.

Whether your diaphragm moves properly or not could be easily discovered by watching the movement of the abdomen. When the diaphragm contracts and its dome-shaped center becomes flattened, it thereby pushes the abdominal contents and makes the abdomen expand. Here the ribs and the intercostal muscles will be at rest. On the other hand, if the abdomen is contracted naturally the diaphragm cannot descend. Therefore the main test here is to watch the abdominal movements and you can easily discover that on inspiration, the dome-shaped diaphragm becomes flattened, thereby increasing the cubic capacity of the chest from above downward. Practice this breathing several times and then compare the result with the following two tests. Count the number of seconds you take to fill the lungs in each of these three tests and also make note of which of these three tests brings maximum air to the lungs.

*Test No. 2.*   Sit erect. Keep your diaphragm still. Do not allow your abdomen to expand, because if the abdomen is expanding during breathing naturally it shows the diaphragm is functioning as stated in test No. 1. Now expand the chest and take a long deep breath. Here the intercostal muscles of the ribs expand the lungs partially and the diaphragm is in neutral position. Therefore the breathing is done absolutely through the actions of the respiratory muscles connected with ribs. Repeat this breathing several times and watch the difference between the No. 1 test breathing and No. 2 test breathing. Watch the duration of time it takes to breathe in and the quantity of air you can take into the lungs while inhaling. If you want to differentiate more clearly between these two breathings, repeat the two tests alternately; first the No. 1 breathing and then No. 2 breathing. See which one of these breathings brings more air into the lungs. The test will show that the Yogic breathing is the correct way of breathing and what is Yogic will be discussed after finding the result of the third breathing.

*Test No. 3.*   Now we know the difference between the No. 1 and No. 2 breathing. Now let us see the difference between No. 2 and No. 3 breathing.

Sit erect as in the previous position. Now contract the abdomen and draw it toward the thoracic cavity. Now take a deep breath by raising the shoulders and collarbones while the abdomen is contracted. Repeat it several times and then compare it with No. 2 breathing and see which one of these two brings in more air.

After the No. 3 breathing test try to find out for yourself the main difference among these three types of breathing and which one of these kinds of breathing brings in more air to the lungs with minimum effort. The result of the test you can see for yourself: that the No. 1 breathing brings more air than the No. 2 and No. 3. No. 2 breathing was inferior to No. 1 breathing and brings less air than by the No. 1 breathing. But No. 2 breathing is better than No. 3. The worst of all breathing is the third one, where the shoulders and collarbones are raised and the abdomen is contracted while inhaling.

Many people breathe this third type of breathing, using maximum energy to get very little air. Many diseases of the vocal organs and the respiratory system are noted in those who use this method of breathing.

I have tested this myself on some of the students who came to my Yoga class with asthmatic complaints. Almost every one of them raised the shoulders and collarbones while breathing and there was only very little expansion of their chests. I noticed in them that there was no downward movement at all of the diaphragm. Many of them recovered from the acute attack of asthma by correcting the breathing habits, along with proper diet.

The No. 1 breathing is known as deep breathing, No. 2 as chest breathing, and No. 3 as high breathing.

During the process of inhalation, the diaphragm plays a great part. This portion of the breathing where the diaphragm plays the major role is the No. 1 breathing, deep breathing, or low breathing. The diaphragm is a great partition muscle, which separates the thoracic cavity from the abdominal cavity. It is dome-shaped or it presents a concave surface to the abdomen at rest. When the diaphragm is brought to use in low breathing, it presses upon the abdominal organs and forces out the abdomen. Naturally, in this type of breathing the lungs are given a freer play than in the other two types.

Though this type of abdominal breathing is the best, yet according to the Yoga system of breathing it is not a complete breathing exercise. The reason is that any one of these breathing methods fills only a portion of the lungs—the low breathing the lower and middle parts, chest breathing the middle and a portion of the upper regions, and the high breathing the upper portions of the lungs.

In the Yoga system of breathing, the first lesson taught is to use all the three methods of breathing simultaneously, starting from the low breathing and continuing to chest breathing and finally finishing with high breathing. Now during this type of inhalation process, the whole respiratory system comes into play and no portion of the lungs is left unfilled with fresh air. This type of breathing is known as Yogic breathing, wherein the entire respiratory organism responds to this method of breathing.

Yogic breathing gives great attention to the process of exhalation; the ratio between inhalation and exhalation is 1:2. If the inhalation is one second the exhalation will be two seconds. The reason for making the exhalation longer than inhalation is to get maximum control over the lungs so that old foul air in the air sacs can be squeezed out.

It will not be out of place here to speak about lungs so that it will be easy to understand why Yogis emphasize exhalation rather than inhalation. As long as the air sacs are filled with old air, no amount of strength applied in inhalation can bring fresh air from the atmosphere. In ordinary breathing we squeeze out a very little volume of air from the apex of the lungs, leaving the base of the lungs almost inactive.

The lungs are spongy, porous, and their tissues are very elastic. The substance of lungs contains innumerable air sacs. The right lung consists of three lobes and the left one two lobes. Each lung consists of an apex and base. The base is directed toward the diaphragm and the apex is situated above, near the root of the neck.

When we breathe, we draw in air through the nose; after it has passed through the nose and the pharynx and the larynx, it passes into the trachea or windpipe, which in turn is subdivided into innumerable smaller tubes called bronchioles. The bronchioles terminate in minute subdivisions in the small air sacs of the lungs, of which the lung contains a great number. Each of these air sacs holds a portion of the inhaled air, from which the oxygen penetrates through the walls of the pulmonary capillaries. Then the blood takes up oxygen and releases carbonic acid gas generated from the waste products that have been gathered up by the blood from all parts of the system. Owing to the contact of the blood, the air sacs are now drained of the pure oxygen and in turn they are filled with carbonic acid gas from the blood. Unless this accumulated foul air is squeezed out from these tiny air sacs, we cannot bring fresh air to them. As long as the air sacs are filled with old air, no amount of strength applied in inhalation can bring fresh air from the atmosphere. In ordinary breathing we squeeze out only a very little air from the apex of the lungs and the base of the lungs lies almost inactive, filled with stagnant air. Some people use only the base of the lungs for breathing, leaving the upper portion idle.

According to medical reports consumption is due principally to lowered vitality attributable to an insufficient amount of air being inhaled. Imperfect exhalation or emptying of the lungs allows a considerable part of the lungs to remain inactive and such portions offer an inviting field for bacilli, which attack the weakened tissues. Good healthy tissue will resist attack and the best and only way to have good, healthy lung tissues is to use the lungs properly by expelling all foul air and refilling with fresh air. This is one of the reasons that Yogic breathing emphasizes long, slow, deep exhalation so that as much as possible of the old stagnant air can be removed and be replaced with fresh air. The more air is squeezed out, the more fresh air rushes into the lungs from the atmosphere, as there cannot be any vacuum in the air sacs.

Therefore, for the practice of Yogic breathing the first lesson is started with inhalation and exhalation, keeping the ratio of 1:2, starting with four seconds of inhalation, double the time for exhalation—that is, eight seconds. Then slowly increase the proportion under the guidance of a teacher. Everybody can in time reach to the higher proportions.

When the students are properly established in inhalation and exhalation, the next step is to retain the breath proportionately. According to the Yogic breathing, the ratio between inhalation and retention is 1:4. Retention is four times inhalation and exhalation is always twice inhalation. Hence the ratio between inhalation, retention, and exhalation is 1:4:2. The minimum schedule to start with is four seconds of inhalation, sixteen seconds of retention, and eight seconds of exhalation, and then slowly work up to five, twenty, and ten, to eight, thirty-two, and sixteen.

It is surprising to see that some persons can retain the breath for a good time but during long slow exhalation they soon are exhausted. This shows their breathing is not properly done. Some persons can take a long deep inhalation but when they are asked to breathe out for double the time of the inhalation, they find it is very difficult. To get maximum benefit from *pranayama* (Yogic breathing), students are always advised to start with inhalation and exhalation under the guidance of an able teacher who knows where the difficulty lies and who himself has gone through the various difficult stages. It is always advisable to do all the breathing exercises under the guidance of a Yoga teacher. The real qualification of a Yoga teacher is that he is very spiritual, kind-hearted, open-minded, and moreover he is absolutely selfless in his teachings and never commercializes his profession. Under the guidance of such teachers only can one make real progress in *pranayama* and spiritual practices. Moreover, a real teacher will not merely teach physical breathing alone.

### PRACTICE OF YOGIC BREATHING FOR THE PURIFICATION OF THE NADIS (SUBTLE NERVES AND PHYSICAL NERVES)

Here I start the purification with a few quotations from well-known authorities on Yoga that have been taken as guides by various classes in Yoga in India.

> The Yogin having perfected himself in the *asanas* (Yogic postures) should practice *pranayama* according to the instructions laid down by his spiritual teacher, with his senses under control observing always a nutritious and moderate diet.

> When the breath wanders, i.e. irregular, the mind is also unsteady, but when the breath is still, so is the mind, and the Yogis live long; therefore one should hold breath.

> A man is said to live only so long as he is breathing; when the breathing ceases he is said to be dead. So one should practice *pranayama*.

> When the *nadis* are full of impurities the breath does not go into the middle *nadi, sushumna;* then there is no arriving at the higher state of mind.

> When all the *nadis* that are now full of impurities become purified then only the Yogin can successfully perform *pranayama*.
>
> *Hatha Yoga Pradipika,* Chapter II, 1–6.

From the above stanzas the importance of purifying the *nadis* is clear. Unless the *nadis* are purified, there will be no real success in *pranayama*. Complete purification of all the *nadis* may be achieved only after a long period of practice of *pranayama*, depending on the individual. Generally it takes at least one to two years.

There are two ways of purifying the *nadis:* (1) *samanu* (the mental process); and (2) *nirmanu* (the physical cleansing, the *kriyas*, described elsewhere in this book).

## Samanu (or the Mental Process of Cleansing the Nadis)

1. Sit in lotus position or *sidhasan,* the adept's position. Meditate on the root syllable (*bijakshara*) of air (*vayu*), *yam*, which is of smoke color. Inhale through the left nostril by repeating six times the root syllable *yam*. This is inhalation. Retain the breath until you repeat *yam* sixty-four times. This is retention. Then exhale through the right nostril very, very slowly while you repeat *yam* thirty-two times.

2. Then draw the breath through the right nostril, repeating sixteen times *ram*, root syllable of fire (*bija* of *agni*) at the navel center. Retain the breath until you repeat *ram* sixty-four times. Then exhale slowly through the left nostril while you repeat *ram* mentally thirty-two times.

3. Fix the gaze at the tip of the nose. Inhale through the left nostril while repeating the root syllable of moon, *tam*, sixteen times. Retain the breath while repeating *tam* sixty-four times. Now imagine that the nectar that flows from the moon runs through all the vessels of the body and purifies them. Then exhale slowly through the right nostril while you repeat the root syllable of the earth principle (*bija* of *prithivi*), *lam*, thirty-two times.

This cleansing is only for advanced students who have been initiated by their teacher. Beginners should not practice this mental cleansing until they practice the following exercises on breathing for a long time.

## Anuloma Viloma Pranayama (or Alternate Breathing Exercise)

We have seen in the previous lessons the importance of *pranayama.* This science of breath has its foundation in the control of *prana* or vital energy. The important starting exercise for every Yoga student is the alternate breathing exercise known as *Anuloma viloma pranayama.* The reason for doing alternate breathing is that the breath alternates between two nostrils. You can easily find this out for yourself by placing your palm near the nostrils. One of the nostrils will always be partially blocked, and the flow of air in and out of the lungs will be mainly through but one of the nostrils. If a person is in normal health the breath will alternate approximately every hour and fifty minutes. This normal period of breath alternation is established only when one has perfected *pranayama,* starting with alternate breathing. In the vast majority of persons this change of the breath from one nostril to the other varies a great deal owing to such conditions as unnatural living habits, wrong diet, diseases, and the lack of proper exercises.

All these wrong habits of living have some effect on the breath, diverting it from its normal flow. According to Yoga the breath in the right nostril is said to be hot, while the flow from the left is cool. Therefore, symbolically, they named the right *nadi* as sun breath or *pingala,* and the left *nadi* as moon breath or *ida.* The energy that flows through *pingala nadi* or sun breath produces heat in the body which is catabolic, efferent, and acceleratory to the organs of the body; while the energy of the moon breath in *pingala nadi* is cooling and is anabolic, efferent, and inhibitory to the body organs.

When the breath continues to flow in one nostril for more than two hours, it is a symptom of derangement caused by excess of heat or cold. So if the *pingala* is more active, the heat of the body increases and there will be mental and nervous disturbances. When the *ida* is more active, the metabolic activity of the body becomes low, thus producing cold and lethargy and a suspended mental activity.

This alternating breathing exercise is mainly for the purpose of maintaining an equilibrium in the catabolic and anabolic processes in the body, and for purifying the *nadis.* According to the Yogis, when breath flows more than twenty-four hours in one nostril without changing, it is a warning that some illness is at hand. The longer the flow of breath in one nostril, the more serious the illness will be. This is because the ganglia of some particular nerve center are being overworked by the abnormal flow of breath, which moves in a particular center for a longer-than-normal period of time.

BREATHING EXERCISE NO. 1. single nostril

Sit in any one of the meditative poses, keeping the spine, neck, and head in a straight line. Close the right nostril with your thumb. Inhale slowly through the left nostril, counting *OM* mentally five times. Exhale through the same nostril while counting *OM* ten times. Exhalation time is always twice the inhalation time. The proportion is 1:2. Repeat this exercise fifteen to twenty rounds through the left nostril, keeping the proportion five seconds inhalation and ten seconds exhalation.

Now close the left nostril with your right ring finger and little finger, and inhale through the right nostril. Count *OM* five times for inhalation. Exhale through the same nostril while counting *OM* ten times. That makes one round. Repeat for fifteen to twenty rounds.

Do not make any sound during inhalation. Apply the basic rules of low, mid, and high breathing during inhalation. In exhalation, try to expel as much as possible of the foul air from the lungs.

You should practice Exercise No. 1 for fifteen days, and slowly increase the proportion to six seconds inhalation and twelve seconds exhalation. Do not try the higher proportion until you are able to do the lower proportion very easily. This is the main rule in every breathing exercise. Always keep within your capacity and never overdo. Get practical guidance from an experienced teacher who practices Yoga himself and not merely teaches Yoga by learning it from a book, something that is done commonly these days.

In Exercise No. 1 there is no retention. The purpose of inhaling and exhaling through one nostril is to correct the wrong breathing habit. Unless one is able to do low, mid, and high breathing perfectly and automatically, he should not attempt advanced *pranayama*. Practice Exercise No. 1 for at least a month, even though some may feel able to extend the time. If the foundation is strong then you can build a strong building. So also if you practice the basic lessons in breathing for a long time, it will be very easy to take up the advanced exercises.

EXERCISE NO. 2. alternate breathing exercise

After a month of practicing Exercise No. 1, take to the alternate breathing exercise. Now you need not practice Exercise No. 1, single nostril breathing.

Close the right nostril with your right thumb and inhale through the left nostril. Now close the left nostril immediately with your right ring finger and little finger. Remove your thumb from the right nostril and exhale through that nostril. This is a half round.

Now, without pausing, inhale through the right nostril. Close the right nostril with your right thumb and inhale through the left, as previously. This makes one full round.

The proportion of inhalation is 1:2, as in exercise No. 1, or six seconds inhalation and twelve seconds exhalation. The same general rules for Exercise No. 1 apply for No. 2 as well. Do fifteen to twenty rounds.

When you are able, without difficulty, to do six seconds inhalation and twelve seconds exhalation, then increase to seven and fourteen seconds, then to eight and sixteen seconds. These increases must be undertaken slowly. You should practice this exercise from two to three months before increasing to eight and sixteen seconds. Within this period you can see tremendous changes taking place in your body and mind. The breathing will become perfect, especially the movement of the diaphragm; and the body becomes very light and the eyes shine. When these signs become apparent, it shows that the *nadis* are being purified.

EXERCISE NO. 3. full alternate breathing

First, for a few minutes, meditate on *OM*, the word that represents the source of all light and knowledge.

In this third exercise we include retention or holding of the breath. This is the only difference between the second and third exercises.

The correct ratio between inhalation and retention is 1:4. But beginners are advised to follow a 1:2 ratio for a few months before taking up the 1:4 ratio. The minimum starting proportion is four seconds inhalation, eight seconds retention, and eight seconds exhalation. After a month increase to 5:10:10. Increase gradually until you reach 8:16:16.

In Sanskrit, inhalation is known as *pooraka*, retention as *kumbaka*, and exhalation as *rechaka*.

Inhale the air through the left nostril while counting *OM* four times mentally. Retain the air while counting *OM* eight times. Exhale through the right nostril while counting *OM* eight times. Now without stopping inhale through the right nostril, retain the breath, and exhale through the left nostril—all in the same 4:8:8 proportion. This is one full round. Practice fifteen to twenty rounds daily.

When you are holding the breath, you must close the right nostril with the right thumb and the left nostril with the right ring finger and little finger. Do not use the index finger for closing the nostril because the magnetic current from that finger is polluted.

When you are able to do 8:16:16 comfortably, change the ratio to 1:4:2. Start with four seconds inhalation, sixteen seconds retention, and eight seconds exhalation. Gradually work up to 8:32:16. It should take eight to twelve months of practice to reach this timing. Do not try to hurry it.

When the *nadis* are purified, certain signs are visible. In the first stage, the body perspires. In the second a tremor is felt throughout the body. In the highest stage, the *prana* goes to the *sushumna nadi* and to the highest center, *sahasrara chakra*. In *Hatha Yoga Pradipika* it is advised to do the following when the body perspires during the *pranayama:* "Rub well on the body the perspiration given out. This gives firmness and lightness to the whole constitution." By such practices the skin also becomes smooth.

There is no other exercise that will bring the purification of the *nadis* as does the alternate breathing. In fact, this is the only *pranayama* for purification. Other *pranayamas*, especially *bhastrika, ujjayi,* and *suryabheda* are for awakening the *kundalini* after the purification of the *nadis* is achieved. *Bhastrika* and *ujjayi,* which will be explained shortly, will bring the best result only when the *nadis* are purified. So students are advised not to jump into higher breathing exercises without spending sufficient time in practicing alternate breathing.

## Kapalabhathi (or Abdominal Breathing, Diaphragmatic Breathing)

In Sanskrit, *kapala* means skull and *bhathi* means shines. Therefore the term *kapalabhathi* means an exercise that makes the skull shine. Here the skull is the nasal passage through which the air passes in and out. Though this is a breathing exercise, it is considered a cleansing exercise and comes under one of the *shad kriyas* or six purificatory exercises. (The remaining five cleansing exercises are explained elsewhere.) This is done before starting the practice of *pranayama*, to clean the nasal passages and to remove bronchial congestion.

One should start this exercise only after practicing alternate breathing, the second exercise, for one or two months. This is because with many people it takes quite a time to get the diaphragm to move in a proper way during breathing. A vast majority tend to move the diaphragm in the opposite to natural direction during *kapalabhathi*. This can be easily noticed by watching the movement of the abdominal muscles. Those who breathe incorrectly contract the abdominal muscles and raise the shoulders while inhaling, which is quite opposite to correct breathing. Therefore, until the diaphragm takes the natural movement, one should not practice *kapalabhathi*.

A few rounds of vigorous practice of *kapalabhathi* will vibrate every tissue of the body. At times it will become more and more difficult to control one's posture, as this exercise is done with more and more vigor. Therefore it is advisable to practice *kapalabhathi* and *bhastrika* in the lotus position if possible; this has the foot lock, which will hold one's seat throughout the practice.

In this exercise, exhalation plays a prominent part. Inhalation is mild, slow, and longer than the exhalation. In other breathing exercises, except *bhastrika,* exhalation is longer than inhalation.

The exhalation should be done quickly and forcibly by contracting the abdominal muscles with a backward push. This sudden contraction of the abdominal muscles acts upon the diaphragm; then the diaphragm recedes into the thoracic cavity, giving a vigorous push to the lungs, expelling the air from the lungs.

This is instantly followed by a relaxation of the abdominal muscles, allowing the diaphragm to descend down to the abdominal cavity, pulling with it the lungs. This allows the air to rush in. In *kapalabhathi,* inhalation and exhalation are done by action of the abdominal muscles and diaphragm. Inhalation and exhalation are performed in quick succession by a sudden and vigorous intake of the abdominal muscles, followed by relaxation of the abdominal muscles. Exhalation takes about one fourth of the time of inhalation. Here exhalation is quick, strong, and short, while inhalation is passive, slow, and longer. Passive inhalation and sudden expulsion of breath follow continuously, one after the other, until a round is completed. In the beginning, a round should have fifteen to twenty expulsions. Beginners are advised to practice three rounds of fifteen expulsions each before practicing *pranayama,* which is practiced twice each day, morning and evening.

Under the guidance of a teacher you can add ten expulsions each week until you reach one hundred twenty expulsions in each round. Between rounds, take a few normal respirations while resting. According to the condition of each individual, the teacher may advise the student to increase the number of rounds. But under no condition should one go beyond one's own capacity.

While practicing *kapalabhathi,* your attention should be concentrated on the abdominal muscles, centered in the solar plexus in the navel, where the vital energy is stored. This practice of concentration must be maintained throughout the practice so that pranic energy will become active in the *sushumna nadi,* which can be felt by a throbbing sensation throughout the spinal column, especially in nerve centers.

This exercise cleanses the respiratory system and the nasal passages and removes spasm in bronchial tubes. Consequently, asthma is relieved and also cured in the course of time. The apices of the lungs get proper oxygenation. Carbon dioxide is eliminated and oxygen is absorbed into the system. This is the best exercise to increase oxygen in the system.

One should learn this *kapalabhathi* thoroughly before learning *bhastrika*. One can learn *bhastrika* in a short time if he knows how to do *kapalabhathi* properly.

## THREE BANDHAS OR LOCKS

After the purification breathing exercises, students of Yoga are taught the three important *bandhas* or locks, which are essential for practicing further advanced *pranayama* for awakening *kundalini sakthi*.

There are three *bandhas*, known as (1) *jalandhara bandha* or chin lock; (2) *moola bandha* or anal contraction; and (3) *uddiyana bandha* or abdominal contraction.

In Sanskrit, *bandha* means a lock. During the practice of *pranayama*, Yogis unite the *prana* and *apana* with the help of these locks. These *bandhas* are also used in the practice of *mudras* or exercises to seal the *prana*.

*Asanas* (postures) stabilize the body and enable *pranayama* or breathing exercises to proceed smoothly. Through *pranayama* the student tries to unite the *prana* and *apana*. *Mudras* seal this union of *prana-apana* so that the union might not be disturbed. *Bandhas* lock this marvelous effect. When the *prana* and *apana* are thus held in union, a great mysterious and powerful spiritual current is generated within, which cannot be described in words, and which has to be experienced by each individual. This power pierces the entrance to the *sushumna*. By *jalandhara bandha* or chin lock the *prana* is prevented from flowing up, and with *moola bandha* or anal contraction, *apana* is prevented from flowing down. Therefore they unite to form an unimaginable power and begin to flow into *sushumna*. Concentration supervenes. Then the *kundalini sakthi* is awakened and taken from lower *chakras* or nerve centers to higher ones, and as the *kundalini* rises upward the Yogi enjoys the bliss of meditation and the *superconscious state*.

### Jalandhara Bandha

The word *jala* refers to the brain and to the nerve passing through the neck. *Dhara* denotes the upward pull.

Press the chin firmly against the chest, into the jugular notch as far as possible. This exercises an upward pull on the spinal cord and on the nerve centers, which in turn work on the brain. *Jalandhara bandha* is practiced during retention of breath.

### Moola Bandha

Sit on a folded blanket. Press the perineum with the left heel and place the right heel on the left thigh as in *sidhasan*.

Now forcibly contract the anal sphincter while the perineum is closely pressed with the left heel. Now along with contraction of the sphincter muscles draw the *apana* upward by contracting the abdominal muscles, and unite the *apana* with the *prana* by means of *jaladhara bandha*. *Jalandhara bandha* and *moola bandha* are practiced simultaneously during *kumbaka* or retention time in order to unite *prana* and *apana*.

These two *bandhas* are applied in the practice of advanced *pranayama*, which will be described shortly. Before applying these *bandhas* with *pranayama*, practice them separately for a few days.

### Uddiyana Bandha

*Uddiyana* should be performed at the end of exhalation when the lungs are empty. This is generally practiced as an independent exercise. Because *prana* or vital energy *uddiyate* goes up the *sushumna* in this *bandha*, it is called *uddiyana* by the Yogis. By a very strong expiration the lungs are emptied and driven against the upper part of the thorax, drawing the diaphragm to the thoracic cavity.

## ADVANCED BREATHING EXERCISES

Yogis practice eight kinds of breathing exercises. They are known as: (1) *ujjayi*; (2) *surya bheda*; (3) *bhastrika*; (4) *sitali*; (5) *sithkari*; (6) *bhramari*; (7) *moorcha*; and (8) *plavini*. The first three are very important for Yogic students.

### Ujjayi Pranayama

"Closing the mouth, draw up the breath through the nostrils till the breath fills the space from throat to the heart (from low to high breathing) with a noise. Perform *kumbaka* or retention with *bandhas* and exhale through *ida* or left nostril. This removes the phlegm from the throat and increases the digestive power of the body. This is called '*ujjayi.*'"

*Hatha Yoga Pradipika*, Chapter II, 51 and 52.

The above quotation from Hatha Yoga Pradipika describes the nature of *"ujjayi"* *pranayama*.

*Practice of Ujjayi.* Sit in any meditative pose. Close the mouth and inhale slowly through both nostrils in a smooth uniform manner. During inhalation partially close the glottis in order to produce a sobbing sound of a low but sweet and uniform pitch. At the end of inhalation, perform *moola bandha,* the anal contraction, and hold the breath with *jalandhara bandha* by pressing the chin against the chest. As long as you can hold your breath, so long should you apply the two *bandhas*. Before exhalation, unlock the *bandhas* and keep the head and neck in a straight position and then exhale the air through the left nostril by closing the right nostril with the thumb. This is one round. In *ujjayi*, inhalation is always through both nostrils and exhalation is through the left one.

To start with, you can practice *ujjayi* five rounds, gradually increasing to twenty rounds in each sitting. If you want to practice only *ujjayi pranayama* then you can even do up to forty rounds in each sitting, under the guidance of a teacher.

*Ujjayi pranayama* removes phlegm from the throat. The practitioner is never attacked by such diseases as nervousness, dyspepsia, dysentery, enlarged spleen, consumption, cough. Perform *ujjayi* to destroy decay and death.

## Surya Bheda Pranayama

*Surya bheda* is the next exercise students are taught to increase the heat of the body. By the practice of *surya bheda* the Yogic student cures such diseases as the pulmonary, cardiac, and dropsical. Practice of this exercise also helps to take the *prana* to *sushumna* and thereby awaken *kundalini.* It also cleanses the frontal sinuses and prevents bodily decay and premature death.

*Practice of Surya Bheda.* Sit in any meditative pose, preferably *sidhasan.* Close the eyes and repeat *OM* mentally while practicing this exercise. Now keep the left nostril closed and without making any sound inhale as long as you can through the right nostril. Then close the right nostril with your right thumb and retain the breath by firmly pressing the chin against the chest (the chin lock or *jalandhara bandha*).

Increase the *kumbaka* (retention) gradually. Then exhale very slowly without making any sound through the left nostril by closing the right nostril with the thumb. In *surya bheda* inhalation is always through the right nostril (*surya nadi pingala*). Start with ten rounds and gradually increase to forty rounds. While practicing this exercise, perspiration oozes from the roots of the hair, which is a healthy sign.

## Bhastrika Pranayama

In Sanskrit, *bhastrika* means bellows. A rapid succession of forcible expulsions is a characteristic feature of this breathing. Just as a blacksmith blows his bellows rapidly, so also you should move your breath rapidly. This is the best exercise Yogis practice to awaken the *kundalini* after purifying the *nadis* and nervous system. If the *nadis* are purified, even a few rounds of *bhastrika* will stir the *kundalini*. Then the Yogi can feel that his whole body is charged with a new energy. The whole spinal cord will pulsate and the *kundalini* rises to higher centers or *chakras*. In whichever center *kundalini* is active, that *chakra* will become like a dynamo generating high voltage of nerve energy. This is the best exercise for the vascular and nervous system and tones the entire nervous system. It increases the circulation all over the body and increases the bodily temperature, which is followed by a reduced bodily temperature owing to profuse perspiration, which eliminates all impurities. When the body is free from physical impurities, the concentration power of the mind increases to a very high degree. The rapid motion of *bhastrika* increases the fresh supply of blood to the brain. After a few rounds of *bhastrika* it is amazing to see how clear the brain is. The wonderful result, both psychic and physical, derived by the practice of *bhastrika*, cannot be understood until one starts practicing it.

*Practice of Bhastrika. Bhastrika* resembles *kapalabhathi* breathing. It is easy to practice if you know how to do *kapalabhathi*. In *kapalabhathi* only the diaphragm moves during the breathing exercise but in *bhastrika* the entire respiratory system is put into full action, though the diaphragm plays a prominent role in it.

Though *bhastrika* resembles *kapalabhathi*, its effect is entirely different from *kapalabhathi*, which is only a cleansing exercise. Moreover, there is *kumbaka* (retention) in *bhastrika*, and all three *bandhas* or locks (*jalandhara bandha, moola bandha*, and *uddiyana*) are firmly and very carefully applied here in order to unite the *prana* and *apana* and awaken the *kundalini.* You should always get the proper technique from a teacher.

Sit in any one of the meditative poses, preferably the lotus pose. Next inhale and exhale rapidly with emphasis on the exhalation, bringing the diaphragm and the entire respiratory muscles into quick action —making a noise that can be felt in the throat and the head.

In the beginning you should start with rapid expulsions of breath, following one another in rapid succession ten times. When the tenth expulsion is finished, the final one is followed by the deepest possible inhalation. Then the breath is suspended as long as can be done with comfort. Then exhale through the right nostril. During retention apply the chin lock and the anal contraction and concentrate on the *kundalini sakthi* at the lowest spinal center, *muladhara chakra.*

This is one round. Rest awhile after the round by taking a few normal breaths. You can gradually increase the number of expulsions from ten to a maximum of thirty in each round of *bhastrika.* Start with three rounds and increase up to eight rounds. Do not overdo this exercise.

*Bhastrika* performed properly breaks the three knots of *grandhis:* (1) *brahma grandhi* of the *muladhara;* (2) *vishnu grandhi* of *manipura;* and (3) *rudra grandhi of ajna chakra.*

These three *grandhis* or knots are the three locations in the *sushumna* in the spinal column. These knots are blocks that prevent the free movement of the pranic current in the *sushumna.* With the help of *bhastrika* these three knots are broken and then the *kundalini* can rise gradually toward the *sahasrara chakra* in the brain.

As soon as *kundalini* has been aroused, *bhastrika* should be practiced more in order to take it to higher centers in the *sushumna.*

MINOR PRANAYAMAS

*Sitali Pranayama*

Protrude the tongue a little way from the lips. Fold the tongue like a tube. Draw the air through the mouth with a hissing sound "Se," hold it as long as possible, and exhale through the nostrils. Practice this fifteen to thirty times daily. This exercise purifies the blood. It helps to quench the thirst. It is a very good exercise to cool the system in summer seasons. *Sitali kumbaka* is an imitation of the respiration of a serpent.

*Sitkari Pranayama*

Fold the tongue so that the tip of the tongue might touch the upper palate and draw the air through the mouth with a hissing sound, "Si-si-si." Then retain the breath as long as you can and exhale slowly through both nostrils. This is also a cooling exercise for the system, and all the effect of *sitali* can be derived from it.

*Bhramari Pranayama*

Inhale rapidly through both nostrils, making the sound of the honey bee. Then exhale rapidly through both nostrils, making the humming sound. Do this ten times and hold the breath comfortably. By the practice of *bhramari* the voice becomes sweet and melodious. It induces meditation.

*Important Instructions for Practicing Pranayama.* You should be regular and systematic in your practice. Do not practice when you are ailing seriously. Do not twist the facial muscles when you do retention, and never suspend the breath beyond your capacity. If you get any aches and pains in the chest, stop the exercise till the pain is relieved. Avoid too much talking, sleeping, and eating such food as meat, fish, etc.

Do not practice *pranayama* mechanically, like other breathing exercises. *Pranayama* requires deep concentration and therefore mind plays a prominent part. Before starting *pranayama,* repeat a few prayers or chant if you know a chant. Salute your spiritual teacher mentally. If the teacher is away, mentally salute and draw his vibration to you and feel that he is guiding you throughout the practice. When you draw his spiritual vibration you are actually tuning yourself to him. He will be able to help you though he is far away, if you are in tune with him. This is very important for spiritual students. For a Yoga student, a *Guru* or spiritual teacher is the visible God who manifests as his spiritual preceptor in the physical world.

A real *Guru* can help the student whether he is near or far away. But the student has to keep his mind pure to receive his instructions. Do not be impatient if you cannot find results by practicing *pranayama* for a few months. If you are sincere and have faith in your *Guru,* surely you will have success. But you yourself must practice if you want the benefit.

Your teacher will show you the path and you walk behind him, and then you will reach the goal. No teacher can do spiritual practices for you and do not think that the mere touch of a master will awaken the *kundalini sakthi.* If any master proclaims that he can use his power for awakening the *kundalini,* do not believe him. He may use some hypnotic suggestions on you for his selfish purpose. Real teachers never do such things. They await the proper time to teach certain things. When you are purified by selfless service, prayer, meditation, he can easily impart higher teachings to you.

Just as, to become a scientist, one has to learn all the alphabets and study for years before graduation, so also Yoga is a mental science that takes years before you get the various psychic results foretold.

When one is attacked by a disease, he says that the disease is due to the practice of Yoga. This is a serious mistake. No one ever gets sickness by following nature's law. Sickness is unnatural and health is natural. Yoga is a natural method of eating, drinking, sleeping, breathing, and exercises. If you get some illness while you practice Yoga, it is due to some other cause and not due to practice of Yoga.

You can consult your teacher and he will help you to find out the cause of your trouble. Even in eating there is danger if man is careless, and food may go to the windpipe instead of the stomach. That does not mean that eating is bad. Therefore you have to use simple caution and common sense everywhere, whether it is in Yoga or eating or walking.

The claim is sometimes made that those who practice Yoga and *pranayama* may go mad. To one making such a claim I say that he is not in good mental condition. If you see mental symptoms in one who practices Yoga, it is because there are many causes other than Yoga. It may be improper food, overexertion, mental and physical tension, family worries, improper knowledge of what is Yoga, and an improper guide or teacher who never instructs the student in what real Yoga means, and its purpose. These causes can be removed if you are under the guidance of a teacher. Even if you do not find one good teacher near you, you can mentally bring your teacher's vibration by tuning yourself, as said before. You will get guidance from within. All your doubts will be cleared away. This experience you can see for yourself. No other proof is necessary.

If you do not find a teacher, do not sit idly waiting for a teacher to come. You can start preliminary studies from books; and advanced students on the spiritual path can help you in the beginning. This will prepare you for meeting a real teacher when the proper time comes. But if you are taking the help of another Yoga student, see whether he practices what he preaches. Nowadays many become teachers of Yoga by reading a few books. They neither practice what they teach nor are they examples of the things they preach. One can become a teacher very easily. To become a student takes a whole lifetime. The easiest thing in this world is to teach something one doesn't know and practice. The most difficult of all things is to practice what one preaches.

Some teachers criticize everything and don't want to know what others are doing. They object that there is no reason for the physical control and breathing exercises to reach God as taught in Yoga. They ask the student just to close his eyes and meditate. Of course everyone can choose the path he likes, but that does not mean others should follow his method.

Nothing is achieved without effort. Nothing man has ever learned has come without mistakes. Those who maintain that physical methods are not necessary are themselves too lazy to practice. If a man can take food, then why not exercise and breathing—which some consider antagonistic to religion and God? If taking care of the body is against religion then taking food, which is also for the body, should be against religion. A real Yoga student keeps his body always neat and clean and free from diseases, because that body is the temple of God, and without it he cannot achieve anything, physical or spiritual. Moreover, he can spend that time and money which he spends for medicine to more useful purpose. Therefore, my friends, do not take any such easy methods, which will take you nowhere, not even toward a normal healthy life.

CONCENTRATION ON SOLAR PLEXUS AND
PRANIC HEALING

The solar plexus is an important center of the nerves connected with the sympathetic nervous system. Yogis consider this one as the main storage house for storing *prana* in the physical body for physical activities. Just as a storage battery stores electricity, so also does the solar plexus store *prana* while you breathe. During Yogic breathing (*pranayama*) the Yogi absorbs a tremendous amount of *prana*, which is stored up in this center.

This plexus is often called the "abdominal brain." It is located in the epigastric region behind the pit of the stomach on either side of the spinal column. It plays an important part in the control of emotions and various bodily functions.

A blow over this powerhouse of *prana* will make a person unconscious. It is composed of white and gray brain matter, and it radiates strength and energy to all parts. Thoughts and *prana*, when directed toward this center through the *pranayama* (alternate breathing exercise), will recharge it. It is constantly discharging *prana* for thinking, acting, and willing. The more *prana* is stored in this center, the more the will power and thought power increase—and vice versa.

Those who practice *pranayama* regularly and recharge the solar plexus can make use of their extra *prana* in healing diseases in others —and again recharge themselves with *prana* in no time by *pranayama*.

Never think that by distributing *prana* to others you will be depleted of *prana;* because the more you give the more it flows from the cosmic source.

When you want to heal others, gently place your hands where the patient feels pain and imagine that the *prana* is flowing from your hands toward the affected part of the patient, just as water flows from higher level to lower level. Mentally connect yourself with the cosmic energy, the power of God, and feel that you are the connecting link to bring the *prana* from the cosmic source to the patient.

The patient will at once feel warmth, relief, and strength. When you send *prana* to liver, spleen, stomach, or any portion of the body, you can mentally speak to the cells and give them orders to do their functions properly. You can command the cells and they will obey your orders.

How could Jesus Christ perform the miracle of giving eyes to a blind man, and curing diseases? They are not miracles as we think. That is the law of God. Christ could connect himself completely with the cosmic energy of God, and he did so absolutely without any selfish motive. My master, Swami Sivananda, one of the greatest living saints today, did many so-called miracles. He did even cure diseases of persons who were far away, through distant healing. All the great saints and prophets of the past did such things. In the future many such miracles will happen. Yet they are ordinary laws of nature. Of course, we cannot perform such great miracles, as we are not able completely to identify ourselves with the cosmic power of God, as Jesus and other saints did. Yet we could do this simple healing, using *prana* to remove various ailments of our brothers.

We must do such healing for the good of the world, and not for selfish gains. Then only such healing will be fruitful. Always think that you are only an instrument in the hands of God for curing and relieving others' suffering. Repeat *OM* when you pass your *prana* to others.

# 9

# ASTRAL BODY, THE MYSTERY OF MIND, AND EXTRASENSORY PERCEPTION

One of the things that has puzzled scientific investigators is the persistent recurrence of stories relating to extrasensory perception. Such stories continue to come to light without proper explanation. There is one where a woman dreamed her son was killed in battle. She awoke, looked at the clock; it was 2 A.M. The next day a telegram arrived stating that her son had been killed at 2 A.M.

Another woman dreamed she was visited by her son who said: "I'm leaving this world and going to a better place and won't be able to see you." She received a message the following day saying that her son had left the physical world.

In trying to interpret these everyday examples, a difficulty arises. The majority of mankind believes only in what their senses perceive. Such persons accept as unquestionable anything that their senses convey to them. They fail to understand that their senses, at best, are imperfect instruments and that the mind is constantly employed in correcting the mistaken reports of the senses. Modern scientific thinking has reached a stage where physicists have been forced to abandon the ordinary world of our experience, the so-called world of sense perceptions. They have crossed the border that divides physics from metaphysics. The theory of Eastern philosophy involving the relationship between observer and reality is now utilized by modern physicists. In Vedanta philosophy the world is described as unreal from the absolute point of view. It has no independent reality without the senses and mind of the observer, and, hence, is true only in relative terms. And the knowledge that we gain through these various senses varies according to the nature of the instrument used to observe the object.

Our senses delude us by bringing knowledge that changes often. We do not have a universal sense that will be a common machine to weigh the reality of the observer. "Common sense" often creates false pictures. A stick plunged into the water appears broken, though in reality it is not so. Sweet and bitter, hot and cold, sun and earth, the whole objective universe of matter and energy does not exist independent of the mind and senses. Even time and space are nothing but the power of the mind. There is nothing to limit man in time and space if there is no mind. All limitations and barriers disappear with the disappearance of the mind.

At our present stage of realization, all our knowledge of the universe is a residue of impressions clouded by imperfect senses. Reality is far away from our present state of consciousness. There are electromagnetic waves such as gamma rays, radio waves, cosmic rays, X-rays that are not visible to the human eye. Yet, through new instruments, we are now aware of such lesser frequency and greater frequency wave lengths. These limitations of man's senses are now studied by modern scientists and lead them nearer to metaphysics.

Now the question arises, if ordinary senses are not reliable, what of extrasensory perception? Is it a fact? Can we believe in extrasensory perception?

From the absolute point of view, the answer is that both extrasensory perception and ordinary sense experience have their limitations and are, therefore, imperfect, because all objective knowledge can be had only through the mind, which is imperfect.

The highest truth is perceived only when we transcend the three-dimensional plane created by the senses and mind, and go beyond time and space.

The ordinary experiences we get through the contact of the body and mind are from the three-dimensional plane, and the so-called unexplained phenomena of the world (so-called extrasensory knowledge) are from the four-dimensional plane.

The ordinary phenomena that happen in our lives are a miracle to those creatures who live in two-dimensional planes. Let us suppose there are creatures who live in the two-dimensional plane. For them there is no awareness of space. Hence, they cannot perceive what happens in space. A railroad track is a one-dimensional space; therefore, a train engineer can describe his position from a single point, a station or a milestone. But the surface of the sea is a two-dimensional world where the captain of a ship fixes his position in latitude and longitude. An airplane pilot has to pilot his craft through a three-dimensional world, i.e., latitude, longitude, and also his height above the ground, altitude, which is space.

Now, for example, let us consider the driver of the train as a man living in a one-dimensional plane, the captain of the ship in a two-dimensional plane, and the airplane pilot in a three-dimensional world. From the point of view of the train engineer, he can go only from one point to another, that is, $A$ to $B$. Both the train engineer and the captain of the ship move in the same direction in a straight line along the coast to the same destination. The captain of the ship can move to his right or left in the sea, away from the straight line, and still arrive at the same place as the train. But when the ship moves away from the train, it appears to the train engineer as if the ship has disappeared from his plane, as he is not aware of the two dimensions. When he sees the ship at the destination, it again appears as a materialized object. But the captain sees both his ship movement and the train, as he can understand latitude and longitude. In the same way, a seaplane and a ship move to the same destination, and it is a strange thing for the captain of the ship when the seaplane disappears from his vision. When the seaplane moves out of sight in space, the ship captain may think of it as dematerialized, and when it reappears in his two-dimensional plane, it looks like the materialization of the plane. The captain of the ship has no idea of space, and hence, whatever happens through space is an unexplained mystery for him. Therefore, a three-dimensional being's action is mysterious to a two-dimensional being. Mr. $X$ is a two-dimensional being who is visited by a Mr. $Y$ from the three-dimensional plane. Mr. $X$ has to carry an object a distance and Mr. $Y$ helps him. Mr. $Y$ brings the object through space. As the object moves into space, suddenly it disappears from the vision of Mr. $X$, and in a few moments it materializes when it is brought down by Mr. $Y$. For Mr. $X$ this is an unexplained mystery and for Mr. $Y$ it is an ordinary thing.

So, in the same way, certain things occurring in a four-dimensional plane are a mystery for the ordinary people of the world. Teleportation, or moving things from one locked room to another through concrete walls, without the help of any physical contact, is a mystery for the earthly people who live in a three-dimensional world. A higher being who lives on a higher plane than ours can do many things that are an unexplained mystery to us. He can move heavy things into his four-dimensional plane and bring them back to the three-dimensional plane. When the object is transferred into the four-dimensional plane, it can penetrate through the solid matter of our world, just as radio waves penetrate the walls. So teleportation, telepathy, and all other things that cannot be explained very clearly are, in reality, phenomena of a four-dimensional world. There are still higher planes that are subtler than our world, and man operates in those higher planes with his astral body, which operates in the astral plane as the physical body operates in the physical plane. Mind and senses are in the astral body, which does not perish when the physical body dies.

The astral body is composed of nineteen elements: five organs of action, five organs of knowledge, the four inner instruments consisting of mind, intellect, egoism, and subconscious mind, and five *pranas* or vital breaths. Some occultists think that it is composed of some semi-fluidic or subtle form of matter invisible to the physical eye. Every human being has an astral body and, in fact, the astral body is nearer to the soul than the physical body. But it must be pointed out here that the soul is encased in these bodies, which are only vehicles of the soul. In waking consciousness, the astral body operates with the co-operation of the physical body. During deep sleep the astral body withdraws to a greater or lesser degree and hovers just above the physical body. The same phenomenon occurs when the individual is under anesthesia or during a trance or fainting. Some occult students can consciously project the astral body away from its physical body and travel about at will. The astral and physical bodies are connected by means of a subtle cord along which vital currents pass. In fact, both of these bodies are connected by this cord, and when it is cut off, death results instantaneously. So, at the time of death, the cord is severed and during sleep the cord is intact.

All the extrasensory perceptions and the so-called unexplained mysteries are the functions of the astral body in a higher dimensional plane. All our experiences in the waking state or in the dream state are the products of the mind and senses, as are also all the various products of the extrasensory perceptions. In fact, nothing can be seen or perceived without the mind, and the mind is everything for us at the present moment. Though the physical body and the astral body are different, both are controlled by the mind.

Yogis give great attention and effort to controlling the mind, and the mental power realized is used to unveil the hidden mysteries of man. The mind is, by nature, unsteady, for at every moment it is being affected by the sight, sound, and so forth, of external objects, which the mind perceives through the agency of the senses. Therefore, the mind must be detached from the objects of the senses, withdrawn from whatever direction it may happen to turn, freed from all distractions, and kept under control to dominate self. The three higher practices known as concentration, meditation, and the superconscious state complete the psychic and mental disciplines. It is very difficult to control and discipline the wandering mind. Therefore, Hatha Yoga prescribes various physical methods to start with, so that the student can manipulate the mind more easily as he advances in his Yogic practices. The great Yogi Swatmarama, author of *Hatha Yoga Pradipika*, the well-known authoritative treatise on Yoga, makes it plain that the object of practicing Yoga is to prepare oneself for attaining communion with one's higher self and not merely to obtain the *siddhis* (physical powers and psychic powers).

Mastery over the mind brings forth various Yogic powers that real Yogis never care to look upon. These powers are often utilized for selfish purposes by less advanced students. These powers are lost if demonstrated to a curious public.

As the physical and astral bodies are intimately connected and the mind is the real master of the body, it is essential to know something about it.

The subtle or astral body is the body of the mind and the senses, out of which proceeds the gross body of matter. Mind and matter are the veiling power of the consciousness of spirit that creates the world. This veiling power is known in Sanskrit as *maya shakthi*, which seemingly makes the whole (*purna*) into the not whole (*apurna*), the infinite into the finite, the formless into forms, and the like. *Maya shakthi* can be termed as the universal mind of the Supreme Being, which in individual beings becomes individual mind, ego, and senses.

MIND AND ITS FUNCTIONS

In the scale of evolution the mind functions in various phases, depending upon the body in which it operates. Thus it goes from subconscious to simple consciousness, gradually evolving to self-consciousness until it reaches universal consciousness. In the lower kingdoms, such as plants and animals, the mind is manifested in a state where consciousness is automatic. This portion of the mind is predominant in plant and animal. Human beings also possess it, and it is a great help in their

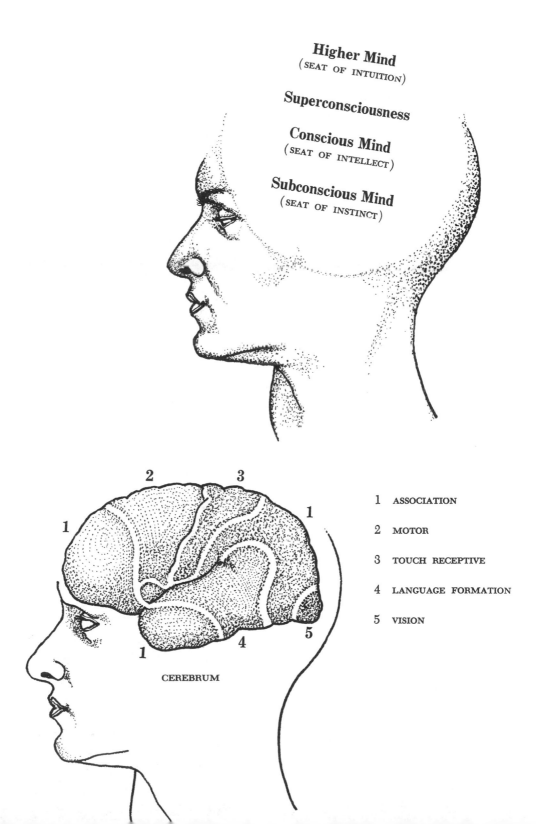

**Higher Mind**
(SEAT OF INTUITION)

**Superconsciousness**

**Conscious Mind**
(SEAT OF INTELLECT)

**Subconscious Mind**
(SEAT OF INSTINCT)

1   ASSOCIATION

2   MOTOR

3   TOUCH RECEPTIVE

4   LANGUAGE FORMATION

5   VISION

CEREBRUM

present stage of development. This mind is known as the subconscious or instinctive mind (in Sanskrit, *chitha*). The mind of man functions on more than one plane. Nowadays psychologists have recognized the varying phases of mentation, and many theories have been advanced to account for them, but psychologists' knowledge of the working of the mind is in its infancy. An interesting picture of the functions of the mind can be gained from Yoga philosophy.

## SUBCONSCIOUS PLANE OF THE MIND

At first sight it would seem that the conscious part of man's mind does most of the work, but a little reflection will show that conscious reasoning of the mind is only a part of its function. In a broad sense, the mind of man functions on the three planes of effort, subconscious, conscious, and superconscious, each plane gradually shading into the planes on either side of it, the one next higher and one next lower, like the colors in a rainbow. Man shares the subconscious plane of the mind in common with lower animals. It is the first stage of mental development in the scale of evolution. The first dawn of the instinctive mind can be traced even in the mineral kingdom. Then, in the plant kingdom, it grows more distinct and higher in the scale. Again, in the animal world, there is an increasing manifestation of the automatic mind from the almost plantlike intelligence of the lowest forms until we reach a degree almost equal to the lowest form of human being. Then, among men, we see it shading gradually into the intellect, the middle principle of the mind. But even the very highly evolved men of today use the subconscious mind and, in varying degrees, are used by it. In fact, we cannot exist without this part of the mind. Though we cannot exist without it, we must learn to use and guide it intelligently. Every one of us has reached the present stage of development after a long journey through 840,000 bodies of various kingdoms, such as mineral, plant, and animal, yet it is only sunrise and the full day is far away. Intellect, the second phase of mind, which civilized man uses at present, has unfolded only to a small degree. For many the intellectual unfolding is only beginning. If we analyze, we can see that many are little better than animals; their minds function almost on the instinctive plane, though it is shaded by the incoming rays of the intellect. The majority of people are led by political leaders and leaders of various communities and tribes. This is nothing but the animal instinct, or herd instinct, where the herd follows the leader. Again, we see that average people think very little; thinking becomes merely automatic in their daily lives.

The lowest phases of the work of the instinctive mind are akin to the same work manifesting in the plant kingdom: birth, growth, decay, and death are automatic processes. This is common to plant, animal, and man. These processes are the functions of the instinctive mind. During the existence of the body—whether the body of plant, animal, or man—the constant work of repair, change, digestion, assimilation, elimination, circulation, etc., is being done by this portion of the mind, all in the subconscious plane, without our conscious knowledge. All the involuntary organs and their functions are under the superintendence of this mind. These involuntary functions are only a small portion of the work of the instinctive mind. In the scale of evolution of the animal, certain things became necessary for its existence. As reasoning powers were not developed to meet exigencies, the wonderful intelligence subconsciously lying unfolded as instinctive mind took the place of intellect. This function of the mind (fighting instinct) in the animal, for its protection and preservation, is still predominant with man. But developed man's intellect holds the fighting instinct in restraint owing to the light obtained from the unfolding higher faculties; undeveloped mind follows the lower natures instead.

The instinctive functions such as making a nest, migrating before the approaching winter, hibernation, nursing the young, are all functions of the subconscious mind, which are essential for the animals' existence. Until the development of the intellect, the instinctive mind takes all the work of the intellect without reasoning. Another function of the subconscious mind is to do things automatically that we have learned through the intellect. When we learn things by heart we have really mastered them on the intellectual plane, and then pass them on to the subconscious plane by mentation. This process is a higher manifestation of the subconscious mind and is due to contact and blending with the developing intellect. Much of our daily work is done automatically, such as walking, painting, sewing, driving, etc. If not, the intellect would tire if it had these everyday tasks to perform consciously or intellectually.

The subconscious mind is also a habit mind or, rather, an obedient servant; as it cannot reason, it often has to be guided by the intellect of the individual or of some other person. Any idea from the intellect consciously or unconsciously comes to it and is carried out faithfully to the very letter. Old notions and tensions lying subconsciously can be corrected and removed through better instructions by the intellect of the individual or of someone else. It is amazing to note how helpful the subconscious mind is; for example, when we have to catch a plane early in the morning, all we have to do is to suggest to the subconscious mind to wake us at a certain time, and it does.

The subconscious mind does not carry out only good instructions from the intellect, but also wrong instructions; so unnecessary fears, anxieties, and worries created during our daily activities are taken on by the subconscious mind and later on projected to the conscious mind. *A shock or fear in childhood will torment a person even when he is old, unless he is helped by countersuggestions.*

Hypnotic suggestions are directed to the subconscious mind. A hypnotist, after giving a severe blow to the conscious mind of the individual, proceeds to manipulate the subconscious mind of his subject. As the individual's conscious mind has temporarily ceased to function, the subconscious is under the control of the hypnotist. Whatever suggestions are given will be carried out implicitly. The technique involved here is a very serious thing to be considered, for the constant blow consciously given by the hypnotist affects the conscious mind of the individual which, in turn, cannot give proper suggestions to itself. This is the main objection to hypnotic suggestion. In some cases, hypnotic suggestion may help the individual if it is done purely by an unselfish person, though such persons are rare. It is rarely advisable to surrender one's own will to another person's will. Moreover, suggestion from one's own intellect is the best way to guide one's subconscious mind. (The Yogic method of achieving control of the lower mind and developing the higher mind is explained in Chapter 9 when we discuss *kundalini* and meditation on *chakras*).

In the subconscious mind or plane lie all the knowledge and impressions received from various sources, not only from this life, but from previous incarnations; it is something like a storehouse having everything known and unknown, which it has received through hereditary and various other sources that it has unfolded within itself. It also contains the knowledge gained by the intellect, as well as the knowledge gained from association with others. It is a common experience that a forgotten passage that was learned in youth suddenly projects from the subconscious mind, even though we have not thought of it for many years. Some persons get the memory of the past life from this mind, though it is very rare. Nature keeps away the mysteries of the past life from the consciousness; otherwise it would increase our mental tensions by reviving past good and bad memories.

Some persons are able to do things that they have not done or learned in this life; some children can paint well or sing well without ever going to school. Others are born orators, authors, and preachers. Knowledge that they have mastered in their previous lives lies in the subconscious mind. Such persons are called geniuses or gifted. In fact, this gift is nothing but the knowledge acquired through constant effort on those subjects in the previous lives. A person who now strives to become a master of a subject might be a genius in his next life, as he carries all the knowledge subconsciously to his next life.

In concluding our discussion on the lower phase of the mind, which we know as the seat of the lower emotions, instinct, passion, desires, appetites, greed, and lust, we should remember also that there are higher emotions, aspirations, and desires for knowledge in advanced man that are from the unfolding spiritual mind and not of the lower mind. The lower mental principle is the grossest and the lowest of the three mental principles and is the one which is ready to bind us closely to the earth and earthly things.

H. H. Swami Sivananda, a great master of Yoga, founder of the Divine Society, of Rishikesh, Himalayas, in his book *The Mysterious Mind,* says

> Emotion is a motive power, like the steam of an engine. It helps you in your evolution. Had it not been for the presence of emotion, you would have passed into a state of passivity or inertia. It gives a push for action or motion. It is a blessing. But you must not become a prey to emotions; you must not allow them to bubble out. You must allow it to rise slowly and subside quietly from the mind ocean. There are certain people who like to hear some new sensational events just to arouse their emotions; they live on emotions; otherwise they feel quite dull. This is a great weakness.

Love, hatred, anger, greed, fear, envy, jealousy are the emotions of the mind. All evil qualities proceed from anger and therefore Yoga students are advised to control anger, and all other evil qualities will then vanish by themselves. Moreover, emotions affect the endocrine glands, which are governed by the nervous system, and cause disorders in the normal functions of the internal organs.

In recent years Drs. Harold Wolff and Stewart Wolff, of the New York Hospital, made a careful and unusual study of the behavior of the stomach and digestion of a patient whose belly was accidentally blasted by a gun, leaving a gaping hole for the rest of his life.

Through this hole in the abdominal wall, doctors could study the mysteries of human digestion.

According to the report of the Drs. Wolff and Wolff, the most damaging emotion is anxiety, which is the cause of ulcers. Investigations showed the patient's stomach was pale pink and relaxed, with many convoluted folds while at ease, but bright red, smooth, and tense when he became angry. Both the face and the stomach turned pale when he was upset by fright. Depression shut off the flow of gastric juices and his stomach was almost incapable of digesting food.

The subconscious or instinctive mind is termed *chitha* in Vedanta philosophy. Much of our subconscious mind consists of submerged experiences, memories thrown into the background but recoverable. As the body grows old, the first symptom is that it is difficult to remember persons and places. It is not hard to find the reason. The mind, as we know, generally remembers through associations. In old age, one can still remember passages that have been read in school and college. But at the same time, one is hard put to remember a passage read the night before. This is because the subconscious mind has lost its power of grasping and storing ideas, as the cells of the brain have degenerated. By the degeneration of the brain cells through overwork, worries, and anxieties, memory power is soon lost and very little impression is put into the subconscious mind.

The reasoning processes are limited to the field of consciousness alone. The field of subconscious mentation is much greater than that of conscious mentation. Messages, when ready, come out like a flash from the subconscious mind. Only a small percentage of mental activities come into the field of consciousness. When we drive a car through a crowded street, even though we are talking to friends in the car or solving some problems, the driving, turning, stopping are done almost subconsciously. When we sit and try too hard to solve a problem we may fail. But during sleep, at times, this kind of problem is solved subconsciously and is projected to conscious mind during wakening. During that period the subconscious mind is working like the man at the wheel while driving.

Even in sleep, this mind works without any rest and solves problems, arranges, classifies, compares, sorts all facts, and works out a proper, satisfactory solution. With the help of the subconscious mind we can remove tension from external and internal organs and give them proper relaxation.

All the involuntary vegetative functions of the body that are below the conscious plane are under the able management of the subconscious mind. Subconscious intelligence as instinct rarely fails. An animal almost instinctively knows a poisonous herb from an edible one, but the work of instinct is limited. It works like a machine. Then comes a higher state of knowledge (intellect), which is fallible and makes mistakes often; its scope is larger. We call it reason. It is much larger than instinct, but instinct is surer than reason. Animals know instinctively what to eat and what not to eat. When they are sick, nature prompts them to fast. When a dog is sick, we see that he does not like to take food. The internal mechanism is controlled by the subconscious intelligence, which prompts the dog to take nature's remedy of removing poison through fasting. This portion of the subconscious mind is still with us, helping us in various ways. But owing to the development of reasoning power, man has lost most of his instinct, though it still plays a great role in our daily life. Even such animals as dogs and cats lose much of their instinct owing to association with man and, subsequently, suffer like man.

Instead of guiding and giving proper suggestions with the developed intellect, man interferes with the natural work of the subconscious mind through wrong suggestions and thus adds miseries to his life.

With the help of the subconscious, we can change vicious nature by cultivating healthy, virtuous qualities that are opposed to undesirable ones. If we want to overcome fear, we must mentally deny fear and concentrate on the opposite quality, courage. The positive always overcomes the negative. Even distasteful tasks and duties can be changed by cultivating a desire and taste for them. All actions, pleasures, and experiences leave subtle impressions on the subconscious mind. Revival of these impressions induces memory. Great Yogis dive deep inside this mind to obtain knowledge of past lives.

Such occult phenomena of the mental world as telepathy, thought-reading, hypnotism, mesmerism, distant healing, psychic healing, etc., clearly prove the existence of extraordinary functions of the mind. From the automatic writing and other experiences of a hynotized person, we can clearly infer the existence of the subconscious mind.

All geniuses have control over the subconscious mind. If an idea is planted in the mind, it grows at night through the operation of the subconscious. Those who know how to manipulate the subconscious mind can turn out tremendous mental work through the automatic process. When the subconscious is at work, the conscious reasoning part of the mind is completely at rest or working only partially, supervising the subconscious mind. Therefore, one feels more relaxed even after hard work. All great individuals have control over the subconscious mind and know how to make it work for them. This ability of the subconscious to operate automatically results from association with the unfolding intellect.

Mind is the greatest force on this earth. He who has controlled his mind, is full of power. He can bring all minds under his influence; one is struck with awe and wonder at the marvels and mysterious powers of the mind of a man.

The subconscious mind manifests varying degrees of consciousness, varying from almost wholly subconscious to the simple consciousness of the highest of animals and the lower form of bushman, who lives almost in an instinctive plane with only a touch of the developing intellect.

Self-consciousness comes to man with the unfolding of the intellect. Cosmic or universal consciousness comes with the unfolding of the intuitional mind or higher mind. This gradual growth of consciousness is a most interesting and important branch of Yoga philosophy.

As we have seen, the lower mind is the seat of appetites, passions, desires, instincts, and emotions of the lower animals. These lower instincts are still with us. Yogis learn to curb and control these lower instincts and subordinate them to developing intellect and higher mind. As we grow spiritually, we can see the lower instincts in us predominant, yet we need not be discouraged by it, because even to know that they are in us is a sign of spiritual progress. Before, when the lower instinct was working, we could not recognize what it was, whereas now it is seen and recognized. As we progress in the spiritual path, the higher mind will obtain mastery over the lower mind, though patience, perseverance, and faith are required for the task.

Though man shares in all the qualities of the animals, that is, hunger, thirst, fatigue, and fear, which belong to the lower mind, he alone has the intellect to control them. This is his superiority over the animals.

Before the development of the intellect, the creature having the lower mind predominant has passions but cannot reason, emotion but no intellect to control it, desires but no self-awareness. Some of the evolved animals, such as monkeys and dogs, have a small touch of their lower mind illumined by the incoming rays of the intellect and show faint reasoning. This is called simple consciousness.

The first sign of the real intellect is noted with the dawn of self-consciousness, or self-awareness; this self-consciousness is also known a "I" consciousness and begins where man starts to compare himself with others and to reason about the comparison.

From here onward man asserts his "I" consciousness everywhere and in everything. He begins to rely upon his mind, rather than blindly accepting that which comes from others.

With the unfolding of the second phase of mind (the intellect) came the beginnings of all the wonderful achievements of the human mind today. At present man thinks that intellect is the highest principle, and what he is not able to grasp he rejects, though as the unfolding of the intellect progresses, it begins to receive more and more light from the next higher phase of the mind, the higher mind. The self-consciousness of "I" consciousness starts when the intellect is the master. This "I" consciousness is called *ahamkara* in Sanskrit. *Ahamkara* is the self-arrogating principle in man. The same mind assumes the form of egoism when man self-arrogates himself. It is under the influence of egoism that man commits evil and wrong actions. To reach spiritual manhood, the soul has to meet new conditions and has many an obstacle to overcome. The soul has to meet many trials and overcome many more obstacles as it progresses, and at times it would seem to retrogress from the onward march.

The awakening of the intellect does not necessarily mean that man is perfect and virtuous. While the unfolding higher intelligence gives an upward tendency to man, it is equally true that some men are so closely wrapped in the animal sheath that they use the awakened intelligence to satisfy their lower animal desires. They use cunning-ness and intelligence with lower instinct instead of curbing them with the awakened intellect. They can plan and scheme when their fighting instinct is awakened, while the beast is governed solely by its instinct.

While the incoming rays of the higher mind pull the intellect toward it, the lower mind or impure mind exerts its power, and man may descend to depths of which a beast never would have thought. This fight between the pure mind and impure mind started even when the intellect was in its infancy, though in many cases the lower mind controls the intellect.

The impure mind or lower mind is the seat of desires, appetite, and passion. The pure mind or higher mind is the seat of intuition, which brings higher knowledge. The intellect is between the two and may be influenced by either or both. If we are rational beings, the choice is with us. Let our developed intellect be on guard and not be drawn back into the animal life that has been passed through. Intuition is a spiritual faculty of the higher mind and is above the intellect. It is the eye of wisdom.

Kant has admitted that there is something beyond reason, something that the reason cannot grasp, and a transcendental something that transcends reason. He also said that the intellect is frail, finite, weak, and impotent, as it is conditioned in time, space, and causation; that it has its own limits, incapable of directly knowing or realizing that all-blissful "thing in itself" which corresponds to the *Brahman* (or supreme being of the Vedanta philosophers).

Reason is a help and a hindrance. It is a help if it serves us in any way to attain the goal of life and to fight the lower instinct. It is a hindrance if it stands in the way of our onward march toward perfection.

When we consider that vast majority of men in whom the intellect has scarcely unfolded and who have taken only a few steps into the land of the intellect, we can understand how difficult it is for people— except the few evolved souls with exceptional spiritual development— to realize even faintly the still higher mind, the intuition.

Intuition, the third and final phase of the mind, does not contradict reason, but transcends reason and brings knowledge and wisdom from its field of consciousness, which the intellect cannot penetrate. Intuition is the way to knowledge of the self-attained through purity of heart brought about by constant, protracted, and intense meditation on the attributeless, timeless, spaceless, birthless, and deathless *atman* or supreme soul. Reason helps us to march to the door of intuition. Reason can give us the information that the experiences of the phenomenal world are unreal when compared with the everlasting experiences of self-realization. Reason has its own definite utility as it helps in the beginning when we start the quest of truth.

Theosophists also have classified reason under two headings, *sudha manas* or pure reason (the higher mind or intellect and *kama manas* or instinctive mind (the lower mind). Kant has made the same classification—pure reason and practical reason. He has given the name "practical reason" for impure reason. Practical reason can help us to carn bread and secular knowledge, and pure reason helps us to attain perfection and higher knowledge. Bergson, the French philosopher, has gone a little farther. He said: "There is something more powerful than reason." That something which is beyond the reach of reason and the senses is the faculty of intuition. With the power of intuition, one can behold the unseen, the unknown.

Every one of us, however undeveloped, possesses the higher principle of the mind, intuition. But only a few have developed the faculty of intuition, while many are aware of the existence of the higher mind.

A tendency toward the Yoga path, the hunger of the soul for more light and knowledge, dissatisfaction with material happiness, are all indications that the higher spiritual mind has started shedding its rays into our consciousness.

Even these little rays of the higher mind can help us to awaken into our spiritual consciousness, though it may be several lives before we attain full spiritual consciousness or universal consciousness.

In the beginning one finds a great spiritual unrest until one is on the right path to knowledge. As man's higher mind begins to unfold, he begins to have an abiding sense of the reality of the supreme power and, growing along with it, he finds the sense of human brotherhood.

Man's growth toward a better and fuller idea of the divine power does not come from the intellect. Reasoning alone cannot give a correct and complete answer toward the growing sense of relationship between man and man. The kindness and love that we preach and practice do not come by the reasoning of the intellect.

In the life of a householder, in the life of the poor man, the rich man, the spiritual man, in everyone's life, it is a great thing to develop intuition.

The greatest power is lodged in the fine, not in the coarse. A heavy-weight champion can lift enormous weights with his powerful muscles yet, if the thin, threadlike nerves that bring them power and impulse are cut, they are not able to work at all. Look at a city with its modern automation, colorful lights, huge factories, electric trains, cinemas, and theaters. Behind it is a single powerhouse that brings life and energy through wires; yet that invisible power with its powerline is the real power behind the hustle and bustle of the city. So it is the fine that is really the seat of power, though we see the movements in the gross. We do not generally see any movement in the fine; occasionally the movement is so intense that we can perceive it. We constantly complain that we do not have control over our thoughts. How can we? When we can get control over the "fine movements," when we can get hold of the thought at the root before it has become thought, before it has become action, only then is it possible for us to control the whole.

Now, if we could advise, investigate, understand, and finally manipulate these finer powers, then would it be possible to control ourselves.

The man who has control over his own mind surely will have control over every other mind, because every mind is connected with the universal mind. That is why purity and morality have always been the objects of religion. Just as one could understand all the clay in the universe by knowing one lump of clay, so by the knowledge of one's own mind one knows the secret of every mind or has power over every mind.

Let us take the childhood of man. Each man in his childhood runs through all the stages through which his race has evolved; though the race took thousands of years to reach its present state, it takes a child but a few. The child at first behaves like a savage man: he crushes a butterfly under his feet, but he quickly passes through these primitive stages of his ancestors and arrives at the level of his race in a short period.

Let us consider all humanity as a race, with his brother animals as one whole. The end toward which the "whole" is moving we call perfection in the highest sense. Some men and women, instead of waiting and being reborn over and over again for ages along with the whole human race, have attained perfection and rush through many stages in a few short years of their life. Yogis claim that we can hasten our process of evolution if we are true to ourselves. If a number of bushmen were brought to a civilized society and given proper education, their progress could be hastened, though their brothers in the bush live in the same savage way. We help the growth of trees and, in the same way, we can use artificial means to hasten man's progress too. We cannot put a limit to this hastening. We cannot say how much a man can grow in a lifetime. A perfect man, the type that is to come of this race millions of years hence, can come today. Such men are prophets, and incarnations of them are those who have achieved perfection in this life. Recently there were such men: Jesus Christ, Buddha, Sankracharya, the great Yogi philosopher, are the names of some.

This hastening process is achieved by developing our higher mind, the fine part of force. One can easily become a psychologist or philosopher. But to study one's own mind and to develop one's own mental powers are only for those determined to curb the lower instinctive mind.

From the higher mind comes all the knowledge of the unknown, and this is the source from which the seer obtains his vision and the prophet his foresight. The scientific knowledge that intellect gets comes from association with the higher mind. Many have concentrated themselves on high ideals in their work and heard their higher mind speaking to them.

Man, by the development of his spiritual consciousness, may bring himself into contact with this higher nature. Many thus become possessed of a knowledge of which the intellect has not dared to dream.

Intuition is the direct perception or immediate knowledge of that which comes from the higher mind. Professor Bergson preached about intuition in France so the people might understand that there was a higher source of knowledge than intellect. In intuition there is no reasoning process at all. Intuition transcends reason but does not contradict it. Intellect takes a man to the door of intuition and returns to wait for the answers that reason is unable to find. It passes down to the intellect certain truths which it finds in its own regions of the mind, and intellect reasons about them. But they do not originate with intellect. Intellect is cold, whereas the higher mind is warm and alive with high feeling, love, and compassion.

As man unfolds spiritually and the higher mind develops, he feels his relationship to all mankind and begins to love his fellow man more and more. It hurts to see others suffering, and when it hurts him enough, he tries to do something to remedy it.

The struggle between the higher and lower mind has been considered by all philosophers. The intellect represents the "I" consciousness of the individual. This "I" has at the bottom the instinctive mind or lower mind, which exerts a negative influence on man, while on the other side is the spiritual mind sending its unfolding impulses into the intellect, which helps him to master and control the lower mind.

In mythologic stories and legends the fight between the lower mind and higher mind is illustrated as that of man being tempted by the devil on the one hand and helped by a guardian angel on the other. The average person reads these stories without knowing their deep philosophical significance. The ego is in a transitional stage and this struggle is painful; yet the growing higher mind enables man to understand the true state of affairs and aids him in asserting his mastery over his lower nature.

From this higher mind comes also the inspiration that philosophers, scientists, writers, preachers, and artists have received in the past and still continue to receive today.

Coming to great leaders, writers, and orators of mankind, we always find that it is the personality of man that counts. This personality is nothing but the power that comes through the development of the higher mind and close association with the pure consciousness or soul. The personality of the man who influences, who does magic, as it were, upon his fellow being is a dynamo of power who can lift his fellow being from this sense world.

Compare the great teachers of religion with the great intellectual philosophers. The philosophers scarcely influenced anybody's inner man, and yet they wrote marvelous books. The religious teachers and prophets with their intuitive knowledge, on the other hand, moved whole countries in their lifetime. The difference was made by personality. In the faint personality of the philosopher there is little touch of inspiration from the higher mind, while the prophet is inspiration itself for those who come to him.

The science of Yoga claims that it has discovered the means of developing the intuition and personality that modern psychologists have yet to learn and understand. While psychologists are still groping in darkness with the workings of the subconscious mind, Yoga science of mind has gone even beyond the higher mind and discovered the source of all knowledge, wherein lie the eternal peace and joy that everyone seeks.

Certain high psychic powers are also open to man in this way, but such powers are rarely obtained until man has risen above the attractions of the lower nature. It is only when man ceases to care for power for his personal use that power comes. This is eternal law.

As man unfolds himself in spiritual consciousness, he relies more upon his inner voice and is able to distinguish it from impulses from the lower planes of the mind. Everybody wishes to be independent. No one likes to be guided by the wishes of others. Almost everyone desires to be guided by his own wishes, and rule over others. No one wishes to have a rival. Does this not indicate that everybody wants something that he cannot obtain merely though intellectual knowledge and material wealth?

With many, the higher or intuitional mind unfolds gradually and slowly, and many feel a steady increase of spiritual knowledge and consciousness. These may not have startling visible changes. But others may get sudden flashes of light of illumination that will lift them out of their prisonlike house of body and mind, where they pass into a higher plane of consciousness and being. When the mind is not ready or prepared, it cannot carry back into consciousness a clear recollection of what it had experienced while in that state of consciousness. An average person who has no idea of anything beyond his ordinary senses would consider these things hallucinations.

These experiences vary materially, according to the degree of unfolding of the individual, his previous training, purity of the mind. Certain characteristics are common to all. The most common feeling is that of possessing almost complete knowledge of all things. This experience may last only for a moment or so, and at first leaves one in an agony of regret at having lost what he has seen. He may again strive hard to glimpse once more that happiness and that knowledge. To some the experience comes as a flashing light that takes complete possession for a few moments or longer and which is accompanied by a sensation of being surrounded by a brilliant and all-pervading light or glow.

Though these experiences may be of short duration, the man who experiences them will never be the same person afterward. The recollection of this experience will afterward prove to be a new source of comfort and strength. When he awakes from that state of ecstasy he thinks, "I cannot be awake, for nothing looks to me as it did before," or else "I am awake for the first time and everything before was a mere dream."

As one cannot communicate what sugar is to a person who has never tasted sweet, or to a man born blind what colors are, so also no one can describe this experience of a Yogi.

Someone describes the inability to express intelligently these things. "When I try to tell the best, I find my tongue is ineffectual on its pivot; my breath will not be obedient to its organs; I become a dumb man."

Yajna Valkya was a great sage and he explained that highest spiritual consciousness to his wife, Maitraya, thus: "Where there are two, one sees another, one hears another, one welcomes another, one thinks of another, one knows another. But when the whole has become that *atman* or soul, who is seen by whom, who is to be heard by whom, who is to be welcomed by whom, who is to be known by whom?" That one idea was taken by Schopenhauer and echoed in his philosophy. Through whom do we know this universe? Through what to know him? How to know the knower? By what means can we know the knower? Because in and through that we know everything. By what means can we know him? By no means. In that experience the knower, the knowledge, and the known are fused, and in that experience past and future merge with the present. In the *Upanishads* this state of experience of the soul is described in negation. "Those who know it, know not and those who know not, know it."

As we progress on the spiritual path, such experience comes to every one of us at the proper time.

In concluding, let us not always be blinded by reason, since intellect is below intuition, and often it fails. But let us not think that intuition, the power of the higher mind, is only for a few gifted persons. Every one of us possesses this, though only a few show the marked development of the higher mind. Devotion, love, purity, an urge to help our fellow men, and selflessness are all the signs of incoming rays of our higher mind in our evolution. The science of Yoga brings this message to every one of us, irrespective of our religion, caste, or nationality, that in man there is an immortal soul wherein lie all knowledge, all wealth, all joy, and peace; and also a practical way to achieve, in a short time, "the kingdom of heaven within us."

To summarize, the mind of man functions on three levels:

1. The subconscious, instinctive, or automatic mind. It controls the involuntary functions of the body; it is the seat of lower emotions and animal instinct, and it also carries on the automatic functions of our daily activities.
2. Conscious mind or intellect. Intellect can control and guide the subconscious and is the basic requisite for the ego or "I" consciousness. Reasoning is the function of the intellect.
3. Superconscious mind, or higher mind. The function of this mind, which is above intellect, is to achieve intuition and higher consciousness. Beyond these three levels of the mind is the pure consciousness known as spirit, soul, or self, which is formless, timeless, changeless, and infinite in its nature.

## MIND, TIME, AND SPACE

The more we analyze time and space, the more it vanishes as nothing but an idea. Time is the motion of the mind. Mind can think only in terms of "before," "now," and "after"—or past, present, and future. According to Yoga philosophy, "reality" is beyond time and space. That means anything we perceive, think, or know is due to the association with the mind: and mind can perform its function only in terms of space and time, just as an artist can draw his pictures only on canvas or similar background.

Without a background a picture cannot be drawn. So also, without the help of time and space, mind cannot think. The moment you try to still the mind, time and space vanish, and come back when the mind starts moving. Therefore, in fact, the mind, time, and space are one and the same. Mind cannot exist independent of time. Nor can space and time exist independent of mind. Mind, time, and space are like the three points of a triangle.

Whatever we perceive in terms of space and time changes and brings different kinds of experiences according to the nature of the mind of the perceiver. Therefore, reality—or God, the substratum behind everything—cannot be known in terms of space and time; for there is no change in God.

How, then, can "reality" or God be known? The answer is that we must transcend the limitation of time and space; that is, we must transcend the mind or still the motion of the mind. When the mind is still, there is no idea of time and space, which means there is no external consciousness except an awareness of self where there is no change.

This awareness of self is called self-realization or God realization, which is possible only when we transcend the mind, time, and space. This awareness of self or God is known as attainment of immortality. Therefore, mortality means externalization of the self, which becomes mind, space, and time.

The self as pure consciousness is the reality that is continuous, constant, and never-changing; but in order to make possible the perception of the self, we must split it into separate moments: imagine it as an infinite series of separate moments out of which there exists for us only one. In other words, when reality is perceived we call it "present." What we did not see and do not see, we call the "past." What we do not quite see at the present moment but are expecting, we call the "future."

Therefore time—past and future—is based on the reality "I," which Hindu philosophy describes as the "eternal now" or "eternal existence."

Now let us analyze our relation to the past, present, and future. Strictly speaking, neither the past, nor the present, nor the future exists for us. And yet we are continuously living on this reality of the present that vanishes before it appears into past, rushing the future into present, only to disappear into past continuously.

Stop here and reflect a moment and you will agree with the Hindu philosophy of nonexistence of the world, the world existing only in some phantasmagoria of illusions, flashing and disappearing in the mind.

We consider the past does not exist as it has passed, disappeared, changed itself into something else. The future also does not exist because it does not exist at this moment: it has not yet arrived. Now what is "the present"? The present is that which does not exist because it has no measurement. The present is that interval of time or moment of time when the future changes into the past. This moment of transition of a phenomenon, from one nonexistence (future) into another nonexistence (past), is the present, which is only a fiction, as the present moment has no measurement. This present moment can never be caught and measured and what we did catch is always the past. So we have to admit here that neither the present nor the past nor the future exists. Therefore the past is that which has disappeared leaving an impression, the present has no existence because that unimaginable time of present moment flashes through the mind before we catch it, into the past, ending nowhere in an endless vicious circle of nothing.

Usually we take no account of this and are constantly fooled by our imaginary reality of the world created by mind. In conclusion, time and space are other aspects of mind.

Conceptions of time differ according to the development of the mind. Animals have their own conception of time, which is absolutely different from our conception. Though animals and birds do not keep a calendar to find out when to migrate before the approaching winter, or when to hibernate, and other such things, they know instinctively all these functions necessary for their existence. Therefore the animals' and birds' conception of time is to perform one action after another as nature prompts them to do. These natural actions of animals in different seasons and time are guided solely by the instinctive mind. Without it there is no time or season for them.

It must be remembered here that the life spans of many animals and birds are much shorter than man, yet for an animal or a bird the short life span will appear as long as ours. Therefore, if the life span of a monkey is twenty years, those twenty years will appear to a monkey as a hundred years appear to us. Within the twenty years of life of a monkey, it will be able to perform all the natural functions from birth to death, etc., which take a hundred years for a man to do. For the mind of the monkey, twenty years may appear as a hundred years because mind can create an illusion of making a hundred years into fifteen and fifteen years into a hundred. Even in our daily life such phenomena occur, though we do not give them much attention. Let us take the condition of a husband who is waiting at the airport for the arrival of his wife, who has been away for a long time. Now let us suppose the plane is an hour late. His mind will create such a condition that each moment will appear as hours. Now let us take the same man's condition after the arrival of his dear wife. His mind now starts functioning in reverse process because he is very happy to see his wife, and the time will pass so quickly that he may not even be aware that hours are passing.

At this happy hour he receives a message that he must go to a distant place the very next day, leaving his wife for some business for a few months. Now every hour will pass as a few moments as the time approaches to leave his wife.

Therefore when there is concentration of the mind or mind is in a very happy mood, time appears to move quickly. But when there is agitation and distraction of the mind owing to worries and anxieties, time appears to move slowly.

Again, in a dream a whole series of the events of twenty years will appear in fifteen minutes, yet in those fifteen minutes time is equal to twenty years in the waking state. For the mind of the man, fifteen minutes of dreamtime is a solid twenty years until he comes back to the waking state. Therefore both waking time and dreaming time are true only in relative terms; and both are false time created by the mind, whether it is in a dream or awake.

Just as for our mind the life span of the animal is very small, so also are there higher beings who live in higher mental planes who consider that our life span of a hundred years is just a day for them.

To illustrate the difference of time in different levels, there is an old story in one of the holy scriptures—the *Srimad Bhagavata.*

Once a great king took his daughter to the plane of the creator, Brahma, to ask the name of a good husband for his daughter. After arriving at the Brahma's court, he waited for a few moments and made his request. To his surprise the Brahma replied, "O King, when you go back to earth you will not see any of your people, friends or relatives—nay, not even your cities and palaces. Though you arrived here only a few moments ago from the earth, these few moments in this world are equal to several thousand years for earth people." [The difference in time of each world is given at the end of this chapter.]

"When you go back now to earth, it is a new age and you will see Lord Krishna's brother, Bala Rama, who will be a suitable husband for your daughter. So a girl born in another age is married to Bala Rama after several thousand years."

When the king returned back to earth after his few minutes of travel to Brahma Loka, he saw a new world, altogether
different in civilization, people, culture, and religion. Several
thousand years had passed on earth, though he was gone for
but a few minutes.

You may consider this only a story, yet ancient Hindus explain,
in this story, one of the great truths of time—a truth that is very near
to Dr. Einstein's theory of the relativity of space and time.

Einstein explained time as a fourth dimension, in his special
theory of relativity. In his theory he discarded the idea of absolute
time—of a steady, unvarying, inexorable, universal flow of time stream-
ing from the infinite past to the infinite future. He explained that the
sense of time is a form of perception, like the color sense. What we
call a year is only a measure of earth's progress in its orbit around the
sun. But for an inhabitant of Mercury, a year and a day amount to the
same thing, because Mercury makes its trip around the sun in 88 of
our days, and in that period rotates just once on its axis. But now we
are aware that all our terrestrial ideas of time are meaningless when
we soar beyond the neighborhood of the sun. According to Einstein's
theory of relativity, there is no such thing as a fixed interval of time
independent of the system to which it is referred; and there is no such
thing as "now," independent of a system of reference.

To translate his basic idea of the relativity of time and space,
Einstein pointed out some hitherto unsuspected properties of clocks
and rods. For example, a clock attached to a moving system slows
down as the system's velocity increases, as compared to a stationary
clock that runs without any motion, though both clocks are of the
same make. Again, a measuring rod made of wood or metal or any
other material, attached to any moving system, shrinks in the direction
of its motion, according to the velocity of the system.

These peculiar changes of the slowing of the clock and the contraction of the rod have nothing to do with the construction of the
clock or the composition of the rod; nor are they mechanical phenomena. According to Einstein's theory of relativity, an observer riding
along with the clock and the rod would not notice these changes. On
the other hand, a stationary observer watching a moving system would
find that the greater the velocity, the greater the contraction, and the
slower the movement of the clock.

For example, a stationary observer will notice that a yardstick
that moves at 90 per cent of the velocity of light has shrunk half its

length; and if the velocity of the yardstick is increased further until it attains the velocity of light, it would shrink away to nothing. Similarly, a clock attached to a moving system that moves with the velocity of light would stop completely. Here it must be remembered that the slowing down of a clock and contraction of the rod are not noticeable in an automobile or airplane, because these changes can be detected only when the velocity of the moving system approaches very near to the velocity of light.

Another important point to be noted is that the contraction of the rod and the slowing down of the clock are entirely relative with respect to the two systems moving with respect to each other. Thus, for example, an observer in a space ship, traveling at very high speed, notices that another space ship moving away from it has shrunk considerably, whereas he would see no shrinking of his own space ship.

Just as speed shortens length, so also speed slows time. These effects are not limited to such mechanical gadgets as clocks and watches. Even biologic, physical, chemical, and mental processes will slow down to the same degree if a person travels with a very high velocity.

Now let us see the conception of time of the crew in a space ship that travels at very high speed approaching the speed of light, compared to the time conception of people on earth. Suppose it takes ten light years to reach from the earth a satellite of another solar system in a space ship that could travel practically with the speed of light; and ten light years back to earth. That makes twenty light years for the round trip. Naturally, we assume the crews in space should be provided with food for twenty years. But according to the law of relativity this precaution of providing food for twenty years is absolutely unnecessary if the space ship is able to travel with a speed approaching the velocity of light. While traveling at the speed of light everything slows down in the space ship, including the heartbeat, respiration, digestion, and the mental processes of crew and passengers. Twenty years on earth would be but a few hours to the people in the space ship. Therefore they would not need to be provided with food for twenty years.

Suppose that in 1960 a passenger ship leaves earth to go to a distant planet in another solar system. The trip takes twenty light years to go and twenty years to return. The space ship will complete its journey and return to earth in the year 2000. One of the crew is twenty years old when he leaves the earth. In 1960, when he leaves, he leaves a wife, age twenty, and a child, age one. When he returns after a few hours from his trip at a tremendous velocity, he will get a big surprise if he had gone on the trip without considering the law of relativity. On arriving home, he will find that wife, child, friends, relatives, have all grown forty years older than himself. But the crewman, and everybody else in the space ship, aged only a few hours. He left at age twenty, and returns forty years later, still age twenty.

Now let us see the similarity between the story of the king who took his daughter to the creator to find a husband and the above illustrations of the law of relativity. When the king returned to earth after a few minutes on the plane of the creator, he found a new age and civilization; just as the passengers of the space ship found everybody on earth had aged forty years while they had aged only a few hours.

The king's method of transportation might be altogether different from our space ship. A developed mind can move without the help of physical transportation. According to the special theory of relativity, the velocity of light is the top limiting velocity in the universe. Nothing can ever move faster than light, no matter what forces are applied. In that case, human beings can never dream of reaching even the nearest star, which is several hundred light years distant. Our life span of a mere hundred years prevents even the possibility of undertaking such ventures.

Yet in ancient Hindu scriptures are descriptions of man traveling to the moon (*chandra mandala*), to the sun (*soorya mandala*), and to the stars (*nakshatra mandala*). The ancients knew a way of traveling the interstellar regions without the help of our so-called modern mechanical devices. Their space ship was the mind.

Generally we think that mind is used only for thinking. Though the limit of man's physical speed is the speed of light, yet with the help of the mind he is able to travel anywhere in the physical universe and beyond the physical universe to the higher astral planes.

Mind is not limited by velocity; it can reach a distant star in a moment; for time and space are creations of the mind.

The ancient Hindus divided time according to the plane of consciousness in which mind functions. In a higher plane of consciousness, several thousand earth years will appear as a few hours, because there the mind functions in a different velocity. In the lower planes of plants and minerals, mind functions in a very low degree of motion, making them appear to be living in a perpetual state of sleep without any conception of time.

As man evolves, he will be able to operate his mind more and more in higher planes, and to transcend his physical limitations. But

Yoga declares that the final liberation from the clutches of space and time is possible only when the mind itself is transcended. For the mind itself is the cause of space and time, whether it is in the physical planes or the astral planes.

In the final stage, when man realizes that nothing is outside and everything is within himself, then he will be able to transcend the limitations of space and time. In Yoga, this stage is known as self-realization or God realization, where there is no difference between the knower, knowledge, and the known; and where the past and the future merge with the present—the eternal "now" of the Hindus.

Real knowledge is possible only when there is no past or future, and where there is no time or space.

In one of the holy scriptures of the Hindus, the *Srimad Bhagavata*, division of time is described thus: the minutest particle of material substance (which cannot be further divided), which has not yet evolved, nay, not even been combined with other similar particles and hence eternally exists (in that causal state) should be known by the name *paramanu*.

It is the combination of more than one such *paramanu* that creates in the mind of men the illusory notion of a unit. Even so the entire range of material substances taken as an unspecified and undifferentiated whole, before it undergoes further transformation, i.e., returns to its ultimate source (*prakriti*), constitutes what is known as the largest size. Just as the minutest particle of a material substance such as earth, metal, gas, and so on leads us to postulate the existence of *paramanu* (atom) and the combination of material substances (the atoms) to that of large size, so can we infer the long and short measures of time which (being a potency of the Lord) is the same as the Lord, all-pervading and unmanifest, and which is the circumscriber of finite objects inasmuch as (in the form of sun) it travels across the large and small dimensions of things. The measure of time that flits across the smallest particle of matter is called *paramanu;* while that which extends over the whole life span of the universe (viz., from the creation to dissolution) is the longest measure of time in relation to the cosmos.

Two *paramanus* make one *anu* (atom); while three *anus* constitute a *trasarenu*. Here the words *anus* and *trasarenu*, though primarily denoting the dimensions of material objects, also signify the measure of time taken by the sunlight to travel across the aforesaid dimensions. The measure of time that travels across a composite of three *trasarenus* is known as a *truti;* a *vedha* consists of a hundred *trutis*, while three *vedhas* constitute what is known as a *lava*. A composite of three *lavas* should be known by the name of *nimesa* (the twinkling of an eye); while three *nimesas* are spoken of as one moment (*kshana*).

The day and night of human beings consist of four *yamas* or quarters each; while fifteen days and nights constitute a fortnight. Both these fortnights, taken together, make one month, which constitutes a day and night of the *pitrs* (manes) who live very near to our physical planes. Two months taken together go to make a *ritu* (season), while an *ayana* is southerly and northerly by turns (according as the sun takes a southerly or northerly course), and the two *ayanas* constitute a year, which is a day and night of the gods in heaven.

A full life span of manes, gods, and human beings has thus been stated in the scriptures as consisting of a hundred years according to the measure of time in each sphere.

Now is explained the life span of other higher enlightened beings who live outside the three worlds of manes, gods, and men—and whose conception of time is different owing to the development of mind.

In order to understand the time conception of the higher enlightened beings, they divided the time as four *yugas* or ages. These four *yugas* are (1) *satya yuga;* (2) *treta yuga;* (3) *dwapara yuga;* and (4) *kali yuga.* According to calculation we are living now in *kali yuga,* which consists of 1,200 celestial years or 432,000 human years. *Kali yuga* is the shortest of all the ages.

The *satya yuga* consists of 4,800 celestial years or 1,728,000 human years, *treta yuga* 3,600 celestial years or 1,296,000 human years, and *dwapara yuga,* 2,400 celestial years or 864,000 human years.

Beyond the three worlds, as far as the abode of Brahma the creator of the universe, one thousand revolutions of the four *yugas* ($4,320,000 \times 1,000$ human years) constitute a day, and equal in length is the night, which is the night of the creator Brahma, who withdraws all the three worlds into himself. This is the dissolution or opposite of evolution or creation. Again the cycle of creation begins at the close of the night of Brahma. The creation of the three worlds commences (as in the preceding *kalpa* or age) and continues for the day of the Brahma. This is the day-to-day creation of Brahma which affects the three worlds alone and in which the subhuman creatures, human beings, manes, and gods are born according to their respective *karma.* Even the Brahma the creator, one of the Trinity, has only one hundred years of his activity and finally he himself merges with the Supreme Being after that hundred years of Brahma's life, along with all the created worlds. The aforesaid period of one hundred years of Brahma, known as two *parardhas,* which is equal to (4,320,000 × 1,000 + 4,320,000 × 1,000) (365 × 100) human years, is figuratively spoken of as the mere twinkling of an eye of the immutable, immortal, beginning-less Lord, the soul of the universe. This all-powerful time, ranging from a *paramanu,* the smallest measure, to the length of two *parardhas* of Brahma, has no control over the all-embracing Lord. It holds sway only on those who have identified themselves with the body and all that is associated with it. Thus the Supreme Being controls, creates, and dissolves under the name of time over which no one has any control as long as one identifies with his body and mind.

The above description of time, according to the ancient scriptures, is given here to illustrate that everyone within the creation is bound by the limitation of time and space, whether he is a human being or an angel.

In conclusion, all our knowledge is based upon the mind, which thinks in terms of time and space. This is limited knowledge, conditioned by time and space. Yoga philosophy declares that there is a timeless state where there is no death or birth or growth, where there is no pain or sorrow, where there is no day or night, nor any distance; and that such a state can be achieved by meditating upon the self within, and realizing that I am everywhere and in everything: "I am the sun and stars. I am the time and space and I am He." This is the end of time and space. When I am everywhere, then where can I move? and when there is no past and future and I am eternal existence, then where is time?

# 10

# THE ABSOLUTE AND EVOLUTION OF *PRAKRITI*

The one question that is most difficult to grasp, the one that will be asked again and again and will always remain unanswered, is "How did the infinite, the absolute, become the finite world?" The one absolute became the universe by coming through time, space, and causation. Time, space, and causation are like colored glass through which the absolute is seen, and when it is seen, it appears as the universe. This absolute and ultimate reality is spirit, or pure consciousness, out of which mind and matter proceed. This spirit or *atman* is one, and its vehicles are mind and body. The spirit or *atman* that is in man is the one spirit, which is in everything. The same spirit is the Lord when it becomes the object of worship.

The nature of the spirit is whole without any section, and mind and matter are parts in that whole that manifest themselves in many degrees and qualities. Spirit is infinite, formless, inactive, unchanging, and witness of the mind. Its power (*sakthi*) expressed in the form of mind and matter, is finite, with form, active, ever-changing.

Mind and matter are considered as unconscious, because all that is not the conscious self is the unconscious object. But according to Vedanta philosophy, there is nothing unconscious; on the contrary, all is essentially consciousness. That which is the object of conscious self we call unconscious mind, and matter. Matter is only the gross portion of the mind. In other words, mind and matter are like the obverse and reverse portions of a coin. The mind is also known as the veiling power of consciousness. Mind limits the consciousness or spirit, so that man experiences only the finite and not the absolute truth as a whole and infinite. Where there is no mind, there is no limitation.

Spirit or consciousness, remaining in one aspect changeless, changes in another aspect as active power (*sakthi*) and is expressed as mind and matter. Therefore, man is the spirit or pure consciousness, the absolute one encased by its veiling power of mind and body. "Man is God playing fool." (Emerson.)

The whole world springs from the active consciousness of the absolute. Owing to the force of *maya sakthi* or the veiling power, man believes in an objective existence beyond and independent of himself. This state of objectivity is felt as long as his consciousness is veiled or contracted by *maya sakthi.*

So, *maya sakthi* or veiling power is that which makes the whole or absolute into the not whole, the infinite into finite, the formless into forms. It is a power that thus cuts down, veils, and negates the absolute.

In the absolute there is neither time, space, nor causation; it is all one and hence cannot be known, because what we call knowledge comes from a mind limited by space and time. When knowledge is beyond the limitation of space and time, it is not knowledge. Now, if the absolute becomes limited by the mind, it is no more absolute, as everything limited by the mind becomes finite. Therefore, to know that one or the absolute is a contradiction in terms. That is why the question, "How does the Infinite become finite?" is never answered. A God known is no more God and, therefore, He is always the Unknowable One and inexplicable.

The ultimate basic experience of the absolute or spirit is possible only when all divergence disappears; for in it lies as undifferentiated mass the experiencer, the experience, and the experienced, or the knower, the knowledge, and the known. When we cannot differentiate the knower from the knowledge and the object to be known, where then is the knowledge, and of what? This again proves the absolute is unknowable.

According to Vedanta, knowledge is of two kinds: (1) *gyana swaroopa,* or the perfect experience of consciousness; (2) *gyana vritti,* the knowledge of objects, or the ordinary imperfect experience of the world owing to the association with the mind.

Sankara's explanation of the relation between the absolute and the finite world is known as *Vivarta Vada,* or superimposition, and is expressed in the story of the snake and rope. In the darkness, one mistakes the rope for a snake. When a light is brought, the illusion of the snake created by the lack of illumination is removed, and once again the rope appears in its true reality. So, also, the world is only a super-imposition on Brahman or the absolute. Owing to ignorance, man thinks of the existence of the finite world like the snake in darkness. When the knowledge of oneness dawns, the world disappears, and once again only the absolute exists.

*Jiva* or the spirit becomes identical with Brahman or the obso-lute when the veil of *avidya* or ignorance drops and the objective world disappears as an object of experience.

## THE EVOLUTION OF THE FINITE WORLD FROM THE ABSOLUTE

1. A transcendent mingled "I" and "this" in which these ele-ments of knowledge have not evolved as such. This is one-ness. Here, "I" represents the consciousness or self, and "this" the objective universe. In this state "I" and "this" are not separated and therefore the objective universe is not evolved. In this state "I" as self and "this" as universe are united like milk and water, which cannot be distinguished when mixed.

   "I" and "this" as oneness.

2. A pure form of knowledge intermediate between the first and the third in which both "I" and "this" are experienced as part of the one "self."

   "I" and "this" as part of the oneself.

3. In the third and last stage of knowledge there is a complete separation between "I" and "this." Here an outer object is presented to the consciousness of a knower, which is other than the subject. There are two divisions in this last stage:

   a. In the first, self experiences a homogeneous universe, though different from himself as *prakriti* or nature. This stage of evolution is like the change of milk into yogurt or curd.

      There is a complete sep-aration between "I" and "this." "I" as knower and "this" as object.

   b. In the second division of the final stage, *prakriti* or nature

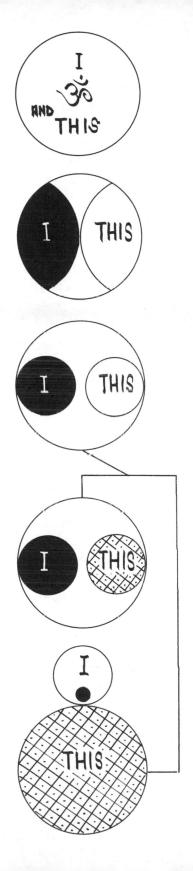

as homogeneous universe is split up into effects (*vikriti*) which are mind and matter and the multitudinous beings of the universe these compose. In this stage of experience the absolute has become the objective universe for the "I" or self. The absolute being, when veiled by its own power or *sakthi*, becomes the universe. Here the one absolute has changed into "I" as the self and "this" as finite world is like buttermilk and butter.

In theology, this pure consciousness "I" is Siva and his active power "this" is *sakthi*. *Sakthi*, the divine power, the mother of the universe, the life force, resides in man's body in the lowest center (*muladhara chakra*) of the spine.

The whole world of five elements (earth, water, fire, air, and ether) proceed from the active power of *sakthi*. Sakthi at first evolves mind and senses and then the five-fold elements of matter.

### EVOLUTION OF PRAKRITI

*Sakthi* as *prakriti* is the unmanifest universe or *avyaktha*, and is like a seed that contains a whole tree. She is of three qualities known as *satwa*, or purity and knowledge; *rajas*, or activity and motion; and *tamas*, or inertia and laziness. The whole world is a mixture of these three *gunas* or qualifications of *prakriti*. Before the evolution of *prakriti sakthi* as the world, these three *gunas* are in equilibrium and do not affect one another. This is the state of *avyaktha* or unmanifest. *Prakriti sakthi* is material but not visible scientific matter. It is the subtle material cause of all things and its effect as visible universe is *vikriti*, which may be divided into two parallel groups: mind and matter. Mind is a manifestation of *sakthi* in the form of force which, in turn, becomes matter, or the five elements of material. Scientists have also come to the same conclusion—that everything is energy itself. "The most intense source of energy is obtained by annihilating matter."

Mind as thought power is a moving force, and mind as matter a lasting, stationary force. Matter is a dense and gross form of the more subtle force of *prakriti*. *Prakriti* or unmanifest force of energy becomes *vikriti* or the manifest force, as mind, senses, and matter. The three bodies (physical, astral, and causal) are evolved from *prakriti*, in which the spirit or pure consciousness is enshrined. The *karana sharira* or causal body is the seed body from which the astral and physical bodies are evolved. The astral body is the body of mind and senses; that which succeeds is the physical body composed of the five elements of matter.

## SAKTHI AS KUNDALINI AND THE EVOLUTION OF THE CHAKRAS

From *prakriti sakthi* evolves the whole universe of five elements. In the individual, *prakriti sakthi* is manifested as *kundalini sakthi*, or serpent power. *Kundalini sakthi* also manifests itself as mind and *chakras*, (astral nerve centers, which correspond to the five elements). Consciousness reaching to the world of enjoyment is contracted and thus becomes the impure worldly experience where subject and object are completely different. Infinite consciousness, while still transcendentally retaining its real nature, becomes *kundalini sakthi* narrowed to the degree that constitutes our experience on the material plane. This process may be represented in the diagram as an inverted triangle. The three dots in the triangle represent the three powers manifested as *icha sakthi* or will, *gyana sakthi* or knowledge, and *kriya sakthi* or action.

Power manifests itself when these three (will, power, and action) are connected. It then resembles a triangle. This *sakthi* is known as *tripura* or triple energy. Within this triangle or triple energy, *kundalini* is manifested as a coiled serpent. Just as the atom consists of a static nucleus around which electrons revolve, so also *kundalini sakthi* is the static force around which the active force of *prana* and mind manifest in the body. Man, physically and psychically, is a limited manifestation of the threefold energies of the *kundalini sakthi*.

Here, the three dots of will, action, and knowledge represent the three revolving electrons around the *kundalini* or coiled power, or static force.

In fact, the whole body is in ceaseless movement around *kundalini*, which is the immobile support of all these operations.

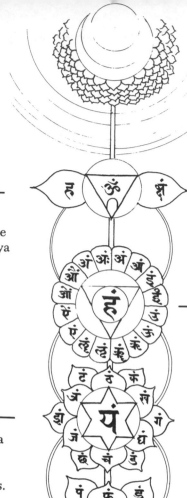

## Sahasrara Chakra
*(Thousand Petal Lotus)*

## Ajna Chakra

Hakini Devi. Sambu. Itara
Linga and Tricona, Mahat. The
Sukshma Prakriti called Hiranya
Garba. Mind. Letters Ham
and Ksham.

## Visudha Chakra

Sakini Devi. Sabda Tatwa.
Hearing (sensation). Ether
principle. Mouth (action).
16 letters. 16 petals. Bija Ham.

## Anahata Chakra

Kakini Devi. Isha. Bana Linga
Trikona. Bija Yam. Air
principle. Sparsatatwa. Feel
and touch. 12 letters. 12 petals.

## Manipura Chakra

Lakini Devi. Rudra on a bull.
Rupa (form and color).
10 letters. 10 petals. Bija
Mantraa Ram. Fire principle.

## Swadhishatana Chakra

Rakini Devi. Vishnu. Varuna
Rasa (sense). Hand (action).
6 petals. 6 letters. Bija Vam.
Water principle.

## Mooladhara Chakra

Dakini Devi. Brahma. Indra
Devata. Earth principle.
Gandha Tatwa. Smell
(sensation). Feet (organ of
action). 4 petals. 4 letters.
Swayambu Linga. Bija Lam.
Kundalini.

# AUTONOMIC NERVOUS SYSTEM

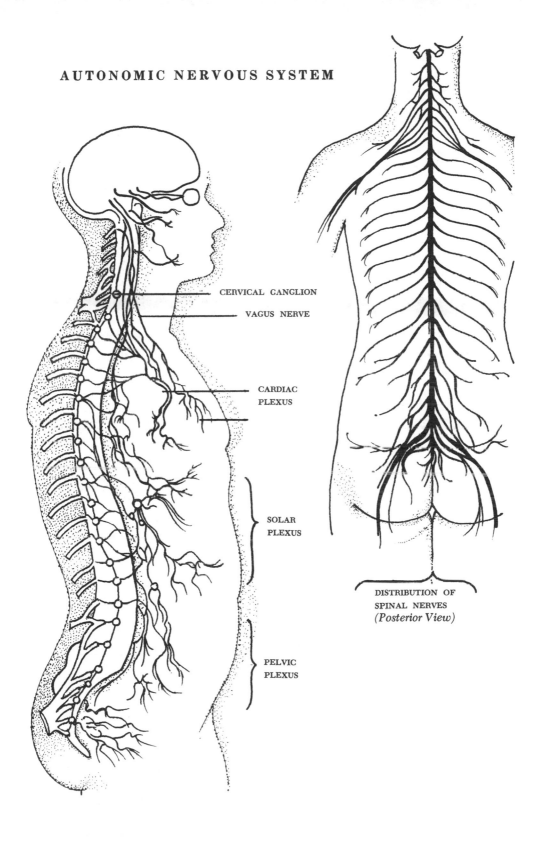

CERVICAL GANGLION

VAGUS NERVE

CARDIAC
PLEXUS

SOLAR
PLEXUS

PELVIC
PLEXUS

DISTRIBUTION OF
SPINAL NERVES
*(Posterior View)*

Siva is always one with his power. He manifests himself through his power in various names and forms. *Sakthi* at first evolves as mind. From the mind evolve the five elements or *bhutas*.

In the second stage of development, *sakthi* becomes the primordial element, the ether or subtle matter from which gross matter emerges. The projecting power of *kundalini* now assumes the gross elements which are represented as *chakras* of different elements.

From *akasa* or the subtle ether of the *sakthi, vayu* (air and gas) was projected; and from the combination of gases, fire and water (liquid); and from liquid, solid matter (earth). When *sakthi* has entered the last and grossest element, the "earth principle," that is, solid matter, there is nothing for her to do. Then her creative activity ceases and the power rests in the last *chakra* of earth principle. Here, power as *sakthi* is coiled and rests from her creative activity and is known as *kundalini sakthi* whose abode is the *mooladhara chakra* represented by the earth principle. This *chakra* and the neighboring astral nerve centers belong to the five elements: earth, water, fire, air, and ether, and the last one, ether or *ajna chakra*, represents the mind.

When *kundalini sakthi* rests or is active only in the lower centers, man has only finite experience. When she is aroused and moves upward, she withdraws into herself the moving powers of her creation, and unites with pure consciousness (Siva) in the *sahasrara chakra* (the thousand-petaled lotus in the brain). This process of the upward movement of *kundalini* and final union with consciousness (Siva) is called *kundalini* Yoga. This is the reverse process of the evolution of mind and the five gross elements. In her creative aspect, *kundalini sakthi* also becomes senses and *prana,* or vital airs.

## ASTRAL TUBE AND SIX CENTERS OF SPIRITUAL ENERGY

In order to have cosmic consciousness, Yogis awaken the *kundalini sakthi,* which now rests in the *mooladhara chakra* in the lower spine, and then slowly, through *pranayama* and meditation, takes her back through the different centers in the *sushumna* (astral nerve tube).

Every portion of the physical body is associated with its astral counterpart. Even after the physical organs are severed, the astral counterpart remains. When a toe or hand is amputated, the astral part of the toe or hand remains. A young man had a chronic ailment in his big toe with severe pain for several years, and finally his toe was amputated. Even after the amputation, the patient had severe pain in the same region where once his physical toe had been. Though psychologists may explain that the pain of the toe is mental, the theory of the Yogis is that pain from the astral counterpart of the toe cannot be removed by the removal of the physical toe alone. Both the physical body and astral body are intimately connected and in the material plane both are interdependent.

All the six nerve centers or *chakras* and the *sushumna nadi* are in the astral body and cannot be seen with the physical eye except during meditation. But in the physical body these *chakras* and *sushumna nadi* are represented as nerve plexus and the spinal column.

There are two astral tubes on either side of the *sushumna,* known as *ida* and *pingala,* through which two nerve currents move. *Ida* and *pingala* are *nadis* (astral nerve tubes) which correspond to the left and right sympathetic cords in the physical body. Through *ida* and *pingala,* the *prana* or vital air flows. When the vital air flows through *ida* and *pingala,* man is busily engaged in manifold worldly activities. The *sushumna nadi,* which corresponds to the spinal column in the physical body, is the main one that Yogis want to operate, because as long as the left and right (*ida* and *pingala*) work, man will be bound by time, space, and causation. When the central *nadi* (*sushumna*) operates, he is beyond the limitation of mind and time. A Yogi tries his level best to make his *prana* or vital air flow in the *sushumna.* The *sushumna nadi* is the most important of all *nadis.* According to Yogic conception, there are 72,000 *nadis,* out of which there are ten principal ones that carry pranic energy. *Ida, pingala, sushumna, gandhari, hasthajihva, pusa, yusasvini, alambusa, kuhuh,* and *sankini* are said to be the ten important ones. Yogis should have a thorough knowledge of these astral tubes and *chakras.*

*Sushumna nadi,* principal of all *nadis,* is also known as *Brahma nadi* or the path toward the Supreme Being. *Sushumna nadi* has two inner linings. The outer is *sushumna,* the second lining is *vajrini,* and the third lining is *chitrini.* Within these three layers is the hollow canal through which the awakened *kundalini sakthi* withdraws herself to her eternal abode, the *parama siva* or supreme consciousness. Yogis can feel the movement of *prana* and the movement of the awakened *kundalini* in *sushumna* during meditation and *pranayama.* When the coiled-up energy (*kundalini sakthi*) passes up along the *sushumna* and is taken from *chakra* to *chakra,* the Yogis experience different kinds of knowledge, powers, and joy. But *sushumna* is generally closed at the base of the spine in the vast majority of people; hence, most minds operate only in the lower planes (material plane) of consciousness.

With the practice of *asan, pranayam, mudras,* and meditation, heat and energy are produced. This concentrated energy is directed toward the *kundalini* herself. After a long period of continuous practice, breathing, and meditation, the *sushumna* is freed of impurities, and the awakened *kundalini sakthi* easily passes upward through the canal of the *sushumna* to the *sahasrara chakra* (thousand-petaled lotus) in the brain.

The awakened *kundalini* that is taken up to the *manipura chakra,* the third nerve plexus situated in the navel, may drop down again to the *mooladhara chakra* (basic center in the spine). It has to be raised again with effort. Only such advanced Yogis as Rama Krishna Paramahansa, Aurobindo, and Swami Sivananda could take *kundalini* to the highest center, that is, to the *ajna chakra* situated between the eyebrows, and above it to the brain center, and retain it for a long time. Only a few Yogis can awaken *kundalini* and take her at will to the *anahata chakra* or heart center for a short period. Some students of Yoga who often speak of *kundalini* only stumbled upon that power, and know neither how to take her to the higher centers at will, nor how to retain her in the higher centers. Nowadays we can see many such people, who after stumbling upon that force, pose as teachers and claim to know everything.

It is said that one should become completely desireless and be full of dispassion before attempting to awaken *kundalini sakthi.* Otherwise, the awakened power will be uncontrollable and inflict a terrible feeling of pain and heat upon the entire body. No doctor can diagnose or cure it, because there will be no noticeable external symptoms. When purity of mind is attained through devotion and selfless service, *pranayama* (Yogic breathing), and meditation, then alone does the awakened *kundalini* move upward and impart different kinds of experience, powers, and *ananda* or bliss.

## MEDITATION ON CHAKRAS OR CENTERS

*Chakras* are centers of spiritual energy that are located in the astral body. They have corresponding centers in the physical body, which are known as plexuses. There are six important *chakras.* They are: *muladhara,* containing four petals, located at the lower end of the spinal column; *swadhisthana* (six petals), at the genital organs; *manipura* (ten petals) at the navel; *anahata* (twelve petals) at the heart; *vishudha* (sixteen petals) at the throat, and *ajna* (two petals) between the two eyebrows. The seventh *chakra* is known as *sahasrara,* which contains a thousand petals, located in the brain.

In the physical body, the sacral plexus tentatively corresponds to *muladhara;* the prostatic plexus to *swadhisthana;* the solar plexus to *manipura;* the cardiac plexus to *anahata;* the laryngeal plexus to *vishudha,* and the cavernous plexus to *ajna.*

Yogis meditate on the five *chakras* while practicing *pranayama.*

*Meditation on Muladhara Chakra:* This *chakra* at the base of the spine represents the *prithivi tattwa* (earth principle) and has the color of orpiment (yellow). The letter *lam* is its secret symbol, or *beeja mantra.* Its form is four-sided (four petals), and Brahma the Creator is its presiding deity. The *sakthi* or power manifested in this *chakra* is *dakini devi.* The four petals are represented by four syllables: *sam, sham, sam,* and *vam.* In the center of this *chakra* there is a triangle, or triple energy, and within it *kundalini sakthi* shines like bright lightning. Meditation on this *chakra* brings steadiness of the body.

*Meditation on Swadhisthana Chakra:* This *chakra* in the genital organs is represented by the *apas tattwa,* or water, and is white like a conch shell. Its form is circular like the moon; the letter *vam* is the seed of this ambrosial element, and Vishnu is its presiding deity. It is six-petaled; it is represented by *bam, bham, nam, yam, ram, lam,* and the power manifested is called *rakini devi.* (Yogis meditate on the bright crescent moon in the center of this *chakra.*)

*Meditation on Manipura Chakra:* This *chakra* is situated at the navel and is represented by the fire element, or *agni tattwa.* Its color is red, its form is triangular, its seed is *ram,* its presiding deity is Rudra. It is ten-petaled, represented by *da, nda, na, ta, tha, de, dhe, ne, pa, pha,* and the power manifested is called *lakini devi.*

*Meditation on Anahata Chakra:* This *chakra* is in the heart region and is represented by *vayu tattwa,* or air principle. The letter *yam* is its seed; its presiding deity is Isa, and the power is *kakini devi.* It has the shape of a twelve-petaled lotus, represented by *ka, kha, ga, gha, ge, cha, chha, ja, jha, je, ta,* and *tha.* It is smoke-colored, and in its center are two triangles, one facing upward and the other downward.

*Meditation on Vishudha Chakra:* This *chakra* of the throat is represented by the first element, ether principle, or *akasa tattwa.* Its color is that of pure sea water; *ham* is its seed, its presiding deity is Sada Siva, and its *sakthi* is *sakini devi*. It has sixteen petals, represented by 16 vowels: *a, aa, e, ee, u, uu, ri, ree, lre, lree, ye, yai, o, ow, am, ah.*

*Meditation on Ajna Chakra:* This *chakra* is situated in the space between the eyebrows. This is the highest *chakra* represented by the mind. This is the place on which Yogis generally meditate to obtain rapid success in controlling the various nerve centers. This *chakra* is the most powerful nerve center, and wonderful spiritual experiences are obtained by the Yogis who meditate upon this. Nobody could prove, in a laboratory, the benefits derived by meditating upon this center, yet one can see in oneself the extraordinary spiritual strength, knowledge, and will power obtained by constant meditation on this center.

This *chakra* is the seat of *sukshma prakriti,* or the primordial power of everything. It has two petals, *ham* and *ksham;* its power is *hakinidevi;* its color is snow white. There is a triangle in its center, or the triple energy; within it the Yogi meditates upon the sacred syllable *AUM.* The higher voice, or intuitional knowledge, is obtained through this *ajna chakra.* This is the mental center and also the seat of the *atman,* or soul, in the form of *pranava* or *OM.* It is here that Yogis consciously keep their *prana* at the time of death when they enter into the supreme primordial being.

With further meditation *Kundalini Sakthi* is taken beyond the *Ajna Chakra* to the thousand-petaled lotus (*Sahasrara Chakra*) in the brain. When *Kundalini* is united with Consciousness (*Siva*) in this center then Yogi is considered to attain complete perfection.

These *chakras* are centers of consciousness and are connected with gross regions of the nerve plexus, which are subject to their influence by meditating on the astral centers (*chakras.*)

The various sounds and alphabets in the different *chakras* are the sound energy of the *kundalini sakthi.* The sound energy, when uttered in human speech, assumes the form of letters, and from the combination of letters, prose and verse result. Hence, spoken letters become the manifested aspect of gross speech or the sound energy of the *kundalini sakthi.* Each manifested letter is a *mantra,* and a *mantra* is the body of the presiding deity. Just as a mother teaches her child the meaning of a word by pointing out an object which is being indicated by that word, so also the Yogic student is taught the *mantra* of a *devata* or *devi* (god or goddess) by uttering the particular *mantra.* But here the Yogic student does not at once see the presiding *devata* of the *chakras.*

The Yogic student is initiated in the chanting of these *mantras* for meditating on the aspect of God connoted by the *mantra* he chants.

With the help of *pranayama* and the chanting of *mantras*, the sleeping *kundalini* power is roused and moves to the next higher center, *swadhisthana*. From there onward, the student with great effort carries the power to the next higher centers in regular ascending order: *manipura, anahata, vishudha, ajna*. Only when the power reaches consciously the *ajna* center in between the eyebrows may it be said that the practitioner has obtained success in controlling and manipulating the *kundalini sakthi*, which appears like a brilliant flash of lightning. Even to reach this state, one has to work hard for several years and follow the method and contemplation taught by one's teacher. Nowadays we can see everywhere pseudo Yoga teachers who proclaim on public platforms that they can awaken *kundalini* with their Yogic powers if students can afford to pay a large amount of money.

Yogic students are warned again and again that *kundalini* can never be awakened by the powers of such teachers, except through long and steady practices of meditation, chanting, and breathing. A true teacher never expects anything from his students, and awaits the proper time—perhaps years—before he teaches everything to them.

The passage of *kundalini* from the lower spinal center to *ajna* in the forehead constitutes the first part of the ascent, and the second is from *ajna* to *sahasrara* (the thousand-petaled lotus) in the brain. Now, the *kundalini* that has been led all the way to *sahasrara* merges with Siva, consciousness, which is called union or Yoga. This is the end of the journey, or the reverse process of the evolution of mind and matter.

Though *kundalini* has reached *sahasrara*, it does not remain there for a long period. There is always a tendency to return, and it does invariably return from time to time to the original abode in the *muladhara*. Only by long and continued practice does *sakthi* make a permanent union, and the aspirant becomes a liberated soul or *sthitha pragnja*. He is no longer bound or limited by time, space, or causation, and all is joy and eternal bliss itself. He is immersed in the ocean of bliss and becomes the possessor of all knowledge and powers.

# 11

# SELF AS EXISTENCE, KNOWLEDGE, AND BLISS

"What is there in this world that remains to be desired to a man who has known the Self? Nothing in all the treasures of the kingdom, nothing in all the charms and beauties of this world can draw his attention. What happiness, what supreme joy, what an ocean of bliss, how indescribable is the Self! That infinite joy, that supreme bliss, that infinite happiness ye are, that is your real Self; that is your *atman*."— Thus declare the *Upanishads*. This *atman* known as soul, or spirit, or self is identical with the all-pervading *brahman* of the absolute. "That which is neither subtle nor dense, neither short nor long, which is unborn, immutable, devoid of form, quality, caste, or name, that should be understood as *atman* or Self" (*Atma Bodha* of Sankara). In *Atma Bodha* Sankara, the great, declares: "Knowledge of Self is the only direct means to liberation. As cooking is impossible without fire, so is liberation without knowledge of Self. Knowledge of Self surely destroys ignorance (I am the body), as light destroys the densest darkness."

For a man who has realized his self, the phenomenal world abounding in worldly emotions is verily like a dream.

"Like the illusion of silver in mother of pearl, the world appears to be real only until the Supreme Self, the immutable reality behind everything is realized."

Where is this self? What is its nature? How can it be realized?

The pure self, when it is reflected through different bodies, appears to assume their respective natures, like a crystal reflecting a blue color. The seers separate the grain of the pure inner self from the chaff of the body by the threshing of reason.

That self is beyond the physical body, which is the place for experiencing happiness and misery; this body is made up of five elements and is obtained as the result of past actions. That self is also beyond the astral body, which is made up of life force (pranic energy), mind, and senses. The astral body is only the second vehicle of the self. Again, the self is beyond the causal body, which is the product of the beginningless indefinable illusion, mistaking the body for the soul. The causal body or seed body is the cause for the astral and physical bodies and is only a third vehicle for the self.

Although the self is at all times and in all things, yet it cannot shine in everything but will shine only in the consciousness, just as a reflection will appear only on polished surfaces. Therefore, when there is no visible reflection of the consciousness or self, we call it unconscious principle, though all manifestation is associated with the unconscious principle, mind and body.

Whatever we see, in the phenomenal world, is a mixture of conscious and unconscious principle and, therefore, there is nothing absolutely conscious or absolutely unconscious. But some things appear to be more conscious and some things more unconscious because the self, which is never absent in anything, whether it is in mineral or man, reflects itself in various ways and to different degrees. However, the degree of reflection is determined by the nature and development of the body and mind through which the self is reflected. The self shines in its own glory without any external agents, as the sun shines on all objects, and yet the reflection of the sun comes only from a polished surface and not from everything. So also the degree of manifestation or reflection of the self is visible only as ascent is made from mineral to man. In the mineral world the self is manifested as the lowest form of consciousness, which may be termed as atomic memory. In the plant kingdom the degree of sentiency is more visible than in the mineral kingdom, though plant life also belongs to the field of limited consciousness. Then comes a stage of development that is in between the plant and animal worlds. This stage of development, which we call microorganisms, has a psychic life different from the plant.

From here onward the development of consciousness becomes more complex. As ascent is made to the animal kingdom, the development of consciousness manifests itself in varying degrees and reaches its fullest degree in man, with all the psychic functions, such as cognition, perception, feeling, and will.

Behind all these particular forms of developing consciousness there is something formless and changeless, different from its manifestation, mineral or man. That something is self or spirit, which remains the same throughout all stages of development. Though the self appears to be developed from the lowest form of sentiency, it itself is not developed or changed. The appearance of development is because the self is now more and now less reflected by the mind and body in which it is enshrined. When the reflection (consciousness) is less, then the self is reflected through dense matter of the mineral and when the reflection is more, then it is reflected by the mind of developed being. However, though consciousness appears to be fully developed in man, it is still only a limited consciousness and this limitation of the consciousness continues as long as one identifies one's self with body and mind. When the self identifies with the body, then it is called individual consciousness, which is only a reflection of the pure self.

When man realizes in himself that self alone illumines the consciousness (mind and senses) as a light reveals objects, that self cannot be illumined by these illuminable objects, and that self is identical with the absolute (I am He—*soham*), then and then alone is man freed from all limitations.

This is called direct realization, or self-realization, which brings liberation of the soul or self from the bondage of mind, time, and space.

How and by what means can the self be realized or known? Just as the perception of things is impossible without light, so knowledge of self cannot emerge by any means other than inquiry. "Who am I?" "How was this universe born?" "What is its cause?" At first the inquiry regards the relation between the observer and the observed or the subject and the object. That which is denoted by the word "I" forever remains the same and transcendental. That which is gross, the objective world, on the other hand, undergoes multiplicity. Owing to ignorance, man thinks "I am the body," "I am Mr. So-and-So." But during inquiry he comes face to face with truth that the "I" is assuredly the perceiver and the body is the perceived, as is evident from the expression "this body is mine," as "this cloth is mine." As the cloth is mine but I am not the cloth, so also the body is mine and I am not the body. How, then, can the body be the self? Again, the self is of the nature of knowledge and pure, while the body consists of flesh and is impure. And yet man identifies the two. This is ignorance.

A dream becomes unreal in the waking state; and the waking state does not exist in a dream. Both dream and waking are absent in deep sleep, and deep sleep, too, is absent in dream and in waking.

Thus, one state is unreal from the other point of view, and therefore all the three states, waking, dreaming, and sleeping are unreal. Then what is the reality? The reality is the "I," the self, the one that is pure consciousness, the witness of these three states.

> Just as one does not see the separate existence of the pot when one knows that it is clay, so, too, one does not see the condition of the individual self when one knows the absolute.

> Just as a pot is only a name of clay, or an earring of gold, so, too, is the individual a name of the Supreme.

> Just as water alone appears as waves and tides, and copper alone as vessels, so does the self alone appear as the universe.

> All phenomenal life is possible for men only by virtue of the Supreme Brahman (God), just as the pot is possible only by virtue of clay. Due to ignorance, men do not know this.

> As the clay alone appears under the name of pot, as the threads appear under the name of cloth, so does the Supreme Brahman appear under the name of the various forms and beings of the world.

> The Self always shines as unconditioned for the wise, and always as conditioned for the ignorant, just as the rope appears as rope to the correct vision and as a snake to the mistaken vision.

> *Aprokshanuboothy* of Sankara, the Great.

Thus, the inquiry brings the knowledge of self: "I am indeed Brahman, or the Absolute," without difference, without change, and of the nature of reality, knowledge, and bliss. I am not the mind and senses because the mind and senses are also instruments of the self. Self can control the mind and senses. Hence they are the instruments of the self and not the "I." When I say, "My mind and senses are not functioning," it is just like saying "My car is not running." Just as the car is "my vehicle," so also the mind and senses are "my vehicle," and I am not the mind and senses. Therefore, the self is the witness of the body, mind, and senses, and because the self shines, the mind and senses reflect the light and appear as consciousness.

The main purpose of this philosophy is summed up briefly. The phenomenal world is created by ignorance and, therefore, unreal. The supreme self is mistaken for the unreal world, in the same way as a rope may be mistaken for a snake in twilight. In fact, the bondage and liberation of the self are illusory, as the soul is never bound. The limitation of the soul is just an illusion and, in relative terms, what we call liberation of the soul is self-knowledge or self-realization.

Sankara, the Great, emphasizes the fact that such knowledge is not merely a theory that can be acquired from books and lectures, but is of the nature of direct realization or experience. Moreover, this knowledge of the self, *Aham Brahmasmi* or (I am Brahma) cannot take place merely by reasoning alone. It can be achieved only by the student whose mind is purified by service and devotion and who hears this truth directly from the mouth of his spiritual teacher. Again, for such initiation and realization of the self, purification of the mind is a prerequisite for every student. It is then and then alone that the disciple realizes in a flash, "I am Brahman, or the absolute," and the individual self is seen in all times and conditions to be one with the supreme self, the absolute being.

From the above point of view, though, it appears as though there were a denial of the personal God. It must be remembered here that spiritual perfection or liberation is impossible without the grace of God and teacher, which is attainable through devotion, prayer, meditation, and selfless service to humanity.

"However, to those whose minds are fully ripe, the above Yoga is by itself productive of perfection." It is easily and speedily attainable by all who have faith in the teacher and in the Lord" (Sankara, the Great). From the above few lines of *Sankaracharya* it is clear that there is need both of a teacher and of devotion to the Lord to attain perfection.

## SELF AS SAT-CHIT-ANANDA

Every one of us, however great or small, saint or sinner, rich or poor, king or beggar, strives for happiness and not for misery. We desire the pleasant and not the unpleasant. Why should we not be happy? It is an instinctive desire to have joy. Now, what percentage of pleasure does man seek? The answer is 100 per cent. How can we get 100 per cent of happiness? Let us take a man who has everything he wants and millions of dollars in the bank, is he satisfied? If he has a million dollars, he will desire two million dollars; and the moment his desire is fulfilled, he will try to multiply two million into four, and goes on endlessly. Is there any limit when he will have complete satisfaction? Why all these possessions and money? The simple answer is for enjoyment. But will he get all the joy he seeks through multiplying his desires? Again there is no answer to how to obtain 100 per cent happiness.

This quest for happiness goes on endlessly because man is vainly searching outside something that he has lost and that he will never be able to find if he continues his pursuit in the world of the senses. That something is the joy of the self or soul.

An old lady lost a gold needle in her bedroom. Though the needle was lost in her bedroom, she went on searching for it outside the house, in the garden. Not only was she looking for the lost needle, but she called her neighbor to help her. When her friend asked her why she was looking for it in the garden instead of in the bedroom, her answer was simple. "Because there is no light in my room. I am searching for the needle where there is light." In the same way, man seeks the lost happiness of his soul in the sense world. This is the cause of man's dissatisfaction, as he is not able to find the inner joy of the soul. Today, tomorrow, or in the next life, every one of us will stop seeking his happiness outside and turn inward to the self or soul.

The pure self is bliss itself; hence there is an inborn desire to be happy. In Sanskrit, this bliss aspect of the self is called *ananda*, and the knowledge aspect is *chit*, and the existence aspect is *sat*. Therefore, the self is known as *sat-chit-ananda* (existence, knowledge, and bliss). This triple nature of the self is expressed in the individual as triple desire: (1) desire to exist; (3) desire to know; (3) desire to have a joyous nature.

Now the question arises, If joy is the nature of the self, then why does man feel miserable? The answer is that the two sources of misery are the sense of "I-ness" in the body and the sense of "mineness." Even the learned man undergoes suffering from disease or assault by mistaking the transient body for the self, and experiences extreme sorrow at the loss of wife, son, or wealth, but not at the loss of an enemy, because there is no "I-ness" or "mineness" in the case of an enemy. The bliss of the self, when it gets clouded over, we call love, attraction for gross bodies, and external things. This is only a distorted manifestation of that blessedness. Pain is not the nature of the soul. The question why water is hot shows the nature of water is not hot, and if it is hot, there is a cause for it (the union with fire). Just as when fire (the cause of heat) has gone, the heat vanishes, and water exists in the original cool state, so also the pain and sorrow caused by "I-ness" and "mineness" vanish as time goes on. Just as heat is not the property of water, so also sorrow is not an inherent property of man. Therefore man will eternally seek only the joy of the self and not the pain of the sense world.

Every man exists; every man must know; and every man is made for love. Real existence is limitless, unmixed, uncombined, knows no change, is a free soul. When it becomes mixed with the mind, it becomes what we call individual existence. When we hear of a person's death, we always ask, "Why did he die?" This question shows that the inherent property of the soul is not death. But when we hear of the birth of a baby, we do not ask, "Why does the child live?" So, living or existence is an inherent property of the self. If a child has two dollars and loses one of them, he asks where the other dollar has gone. Even a child does not believe that an existing thing cannot exist. Therefore, the nature of the self is eternal existence, and there is no death or birth for the self, as its nature is existence itself.

The third aspect of the self is knowledge. Everyone wishes to be independent and a scholar; everyone wants to be a teacher. Nobody wants to be guided by others. Everybody, in his heart, really wishes to be a knower of everything, if only he could. Nobody wants to believe that there is anybody who knows more than he does. Whatever he thinks, his religion, philosophy, science, or God is the greatest knowledge. The real cause of such thinking is that his pure self is knowledge itself, and when this pure knowledge is associated with the mind, it becomes objective knowledge. Again, just as the man in quest of eternal enjoyment in the outside world finds that joy is within himself, so also man's quest for knowledge will never be complete until he turns his vision inward. Is there any limit to man's knowledge? Scientists, day and night, unveil the mystery of nature and man is growing in knowledge and strength day after day. Some scale Mount Everest to learn, and others navigate under the Arctic Ocean, while others fly to outer space. Some retire from the world and hide in Himalayan caves, while others wander from place to place—all in search of knowledge. But from where does man get complete knowledge? The *Upanishads* declare that all knowledge is in the self and, in fact, knowledge itself is self. This is the end of knowledge, or Vedanta. That eternal knowledge of the self when reflected through the mind and brain of man becomes intuition, reason, and instinct. Its manifestation varies according to the medium through which it shines. In lower animals it is manifested as instinct, in man as reason, and in advanced man as intuition. Individual existence is a manifestation of the real existence of the self, and the bliss that is manifested as love or attraction is a reflection of the all-blissful self. Absolute bliss, knowledge, and existence are not qualities of the self but are one and the same.

The pure self is conditioned by the mind, and when that limitation is destroyed, the unconditioned self shines, as *sat-chit-ananda* (existence, knowledge, and bliss), like the sun when the clouds have disappeared. Even a little theoretical knowledge of the self brings great joy and courage to those afflicted by pain and miseries of the world. Then what would be the state of joy and bliss by realizing the self as *sat-chit-ananda*? Though the absolute realization of self for ordinary people at the present state of evolution may take a long time, one could get great joy and comfort by following the path of Yoga and Vedanta while doing his worldly duties. Although dwelling in the house as the head of the family doing his duties, a wise man remains there like a guest of honor, unaffected. So also one feels neither happiness nor misery if one lives as a master while residing in the body. This nonattachment with the body and identification with the absolute being under all circumstances are the real knowledge, which brings real happiness.

# 12

# CONQUEST OF DEATH

Among the strongest motive powers of religion and religious life are the thought of death and the fear of hell. The common man is afraid of death. He would like to live forever. He wants to know where he is going, even after the dissolution of his body. This is the starting point of real philosophy, which inquires into the wonders of death.

Great philosophers, prophets, and religious leaders agree that a clear understanding of man's·relation to God and the universe is the only way to escape the fear of death, and, in the spiritual sense of the word, to escape death itself. When man realizes that the immortal self is identical with the supreme self or God, what, then, is death and where is fear? The one theme of the Vedanta philosophy is the search after the unity of the individual self with the universal self or God. When this unity is achieved, no fear or death can remain.

Now let us see what death means in ordinary terms and what happens to the soul after death. Mortality means decomposition, and decomposition is possible only for things that are the result of composition; anything that is made of two or three ingredients must become decomposed. Not so the soul, which is not the result of composition, but is a single entity apart from mind and body. It can, thus, never become decomposed and can, therefore, never die. It is immortal. It has existed throughout eternity and was not created. Never has anything come out of nothing. Whatever we know of creation is the combination of already existing things into newer forms. That being so, the soul of man, which is not a combination of anything, must have been in existence forever and will continue to exist forever.

When the body dies, the vital forces of man go back to his astral body, and the soul of man is again clothed in this astral body composed of mind, senses, and vital forces.

In this astral body lie all the *samskaras* (impressions) of man. What are the *samskaras* or impressions? The mind is like a lake, and every thought is like a wave upon that lake. Just as waves rise, fall, and disappear, so these thought waves are continuously rising in the mental lake and then disappearing, but they do not disappear forever. To use a different metaphor, it is as though they remained in the form of seeds, ready to sprout up once more when called upon to do so. Memory is simply calling back these submerged seed thoughts that have been buried deep in the subconscious. Thus, everything man has thought or done is lodged in the subconscious in the seed form, and when the body dies, the soul moves into its finer vehicle, the astral body, with all these seeds of impressions and the soul is guided by the force of these impressions. According to these forces of thought and actions of the past, there are three different roads for the soul to travel in its temporary astral existence. When they die, the souls of those who are truly and completely spiritual follow the solar rays and reach the solar sphere and finally meet another soul on its journey that is already blessed, and this soul guides the newcomer forward to the highest of all spheres, which is called the sphere of Brahma. There, these souls attain omniscience and omnipotence and live forever, according to dualists; or, according to nondualists, they become one with the universal being at the end of the cycle. This is called progressive liberation or *kramamukthi.*

The souls of the next class of virtuous people, those who have done good work but with selfish motives, are as the result of their good works carried when they die to the lunar sphere, where there are various heavens in which they acquire fine bodies—the bodies of gods or angels. There they live enjoying the blessings of heaven for a long period until the merit of their good actions, which entitled them to live in this heavenly sphere, is exhausted. They then fall back to earth or material plane and are born again as human beings. Thus, heaven is only a temporary period of rest where the soul enjoys the fruits of its good actions as long as its merits last, but cannot have a permanent abode. Once again the soul in a new body must strive to achieve its further evolution. It cannot evolve to a higher level in the astral worlds or heavenly worlds, since they are for enjoyment only and not for fresh actions. For its progress onward, the soul must put on a new physical body. This process is called the birth of a new soul, although the soul is always the same and carries within itself all the impressions and knowledge of its previous physical existences. This cycle of birth and death goes on endlessly until the soul is finally liberated from the law of *karma* or actions and reactions; for good actions bring good fruit and bad actions bring bad fruit.

It should here be made clear that "good" and "bad" as used in this connection, and indeed in all Vedanta philosophy, are relative terms. There is no action that is either good or bad in itself: its quality depends upon the motive behind it. Even charity itself, if performed for the selfish purpose of gaining prestige or power, cannot be determined to be wholly good. By the same token, even killing a man, if done with a selfless motive, as for example by a policeman to protect the innocent from a murderer or by a soldier in defense of his country, cannot be deemed bad. The soldier or the policeman is only carrying out his duties and hence there is no selfishness. So in all things the motive determines the virtue or vice of the deed.

But ultimately, all actions, whether good or bad, are like chains that bind the soul to the wheel of birth and death. Good actions bind the soul with gold chains and bad actions with iron chains. But as long as the soul is bound, be it with gold or with iron, or both, it is still a prisoner. The only way for man to break the chains is for him to give up all thought of enjoying the fruits of his actions. By this renunciation the soul is liberated from the cycle of birth and death. This great philosophy is stated very clearly and simply in the Old Testament story of Adam and Eve.

The Lord asked Adam and Eve not to eat the fruit from the tree. What was that tree? The tree was *aswadha*, the sense world, which bears only two kinds of fruits—good fruit from good actions and evil fruit from evil actions. As long as Adam and Eve (the souls) were not interested in enjoying the fruits of their actions, they were not bound by the law of Karma. But as soon as they associated with *kama nanas* or lower mind, as represented by the serpent, the souls (Adam and Eve), wanted to enjoy and to know the sense world, rather than to heed the voice of the pure self or God within. Thus, the soul in its pure form without any sin, when tempted by the lower mind (the serpent), becomes a sinner or individual limited by *karma*, the law of action and reaction. To enjoy the fruits of actions, a physical body is essential. Thus, only when Adam and Eve ate the fruit did they realize they were naked, which means that they were born again as human beings subject to the miseries and pains of the physical world. These miseries and pains are the curse of God, or of the pure consciousness.

Thus is expressed in the Bible the same wisdom as is expressed in the *Gita* when Lord Krishna instructs Arjuna: "Do your duty or work but do not expect any fruits from your actions." The lesson of both is that there is only one way to be pure souls without sins. This is by heeding the voice of the inner soul or God, and abandoning the desire to enjoy, thus freeing oneself from the cycle of birth and death.

Now comes the last class of people, namely, the wicked. When they die, their souls become ghosts or demons and live somewhere midway between the lunar sphere and this earth. Some try to disturb mankind as they did while they were in their physical existence. Some are friendly, and after living in the mid-sphere for some time, they also fall back, as the souls from the heavenly sphere do, either into an animal body or into a lower type of undeveloped bushman. After living for some time in an animal body, they come back again in a human body, once more to work out their salvation.

The souls of those people who are most highly evolved spiritually go to the *brahma loka* waiting to be one with the Supreme Being; the souls of those who, by reason of their virtuous actions, are in the middle stage of evolution, go to heaven; and the last type go to the lower sphere. However, it must be remembered here that the soul or the self is the same whether it be that of an advanced man or a sinner. Actions can only cloud the soul, which shines like the sun. When the soul is clouded with a thick cloud, we call man a sinner, and when it is less clouded, a good man. But, however virtuous and pure an act may be, it is still tainted by impurity, as good and bad are only relative terms. All actions are products of the mind and so of the world. In the physical world, man enjoys all objects with his body, mind, and senses. Without the mind there is no world. This philosophy applies to the astral spheres too, because heaven and hell are also the products of the mind. Without the mind, one can neither enjoy heaven nor suffer in hell. So when the mind is pure through virtuous actions, man feels enjoyment. This state of mind in the astral sphere is called heaven. In the same way, when the mind in life is dense and dark because of brute actions, then after death the mind functions on lower planes, which we call hell.

Man, therefore, according to the Vedanta philosophy, is the greatest being in this universe, and this world of work (*karma bhoomy*) the best place in it, because only herein is the greatest and the best chance for him to become perfect and conquer death.

Vedanta declares that this entire world, including heaven and hell, and all the bodies in this world have no existence except in the imagination of the mind of man. It is the imagination and the current of thought turning in the wrong direction that brings all sorrow, pain, anxiety, and death. It is the mind turned in the wrong direction that mistakes the body for the immortal self and binds the soul; and the mind directed in the right channel that liberates the soul from the cycle of birth and death.

The ladder from which one falls, so to speak, is the same ladder that leads one up. One must retrace one's steps by the same road down which one descends to this mortal world. The kind of imagination that Vedanta recommends for the liberation of the soul is just the opposite of the imagination that produces base worldly thoughts, enslaves, binds, and keeps one at the mercy of all sorts of circumstances.

A man dreams, and in his dream all sorts of things appear. Those things in the dream are mere ideas, mere thought and imagination, yet for the person dreaming, a tiger or a lion in a dream is as real as a living one, and he is startled and awakened. But as soon as he is awake, fear of the tiger or lion vanishes and without further explanation he knows that all the objects in the dream world were unreal.

Similarly, the whole world is a dream. The pictures of birth and death, big and small, rich and poor, good and evil, pain and pleasure are nothing but false imagination. The practice of Yoga and Vedanta leads one to that place where all imagination ceases, where all language ceases, in which there remains only that one indescribable reality. In that state there is no more birth or death for the soul, and the soul shines in itself.

Now there comes the objection from the vast majority of undeveloped souls. "If we are landed into this superconscious state where all consciousness and thought cease, is that not a state of vacancy or emptiness? Is it not a state of senselessness? Is it not self-hypnotism? What is the use of taking all the trouble to enter into a state of unconsciousness?

To this objection, Vedanta replies that there is a whole world of difference between the state of realization or superconsciousness and the state of unconsciousness, though one thing is common to both —all thought stops.

We all know that a ray of the sun passed through a prism produces seven visible colors. But on either side of the spectrum there are invisible rays that our naked eyes cannot detect—on one side infrared and on the other ultraviolet. Because both of these rays are invisible to the naked eye, it does not mean they are one and the same. The difference is that infrared rays are invisible because their wave length is too long, and ultraviolet because their wave length is too short to excite the retina. Similarly the superconscious state is one kind of suspension of thoughts, where the past and future merge with the present; and the unconscious state is another kind, where there is no thought but only a state of blankness. The unconscious state, when the mind stops thinking because of lack of activity, resembles death; but the superconscious state, or state of realization, is all energy, all power, all knowledge, all bliss. Again, in the absence of light, one cannot see, and when there is excessive light, it is also impossible to see. Darkness caused by lack of light is one thing, and darkness caused by excessive light is another thing. Similarly, cessation of thought in the state of realization of the self (superconsciousness) is the opposite of the cessation of thought in an unconscious state or state of deep sleep.

Those who think that Vedanta teaches pessimism are mistaken. What Vedanta teaches is how to keep the whole world and oneself under control. Vedanta does not mean that we should live a life of inactivity. A real Vedantin has more love toward his brothers than the so-called humanitarians. He sees himself in everything and feels himself to be one with everything. It is not merely a philosophy but a living experience for him. He cannot tolerate the suffering of other beings, as they are all as his own self.

For the Vedantin the whole universe is made up of one infinite ocean of love. This infinite love manifested in the material world is finite human love. When in the material world this infinite love is broken down and limited to anything less than the entire world, say to family, friends, and even neighbors but not to every single creature and object as an extension of oneself, then it is known as finite or human love. Finite love is always associated with its opposite, hatred. In the infinite love of a God-realized soul there is no hatred. Gravitation is attraction, and that is love. The stars are held together by gravitation, which is the manifestation of the great attraction. There is love between atom and atom, which makes molecules. In fact, Yogis envisage the whole world as the waves of one great ocean of love. All desire is love, and God is love and "God ye are." Realization of this love and oneness with God is superconsciousness.

Now the question is raised: Is this state not caused by self-hypnotism? Vedanta answers that question: It is not self-hypnotism but rather dehypnotization. Every day man hypnotizes himself by identifying himself with the perishable body. He expresses this as he says,

"I am Mr. So-and-So." To overcome this state of hypnotic suggestion, Vedanta seeks to evoke opposite thought currents to help man to rise above his consciousness of body.

## VEDANTIC MEDITATION TO CONQUER DEATH AND DEVELOP INTUITION

In Vedantic meditation the most important thing is to realize that one's real self is the sun of suns, the light of lights. In the state of meditation one can rise above the body and above the mind and dehypnotize onself into the light of lights, into the sun of suns.

Meditation should be started after a few rounds of breathing exercise and a few minutes of chanting of the name of the Supreme Almighty who resides in the heart of hearts as the self or *atman,* and when the mind obtains some exaltation or is elevated to a certain height, it becomes very easy to make it soar much higher and even to great heights. One must make the mind rise into the higher regions by humming the syllable *OM (AUM).* The meaning of the syllable *OM* is different to different persons. Everyone in his own stage of spiritual development has to give it the meaning that suits him best. Some people meditate on *OM* as the sun of suns shining within their hearts, while others meditate upon the *ajna chakra* (space between the eyebrows) while chanting *OM.* One can choose and meditate on either of these places (the heart or the space between the eyebrows.)

While chanting *OM* one should meditate on the meaning attached to it, as follows:

> I am the light of lights; I am the sun; I am the real, real sun; the apparent sun is my symbol only. [In dreams we see objects not by the light of a lamp, nor by the light of the moon, sun, or stars, and yet we see them. If without light we cannot see, then with what light do we see light?] It is the light of my real self; it is the light of my *atman,* and it is my light that makes everything visible in my dreams.
>
> I am a monarch of monarchs. It is I who appear as all the beautiful flowers in different gardens. In me the whole world lives, moves, and has its being. Everywhere it is my will that is being done. I am manifested everywhere, I feed every being, from the smallest microbes to man. I existed before the world began.

Evil thoughts and worldly desires are things concerning the false body and the false mind, and are things of darkness. In my presence they have no right to make their appearance. I am not bound by any actions; I command elements. I am all-pervading, like supreme ether. Like light and invisible rays, I permeate and pervade every atom and every object. I am the lowest; I am the highest; I am the spectator, I am the showman, I am the performer. I am the most famous people, and most disreputable, ignominious; I am the most fallen. Oh, how beautiful I am! I shine in the lightning; I roar in the thunder; I flutter in leaves; I hiss in the winds; I roll in the surging seas. The friend I am; the foe I am. To me, no friends, no foes. Whatever be the state of this body, it concerns me not; all bodies are mine. I am the whole universe; everything is in me; I am limitless, eternal, all-pervading. I am in each and all. I am in you; you are in me. Nay, there can be no you and I, no difference. *Soham, Soham, Soham.* I am that, I am that, I am that. *OM OM OM.*

To realize his self, a beginner gets great help from the chanting of the syllable *OM* while meditating on its meaning. With this kind of meditation, one frees oneself from the clutches of death and attains immortality. No action can bind one, as there is no agency or "enjoyership" in one's actions. One always identifies oneself with the all-pervading self by removing "I-ness" and "mineness."

Before beginning this kind of meditation, students are advised to remove the three impurities of the mind: *mala* or selfishness; *vikshepa* or tossing of the mind; and *avarana*, or the veiling power, if they wish to achieve quick results. These three impurities of the mind may be described as follows:

1. *Mala*, or selfishness, is the grossest impurity. It is to be found in all men, in varying degrees and intensities, according to the degree of spiritual development of their souls; and it can be removed only through selfless service. Therefore every student, low or evolved, should spend some time in serving others without thought of reward before proceeding to deeper meditation.
2. The second impurity is known as *vikshepa sakthi*, or tossing of the mind. Mind becomes unsteady because of this impurity, and concentration becomes difficult. The Yogi method

of stopping this tossing is through Yogic breathing (see Breathing, Chapter 8), devotion, and chanting.

3. The last is the subtlest of all impurities, known as *avarana sakthi*, or the veiling power of the mind. This *avarana sakthi* clouds the pure consciousness or self, and produces body consciousness. This is the most difficult impurity (the idea of body consciousness) to get rid of. Vedantic meditation and the inquiry, "Who am I?" removes this veiling power. Only then can the self shine of itself.

## THE PHILOSOPHY AND MEANING OF THE SACRED SYLLABLE OM

Several volumes have been written to explain the meaning of the great syllable *OM*. In fact, all Vedanta and all Hindu philosophy is simply an exposition of this syllable *OM*. *OM* covers the whole universe. There is not a law, a force, or an object in all the world that is not comprised within the syllable *OM*. We shall try to explain how all the planes of being, all the worlds, all phases of existence are encompassed by *OM*. The importance of this syllable will be explored from various points of view in order that people may attempt to grasp it with their minds as well as accept it with their whole hearts. As we are all rational beings, we should not take up anything unless it appeals to our intellect.

The literal meaning of Vedanta is the end of knowledge, the end of speech; and the whole of Vedanta is represented by *OM*. *OM* consists of *A, U, M*, and according to the rules of Sanskrit grammar, *A* and *U* when joined together become *O*, and thus *A, U, M*, produces the sound *OM*. The sound of *OM* is the most natural sound that can be uttered; even a mute can produce this sound. Observe boys in a playground when they are very happy; their overflowing joy finds natural expression with a prolonged sound of *O*, which is simply *OM* cut short. Not only children, but all people use this sound on occasions when they feel exhilarated, whether it is at a football game, a horse race, or a party. It is common to note that many people answer "Oh, yes," or "Oh, my God!" When one is sick in bed or in trouble, when one is suffering from extreme pain, this sound of *oh* or *um*, which is a corrupted expression of *OM*, comes from one's lips. The Hebrew, Arab, and English prayers end with "Amen," which most remarkably resembles *Aum*.

Why should this sound be so prominent in everybody's life? The answer is because it is a natural sound; it brings relief from pain for a sick person; it expresses mental moods in the form of sounds, which in turn bring peace and harmony. If one gets a little relief from pain by uttering this sound incorrectly, then may it not bring more peace and harmony if it is chanted in the right way? This *OM* is also known as *pranava,* or that which pervades life or runs through the *prana* or breath. Even the sound of bells, the noise of a flowing river, the whistling of the wind, or blowing of a conch shell produces the sound *OM.*

All thought is related to language as the obverse and reverse sides of the same coin. One cannot exist without the other. Can anyone see an object without thinking of it? Nothing is perceived without thinking accordingly. The very word "perceive" signifies mental thought. Thought and language are the same, and one cannot think without language.

Absence of language occurs primarily in two cases: in intuitive perception and intuitive ideation. Intuitive ideation is the formation of a mental image of an object. I see a tree and close my eyes and see it again in mental image. Every form is associated with a name and utterance of a name brings forth the picture of the object. When I say "chair," immediately the form of a chair appears in my mind. Though many mental images of sights and sounds occur that do not always bring up their names, and though this intuitive process may actually take place without language, yet in description, analysis, classification, judgment, and other mental elaborations, language is indispensable. One can look at the moon without remembering the name of the moon, but when one analyzes and thinks of what it is, then language comes. Therefore, nothing is perceived in this world without thought, and there can be no thought without language. Thus the world is related to language; language, to thought; and thought, to the world

In the Bible it is said: "In the beginning was the Word, and the Word was with God, and the Word was God." The word or language is not something arbitrary or invented. No man ever invented language because the word itself is God. The Vedic language (the original language) was revealed by God directly to the mind and when it was corrupted, it was called human language. Now we want to have a single word or sound that will represent the whole world. In all languages we have some sounds that come from the throat, others that come from the palate, and others from the lips. There is not a single sound in any language that comes from organs below the throat, as the throat is the one boundary of the vocal organ, and none come from outside the lips as the lips are the other boundary. Now we have A, U, M. The sound A is guttural; it comes from the throat. U (oo) proceeds exactly from the middle of the vocal region, the palate. M is labial and nasal, which comes from the extremity of the vocal organ or lips.

Thus, A represents the beginning of the range of sound; U represents the middle, and M represents the end. It covers the whole field of the vocal organs. Thus OM represents all language and, since world and language are interrelated, it represents all the world.

Sounds are of two kinds: articulate or *varnatmak* and inarticulate or *dhvanyatmak*. *Varnatmak* sounds are capable of being written, while *dhvanyatmak* cannot be expressed by characters or by written words. Ordinary language is *varnatmak*, and the language of feeling, such as laughter and weeping, is *dhvanyatmak*. Laughter cannot be expressed in written language.

The articulate or natural language (*dhvanyatmak*) has a purpose that cannot be served by *varnatmak*. Suppose a foreigner who does not know the language of another country wants some food, and people cannot understand his language. He may then start weeping because of hunger; this language of feeling (weeping) can be understood and people give him food. When you laugh, everyone understands that something pleasant has happened. The language of music is also *dhvanyatmak*. The language of music is different from the language of thought. In melodious music there is a charming effect upon the mind. Similarly, OM chanting has a charm about it that brings the mind of one who chants under control and directly brings the feeling of peace and rest to the mind. In that state the individual is one with God. Though the effect of the chanting of OM cannot be scientifically proved, it is nonetheless experienced by all who practice it sincerely. There is no denying the changes within oneself when they take place.

Now let us discuss the philosophy of AUM. The sound A, according to the teaching of Vedanta, represents the so-called material universe, the world of the gross senses, that which is observed in the waking state. All the experience of the dream world and the world of spirits, the astral plane, and heaven and hell are signified by U. M represents the unknown, the deep-sleep state and all those things which are beyond the comprehension of the intellect.

Thus, AUM (OM) covers all the threefold experience of man (waking, dreaming, and deep sleep).

It is a common thing to note that generally the philosophy of the West is based on experience in the waking state and takes little or no notice of the experience of the dream or of the deep-sleep state. Vedanta says that in order to find out the reality or truth, one must analyze all three states of experience of man; otherwise the data will be incomplete. Most philosophers limit themselves to the waking state, and all their discoveries and investigations are based on the waking state alone. Vedanta considers all the data from the threefold experiences. The world of the waking state disappears entirely in the other two states, dreaming and deep sleep.

In dreams, though the external world disappears, it is the same "I" which perceives. The intellect and personal consciousness vanish entirely in the deep-sleep state and yet the real "I" or self remains the same. Thus "I" or self is the same in all these three states, and this self is the underlying reality that experiences all these states. This unchangeable and immutable principle, this reality that remains constant through the threefold worlds, is the true self or *atman*. This is *OM*.

How do we know that the world exists? How do we know there is a universe? Because we touch, hear, see, smell, and taste things; that is the only proof. Our senses are the only direct or indirect proof of the existence of this world.

Sensation is the primary cause of all perception, intellectual understanding, etc., and it is not limited to our waking state alone. In the waking state our senses are in the gross form and we perceive objects. But we perceive in our dream state also. The sense organs operate in the dream state even though the external ears and eyes are not functioning. Thus in effect the dreaming mind evokes simultaneously both the object and the sense organs that perceive the object. So in dreamland the senses and the objects sensed are like the positive and negative poles of the same object. In dreams the subject and the object spring up together. Both the subject and the object of dreams are represented by the sound *U* in *AUM*, and the underlying reality, in which both the subject and the object appear as waves in the ocean, is the pure self or *OM*.

Although objects in dreams are produced simultaneously with the corresponding perceiving senses, they appear to have a long past of their own and as long as one is dreaming, so long is the dream reality for one's consciousness. When we say that this solid, rigid world is real, the statement is entirely founded on the evidence of perceiving senses and is equivalent to the dreaming person calling the object of the dream real whereas in reality both waking and dreaming states are unreal.

The senses themselves exist only by virtue of the elements they perceive. Without the objective world of the elements, the senses could not perceive whether they were in a dreaming or a waking state; so for the existence of the senses the objective world is essential. In the same way, for the existence of the world the senses are essential. Is that not reasoning in a circle? It is, indeed, and serves only to prove the illusory nature of the world in the waking state as in the dream state. The objects of dreams are real as long as the dream lasts. Those objects are no more when one wakes. In the deep-sleep state, what happens to the solid world of the waking state? Everything disappears. Thus we see that there is no reality to the world either in the waking state or in the dream state.

Vedanta defines reality as that which persists in all circumstances. That which appears as reality at one time and disappears like a mist after awhile must be an illusory phenomenon. The dreamland we call unreal because when we are awake it is not there. Just so the solid must be unreal because it also vanishes in the dream and deep-sleep states.

Then what is reality? The sound A in AUM represents the apparent subject (senses) and object (elements or world) of the waking state as mere manifestations of the underlying reality, me. The only hard reality is the Self or "I," which never changes in any state. That "I" is the witness of the waking, dreaming, and deep-sleep states. Thus Vedanta comes to the conclusion that all the three states of man, waking, dreaming, and deep sleep, are unreal and the real self, which is knowledge absolute, existence absolute, and bliss absolute, is the only stern reality, before which the apparent reality of the world melts away.

Many do not like to accept this conclusion because it is derived from considering the dreaming and deep-sleep states as rivals of the waking state. If we analyze our lives, almost half of the time we are either in a dreaming or a deep-sleep state. There being night at any time over half the surface of the earth, almost half the population is always in the dreaming or deep-sleep state. Thus a man spends almost half of his life either in sleep or in dream. Childhood is a long dream. If we count the time, the hours spent in the waking state are almost equal to the time spent in sleeping and dreaming. Therefore we cannot consider only those things that take place in the waking state as all of reality and the other states as unreal. Even the strongest man or wisest man without exception is bound by the law of sleep, and the inexorable power of sleep takes no account of his ardent desire to stay awake and enjoy the sense world. Since the dream and deep-sleep states are as powerful as the waking state, we cannot neglect these former two states and consider only the latter. That is why Vedanta philosophy delves deeply into all the threefold states of man to find out the underlying reality. Again there are plants in a state of perpetual deep sleep and there are animals in a constant state of dreaming. To them our world is different. To the eyes of an ant, a frog, an elephant, a fish, or an owl things are very different. How dare we disregard their experience and consider the waking state of man alone as real?

Thus in *OM* (*AUM*) the first letter *A* stands for this reality, the self, as underlying and manifesting the illusory material world of the waking state. *U* represents the dream and the psychic or astral worlds, and the last letter, *M*, denotes the absolute self underlying the chaotic state and represents all the unknown, the deep sleep. Thus *OM* means the underlying reality behind the scenes, the eternal truth, the indestructible self that one is, and when *OM* is chanted one must throw the body and mind into the true self and melt into the real *atman* or pure consciousness.

A Yogi through *pranayama* and meditation on *OM* transcends one by one all the planes and finally reaches the seventh and the last stage, where the soul is freed from all bondage and merges with the cosmic consciousness. The development of the mind determines which one of the seven stages to conquer death a Yogi has achieved, how far or how near he is to his higher self. The seven stages may be described as follows.

The first stage is *subhecha* or a longing for the truth. One who has rightly distinguished between the permanent and impermanent, who has cultivated a feeling of dislike toward worldly pleasures, who having acquired full mastery over his *physical body* and *mind* feels an insatiable longing to free himself from this cycle of birth and death, has attained this first stage.

The second stage is *vicharana* or right inquiry. He who has pondered over what he has read and heard and has realized the truth in his life has attained the second stage. This is not an intellectual understanding. He knows the truth by realizing it in himself through constant practice and not by blind faith.

The third stage is *tanumanasa* or the fading of the mind. When the mind, having abandoned the many (the external world), remains steadily fixed on the one (supreme being), it has attained the third stage.

The fourth stage is *satvapatti* or attainment of the state of *sattva* or purity. Having reduced his mind by the three previous stages to a state of pure *sattva* or purity, when man knows directly in himself the truth (I am Brahman or God), he is in the fourth stage. This is a direct experience and not an intellectual understanding that "I am Brahman." In this stage intuition takes the place of the intellect; it is above the intellect, as the intellect is limited.

In these first four stages man practices *samprajnata samadhi* or contemplation, where the consciousness or duality still lingers. He feels the separation from the object of contemplation. In this state of consciousness he is not completely identical or one with his higher self as duality still lingers in his consciousness. Up to this stage he is considered to be a practitioner or student.

The three remaining stages beyond the *samprajnata samadhi* are knower, knowledge, and known. Here the individual self merges with the higher self. Hence there is nothing to be known or meditated upon; with nothing to be meditated upon, there cannot be any objective knowledge. As the individual self or "I" consciousness merges with universal consciousness wherein man sees nothing external to himself, there cannot be any knower either. These three stages are known as: (1) *asamsaktha*, being unaffected by anything; (2) *pararthabhavina* where the external things do not appear to exist; and (3) *turya*, where the Yogi sees nothing but God everywhere.

When the Yogi is unaffected by the psychic powers (*sidhis*) that manifest themselves at this stage, he attains the stage called *asamsaktha* or being unaffected by anything. This is the fifth stage.

In the sixth stage the external things to the consciousness of the Yogi do not appear to exist; hence this stage is known as *parartha-bhavina*.

The seventh stage is called *turya*. The Yogi sees nothing but Brahman or God everywhere. In this state a Yogi neither performs his daily duties himself nor is prompted by others, but remains in a state of perpetual *samadhi* or superconsciousness. This state of experience of a Yogi wherein he knows in himself bliss absolute, knowledge absolute, and existence absolute can never be explained by ordinary human language. Here individual self merges with the all-pervading supreme self as a drop of water merges with the ocean and becomes one with it.

For undeveloped minds, this idea of losing the individual consciousness is frightening. This is only because of the veiling power of the mind, which limits the consciousness and brings false pictures and ideas, which frighten him. Yogi philosophy declares that self-realization or God realization alone can bring real peace, joy, and liberation of the embodied souls. Yogi realizes that the self alone exists, which is manifest as the universe. Everything in the universe is that one self, appearing in various forms. He realizes that the self, when it appears behind the universe, is called God and that the same self when it appears behind this body is the individual soul or *jiva*.

Yogi realizes "I am Brahman." The whole universe is myself. Whatever exists, I am. "I am neither the body, nor the organs, nor was I the mind; I am existence, knowledge, and bliss absolute; I am he." Where is knowledge for me? I am knowledge itself. I am the free one. Where is joy for me? I am bliss itself. This is the knowledge or realization that a Yogi attains: this knowledge brings freedom and freedom is the goal of all nature. Bondage of the soul is death and freedom of the soul is the liberation or conquest of death.

## OM TAT SAT

# TRAINING TABLES

The training tables which follow are based upon my many years of teaching and research with individuals of various age groups. The exercises contained herein may be practiced with safety and are ideal for everyone wishing to attain spiritual perfection and perfect health of body and mind.

In the event that a given portion of the instructions is not clearly understood, the student is encouraged to consult the text of the book for more explicit directions. He is, moreover, advised to select the table appropriate for his age and physical condition.

If the student finds that he does not have sufficient time to practice all of the exercises recommended for him, it is suggested that he perform as many of the basic exercises from each of the groups as are convenient for him to undertake. For example, the exercises in Table 3, Lesson III require from one to two hours to complete, in which case, because of insufficient time, the matter of selectivity arises. In this event, it must be remembered that the principal rule in the performance of any exercise is that it is to be countered with a performance of its direct opposite, since counter-exercising is related directly to the spine. Therefore, if a forward bending exercise is selected, it is imperative that a backward bending exercise is performed to offset it.

In expanding the subject of counter-exercising, and using Table 3, Lesson III once again to demonstrate it, the student will note that in the backward and forward bending exercise groups there are several poses recommended for practice. Here, an advisable approach would be to select and perform two or three of these exercises from each group the first day and then, on the following day, complete the exercises previously omitted. In this way, within a few weeks, the body will have undergone a complete cycle of exercises.

In regard to exercising it is urgent that such essentials as the headstand, shoulderstand, sun exercises, and breathing, relaxation, meditation, etc., are practiced daily in addition to the other recommended exercises, whenever possible within the student's time limit.

Because of space limitations, the order of exercise is not given in the training tables and is presented here in numerical sequence for easy reference:

1) Prayer before beginning exercises
2) Sun exercises
3) Relaxation (two to three minutes; longer if required)
4) Headstand
5) Shoulderstand
6) Fish pose (to be followed by a brief period of relaxation)
7) Forward bending exercises
8) Backward bending exercises
9) Twisting exercises
10) Balancing exercises
11) Leg and foot exercises (sitting)
12) Exercises in standing position
13) Complete relaxation for ten to fifteen minutes (end of physical exercises)
14) Abdominal exercises
15) Breathing exercises
16) Meditation

Breathing and meditation may be performed separately (during the morning hours, with exercises performed in the evening, or viceversa); cleansing exercises should be done separately in the early morning along with care of the teeth and body. Meditative positions need not be practiced separately, as they are part of the breathing and concentration exercises.

Students unable to obtain a competent teacher may safely practice the exercises given in Training Tables 1 and 2, since they are mild, but extremely effective. The training tables and the text will serve as teacher and guide throughout your practice at home.

## TRAINING TABLE 1

Yogic Exercises for Very Old People and Sick People

NOTE: *Physical and breathing exercises may be intensified and extended upon the advice of your teacher*

| Yogic discipline of body and mind | Lesson I—2 to 6 weeks, or more |
| --- | --- |
| HIP AND LEG EXERCISES | *Pavana Mukthasan* (liberated pose), Plate 15, six to twelve times |
| FORWARD BENDING EXERCISES | |
| BACKWARD BENDING EXERCISES | *Bhujangasan* (cobra pose), with deep breathing; Variation 1: Plate 76, three to four times |
| TWISTING EXERCISES | |
| BALANCING EXERCISES | |
| FOOT EXERCISES | |
| MEDITATIVE POSITIONS | |
| ABDOMINAL EXERCISES | |
| SPECIAL EXERCISES | |
| RELAXATION | Ten to fifteen minutes |
| DIET | Fast once a week; drink only fresh fruit and vegetable juices and four to five glasses of fresh water daily |
| CLEANSING EXERCISES | |
| BREATHING EXERCISES | Deep breathing in lying position, five to ten minutes |
| CONCENTRATION AND MEDITATION | Read religious or philosophical books, approximately fifteen minutes each day |

| Lesson II—2 to 6 months, or more | Lesson III—1 to 2 years, or more |
|---|---|
| Same as in Lesson I | Same as in Lessons I and II |
| *Paschimothan Asana* (head-knee pose), Variations 1, 2, 3, 4: Plates 55, 56, 57, 58, three to six times each | Same as in Lessons I and II |
| *Bhujangasan* (cobra pose), Plates 76, 77, 78, three times each, and *Ardha Salabhasan* (half locust pose), Plate 80, four times | Same as in Lesson II, plus *Salabhasan* (locust pose, full), Plate 81, and *Dhanurasan* (bow pose), Plates 84, 85, 86, 87, two to six times each |
| *Sarvangasana* (shoulderstand), Plates 42, 43, thirty seconds to three minutes, followed by *Matsyasan* (fish pose), Variation 1: Plate 45, two minutes | *Sarvangasan* (shoulderstand), Variations 1, 2: Plates 42, 43, three minutes, followed by *Matsyasan* (fish pose), Variation 1: Plate 45, one minute |
|  | *Sukhasan* (easy pose), Plate 19, and *Siddhasan* (adept's pose), Plate 14, three to thirty minutes each |
|  | *Agni Sara Kriya* (breathing and abdominal manipulation), page 21, three to six rounds |
| Ten to fifteen minutes | Ten to fifteen minutes |
| Avoid sweets and fried foods. Fast once a week; drink vegetable juices and four to five glasses of fresh water daily | Eat only natural food; avoid meat, liquor and smoking. Fast on water one day every week |
|  | Nasal and throat cleansing with salt water |
| Same as in Lesson I | Alternate breathing exercises, fifteen to forty rounds |
| Same as in Lesson I. In addition, devote ten minutes to your religious prayers | Same as in Lesson II, plus candlelight gazing, Plate 4, five to fifteen minutes. Increase prayers and reading. Observe silence one hour daily |

# TRAINING TABLE 2

Yogic Exercises for People of Normal Health and Between the Ages of 40 and 60

(*Training Table 1 for very old people and sick people*)

| Yogic discipline of body and mind | **Lesson I—2 to 6 weeks** |
| --- | --- |
| HIP AND LEG EXERCISES | *Pavana Mukthasan* (liberated pose), Plate 15, six to twelve times |
| FORWARD BENDING EXERCISES | *Paschimothan Asana* (head-knee pose), Variations 1, 2, 3, 4: Plates 55, 56, 57, 58, three to six times each |
| BACKWARD BENDING EXERCISES | *Bhujangasan* (cobra pose), Variations 1, 2, 3: Plates 76, 77, 78, three times each, and *Ardha Salabhasan* (half locust pose), Plate 80, four times |
| TWISTING EXERCISES | |
| BALANCING EXERCISES | *Sarvangasana* (shoulderstand), Variations 1, 2: Plates 42, 43, and *Matsyasan* (fish pose), Variation 1: Plate 45, one to two minutes each |
| FOOT EXERCISES | |
| MEDITATIVE POSITIONS | *Sukhasan* (easy pose), Plate 19, five to fifteen minutes |
| ABDOMINAL EXERCISES | |
| SPECIAL EXERCISES | |
| RELAXATION | Ten to fifteen minutes |
| DIET | Fast once a week on fresh water only. Avoid sweets and fried foods. Drink four to five glasses of fresh water daily |

| Lesson II—2 to 6 months | Lesson III—1 to 2 years |
|---|---|
| Same as in Lesson I | *Padmasan* (lotus pose), Plate 13; *Mandukasan* (frog pose), Plate 121; *Vajrasan* (kneeling pose), Plate 16; *Padangushtasan* (tiptoe pose), Plate 123, one to ten minutes each |
| *Paschimothan Asana* (head-knee pose), Variations 1, 2, 3, 4: Plates 55, 56, 57, 58, six times each, and *Halasan* (plough pose), Plates 50, 51, 52, three times each | Same as in Lesson II, plus *Janu Sirasan* (head-knee pose), Plates 61, 62, 63, 64, 65; *Karna Peedasan* (ear-knee pose), Plate 53; *Paschimothan Asana* (head-knee pose), Plates 55, 56, 57, 58, two times each |
| *Bhujangasan* (cobra pose), Variations 1, 2, 3: Plates 76, 77, 78, three times each, and *Salabhasan* (locust pose), Plates 79, 80, 81, 82, 83, three times each | *Bhujangasan* (cobra pose), Plates 76, 77, 78; *Salabhasan* (locust pose), Plates 79, 80, 81, 82, 83; *Dhanurasan* (bow pose), Plates 84, 85, 86, 87, three times each |
| *Ardha Matsendrasan* (spinal twist), Variation 1: Plates 101, 102, twice on each side | *Ardha Matsendrasan* (spinal twist), Variations 1, 2: Plates 101, 102, 103, two times each |
| *Sarvangasana* (shoulderstand), Variations 1, 2: Plates 42, 43, four minutes, followed by *Matsyasan* (fish pose), Variations 1, 2, 3, 4: Plates 45, 46, 47, 48, two minutes each | *Sirshasan* (headstand), Plates 32, 33, 34, 35, 36, one to ten minues; *Sarvangasan* (shoulderstand), Variations 1, 2: Plates 42, 43, eight minutes (PEOPLE WITH HIGH BLOOD PRESSURE SHOULD NOT DO HEADSTAND) |
| Walk barefooted whenever possible | Walk barefooted whenever possible |
| *Siddhasan* (easy pose), Plate 19, five to ten minutes | *Padmasan* (lotus pose), Plate 13, five to fifteen minutes |
| | *Agni Sara Kriya* (breathing and abdominal manipulation), page 21, three to six rounds, with twenty to twenty-five pumping |
| *Soorya Namaskar* (sun exercises), Variations 1 through 12: Plates 20 through 31, three to eight rounds | *Soornya Namaskar* (sun exercises), Variations 1 through 12: Plates 20 through 31, eight rounds; *Trikonasan* (triangle pose), Plates 135, 136, 137, 138, two times each; *Matsyasan* (fish pose), after shoulderstand, Plates 45, 46, 47, 48, two minutes each |
| Ten to fifteen minutes | Ten to fifteen minutes |
| Fast once a week on fresh water alone. Avoid meat and fried foods. Drink four glasses of water daily (overweight people should fast two weeks on vegetable juices) | Same as in Lesson II. Avoid meat, fish, eggs. Live on a natural diet |

| | |
|---|---|
| CLEANSING EXERCISES | |
| BREATHING EXERCISES | Alternate breathing exercises without retention, fifteen rounds |
| ERADICATING BAD HABITS | Avoid drinking excessive coffee or tea; do not indulge in soft drinks and candies |
| CONCENTRATION AND MEDITATION | Read religious or philosophical books, approximately fifteen minutes each day |
| DEVELOPMENT OF THE SPIRITUAL HEART | |

| | |
|---|---|
| *Neti* (nasal cleansing) with water, Plates 2, 3; in addition, observe daily dental cleansing | *Neti* (nasal cleansing), Plates 2, 3, and *Dhauti* (cleansing), with water only, pages 25, 26. (*Dhauti* SHOULD BE PRACTICED ONCE A WEEK) |
| *Kapala Bhathi* (diaphragmatic breathing), page 20; practice until you achieve eight seconds inhalation and sixteen seconds exhalation | *Kapala Bhathi* (alternate breathing exercise), page 20, three to six rounds; with retention, fifteen to twenty-five rounds |
| Avoid smoking and alcoholic beverages | Start eliminating a bad habit you would like to do away with |
| Read from the Gita or the Bible or any other preferred religious work for approximately fifteen minutes daily | Same as in Lessons I and II, plus candlelight gazing, Plate 4; and chanting of OM, ten to fifteen minutes or more |
| Once a week, work with some religious or charitable organization, or lend your help in some similar way | Same as in Lessons I and II |

# TRAINING TABLE 3

Yogic Exercises for People of Normal Health and Between the Ages of 30 and 40 (Excessively obese or stiff people, use Table 1)

(*Training Table 1 for very old people and sick people*)

NOTE: *Physical and breathing exercises may be intensified and extended upon the advice of your teacher*

| Yogic discipline of body and mind | **Lesson I**—2 to 6 weeks |
|---|---|
| HIP AND LEG EXERCISES | *Pavana Mukthasan* (liberated pose), Plate 15, six to twelve times |
| FORWARD BENDING EXERCISES | *Paschimothan Asana* (head-knee pose), Variations 1, 2, 3, 4: Plates 55, 56, 57, 58, three to four times each |
| BACKWARD BENDING EXERCISES | *Bhujangasan* (cobra pose), Plates 76, 77, 78, and *Salabhasan* (locust pose), Plates 79, 80, 81, 82, 83, three to four times each |
| TWISTING EXERCISES | *Ardha Matsendrasan* (spinal twist), Variation 1: Plates 101, 102, twice on each side |
| BALANCING EXERCISES | *Sarvangasana* (shoulderstand), Variations 1, 2: Plates 42, 43, three minutes, and *Matsyasan* (fish pose), Plates 45, 46, 47, 48, one minute each |
| FOOT EXERCISES | Walk barefooted whenever possible |
| MEDITATIVE POSITIONS | *Siddhasan* (adept's pose), Plate 14, five to ten minutes |
| ABDOMINAL EXERCISES | |

| Lesson II—2 to 6 months | Lesson III—1 to 2 years |
| --- | --- |
| *Sethu Bandhasan* (bridge pose), Plate 44, one to two minutes | Same as in Lesson II |
| *Halasan* (plough pose), Variations 1, 2, 3: Plates 50, 51, 52, three to four times, and *Paschimothan Asana* (head-knee pose), Plates 55, 56, 57, 58, three times | *Halasan* (plough pose), Plates 50, 51, 52; *Paschimothan Asana* (head-knee pose), Plates 55, 56, 57, 58; *Janu Sirasan* (head-knee pose), Plates 61, 62; *Pada Hasthasan* (foot-hand catch pose), Plates 133, 134, three times each |
| *Bhujangasan* (cobra pose), Variations 1, 2, 3: Plates 76, 77, 78; *Salabhasan* (locust pose), Plates 79, 80, 81, 82, 83; *Dhanurasan* (bow pose), Plates 84, 85, 86, 87, three times each | *Bhujangasan* (cobra pose), Plates 76, 77, 78; *Salabhasan* (locust pose), Plates 79, 80, 81, 82, 83; *Dhanurasan* (bow pose), Plates 84, 85, 86, 87; *Supta Vajrasan* (kneeling pose), Plates 88, 89, 90; *Chakrasan* (wheel pose), Plates 95, 96, 97, 98, 99, three times each |
| *Ardha Matsendrasan* (spinal twist), Variation 1: Plates 101, 102, twice on each side | *Ardha Matsendrasan* (spinal twist), Variations 1, 2: Plates 101, 102, 103, two times each |
| *Sirshasan* (headstand), Plates 32, 33, 34, 35, 36, two minutes, and *Sarvangasan* (shoulderstand), Variations 1, 2: Plates 42, 43, five minutes, and *Matsyasan* (fish pose), Plates 45, 46, 47, 48, two minutes | *Sirshasan* (headstand), Plates 32, 33, 34, 35, 36, five minutes; *Sarvangasan* (shoulderstand), Plates 42, 43, ten minutes; *Matsyasan* (fish pose), Plates 45, 46, 47, 48, two minutes; *Mayoorasan* (peacock pose), Plates 105, 106, 107, 108, 109, two minutes |
| *Gomukhasan* (cow head pose), Plate 122, one to two minutes, and *Mandukasan* (frog pose), Plate 121, one to two minutes | Same as in Lesson II, plus *Bhadrasan* (ankle-knee pose), Plate 116, and *Gorakshasan* (ankle-knee pose), Plate 117, two minutes each |
| Same as in Lesson I, ten to fifteen minutes during breathing exercises and meditation | Same as in Lesson I, fifteen to thirty minutes during breathing exercises and meditation |
| *Agni Sara Kriya* (breathing and abdominal manipulation), page 21, fifteen pumping in each round—three rounds | *Sgni Sara Kriya* (breathing and abdominal manipulation), page 21, four rounds—fifteen pumping, and *Uddiyana Banda* (abdominal contraction), Positions 1, 2: Plates 7, 8, three times each, and *Nauli* (manipulation of the abdominal muscles), Plates 9, 10, 11, 12, three times |

| | |
|---|---|
| SPECIAL EXERCISES | *Vajrasan* (kneeling pose), Plate 16, three [to] five minutes, and *Supta Vajrasan* (kneelin[g] pose), Variations 1, 2, 3: Plates 88, 89, 90, o[ne] to two minutes each |
| RELAXATION | Ten to fifteen minutes |
| DIET | Fast once a week on fresh water only. Avo[id] excessive sweets and fried foods. Drink fres[h] fruit juices. Daily water intake: four to fi[ve] glasses |
| CLEANSING EXERCISES | *Neti* (nasal cleansing), with water, Plates 2, [3] once each day |
| BREATHING EXERCISES | Alternate breathing exercise without reten[ta]tion (fifteen rounds). Increase proportio[n] gradually |
| ERADICATING BAD HABITS | Avoid excessive coffee or tea. Do not tak[e] candy or soft drinks |
| CONCENTRATION AND MEDITATION | Recite your favorite religious prayers ten [to] fifteen minutes daily (morning and evening[)]. Read religious and philosophical works |
| DEVELOPMENT OF THE SPIRITUAL HEART | Once a week, work with some religious [or] charitable organization, or lend your help i[n] some similar way |

| | |
|---|---|
| *Soorya Namaskar* (sun exercises), Variations 1 through 12: Plates 20 through 31, four times, and *Trikonasan* (triangle pose), Variation 1: Plate 135, two times | *Soorya Namaskar* (sun exercises), Variations 1 through 12: Plates 20 through 31, six rounds, and *Trikonasan* (triangle pose), Plates 135, 136, 137, 138, three times |
| Ten to fifteen minutes | Ten to fifteen minutes |
| Fast once a week. Avoid salted foods one day per week. Do not eat excessive sweets and starchy foods. Drink four glasses of water daily | Cultivate new, beneficial eating and drinking habits; live on a natural diet, avoid meat and fish |
| *Neti* (nasal cleansing), Plates 2, 3, with salt water. Other cleansing exercises may be practiced with guidance of teacher | *Neti* (nasal cleansing), Plates 2, 3, with water; *Dhauti* (cleansing), pages 25, 26, with water. (Other cleansing procedures may be done under the guidance of a teacher) |
| Alternate breathing exercises with retention, fifteen rounds, ratio 1:2:2 (See chapter on Breathing) | *Kapala Bhathi* (alternate breathing exercise), page 20, twenty to forty rounds, ratio 1:4:4. (All other breathing exercises may be practiced with the help of a competent teacher) |
| Avoid excessive coffee, tea and other liquid stimulants; Reduce smoking | Same as in Lesson II. Avoid smoking completely; abstain from all alcoholic beverages |
| Same as in Lesson I, plus candlelight gazing, Plate 4, or read from religious or philosophical works fifteen minutes daily | Same as in Lesson II. Meditate on and chant OM. (Refer to chapter on OM) |
| Same as in Lesson I. If possible, devote more time to giving of yourself with a religious or charitable organization | Same as in Lessons I and II. Try to associate with people with recognizable good personality and character traits |

## TRAINING TABLE 4

Yogic Exercises for People of Normal Health and Between the Ages of 18 and 30 (People with abnormal conditions of the spine and other regions of the body should follow Training Table 1 under the guidance of a competent teacher before attempting more advanced exercises)

(*Training Table 1 for very old people and sick people*)

NOTE: *Physical and breathing exercises may be intensified and extended upon the advice of your teacher*

| Yogic discipline of body and mind | **Lesson I**—2 to 6 weeks, or more |
|---|---|
| HIP AND LEG EXERCISES | *Pavana Mukthasan* (liberated pose), Alternate leg raising, three times |
| FORWARD BENDING EXERCISES | *Halasana* (Plough pose), Variations 1, 2, 3: Plates 50, 51, 52, three to four times each |
| BACKWARD BENDING EXERCISES | *Bhujangasan* (cobra pose), Variations 1, 2, 3: Plates 76, 77, 78, three to four times each, and *Ardha Salabhasan* (half locust pose), Variation 2: Plate 80, three to four times |
| TWISTING EXERCISES | *Ardha Matsendrasan* (spinal twist), Variation 1: Plates 101, 102, twice on each side |
| BALANCING EXERCISES | *Sarvangasan* (shoulderstand), Variations 1, 2: Plates 42, 43, three to five minutes, and *Matsyasan* (fish pose), Variations 1, 2, 3, 4: Plates 45, 46, 47, 48, one minute each |
| FOOT EXERCISES | *Padangushtasan* (tiptoe pose), Plate 123, two to three minutes |
| MEDITATIVE POSITIONS (AND SITTING EXERCISES) | *Siddhasan* (adept's pose), Plate 14, three to five minutes, and *Padmasan* (lotus pose), half position, Plate 13, three to five minutes |

| Lesson II—2 to 6 months, or more | Lesson III—1 to 2 years, or more |
|---|---|
| *Sethu Bandhasan* (bridge pose), Plate 44, one to two minutes, and *Karna Peedasan* (ear-knee pose), Plate 53, one-half to one minute | *Anjaneyasan* (split pose), Plate 100, ten to thirty seconds |
| *Halasana* (plough pose), Variations 1, 2, 3: Plates 50, 51, 52, three times each, and *Paschimothan Asana* (head-knee pose), Variations 1, 2, 3, 4: Plates 55, 56, 57, 58, three times each | Same as in Lesson II, plus *Janu Sirasan* (head-knee pose), Variations 1, 2, 3, 4, 5: Plates 61, 62, 63, 64, 65, three times each, *Kurmasan* (tortoise pose), Plate 59, three times |
| *Bhujangasan* (cobra pose), Plates 76, 77, 78; *Salabhasan* (locust pose), Plates 79, 80, 81, 82, 83; *Dhanurasan* (bow pose), Plates 84, 85, 86, 87; *Supta Vajrasan* (kneeling pose), Variation 1: Plate 88; *Chakrasan* (wheel pose), Variation 1: Plate 95, two times each | *Poorna Supta Vajrasan* (diamond pose in full kneeling position), Variation 3: Plate 90, ten seconds, and *Chakrasan* (wheel pose), Plates 95, 96, 97, 98, 99, ten to thirty seconds |
| *Ardha Matsendrasan* (spinal twist), Variations 1, 2: Plates 101, 102, 103, twice on each side | *Poorna Matsendrisan* (full spinal twist), Variation 3: Plate 104, two times |
| *Sirshasan* (headstand), Plates 32, 33, 34, 35, 36, two minutes; *Sarvangasan* (shoulderstand), Variations 1, 2: Plates 42, 43, five minutes; *Matsyasan* (fish pose), Plates 45, 46, 47, 48, two minutes; *Mayoorasan* (peacock pose), Plates 105, 106, 107, 108, 109, two times each; *Kakasan* (crow pose), Variations 1, 2: Plates 110, 111, two times each | *Sirshasan* (headstand), Plates 32, 33, 34, 35, 36, five minutes; *Sarvangasan* (shoulderstand), Plates 42, 43, ten minutes; *Matsyasan* (fish pose), Plates 45, 46, 47, 48, two times each; *Mayoorasan* (peacock pose), Plates 105, 106, 107, 108, 109, two times each; *Kakasan* (crow pose), Plates 110, 111, two times each |
| *Bhadrasan* (ankle-knee pose), Plate 116; *Gomukhasan* (cow head pose), Plate 122; *Mandukasan* (frog pose), Plate 121, one to two minutes each | Same as in Lessons I and II |
| *Padmasan* (lotus pose), full position, Plate 13, three to ten minutes | *Kukudasan* (cock pose), Plate 114, one to two minutes; *Yoga Mudra* (lotus pose), with forward bending, Variation 1: Plate 128, three times; *Bandha Padmasan* (bound lotus pose), Variation 3: Plate 130, three minutes |

| | |
|---|---|
| ABDOMINAL EXERCISES | *Uddiyana Bandha* (abdominal contraction), Positions 1, 2: Plates 7, 8, three to six times |
| SPECIAL EXERCISES | *Soorya Namaskar* (sun exercises), Positions 1 through 12: Plates 20 through 31, six times |
| RELAXATION | Ten to fifteen minutes |
| DIET | Fast once a week on fresh water only. Drink vegetable and fruit juices. Avoid candies and soft drinks |
| CLEANSING EXERCISES | *Neti* (nasal cleansing), Plates 2, 3, with salt water; *Dhauti* (cleansing), with water only, pages 25, 26. (See instructions in the text) |
| BREATHING EXERCISES | Alternate breathing, without retention, fifteen rounds |
| ERADICATING BAD HABITS | Avoid excessive coffee and tea. Refrain from using abusive language |
| CONCENTRATION AND MEDITATION | Recite your favorite religious prayers ten to fifteen minutes daily (morning and evening). Read from the Gita or the Bible (about fifteen minutes); concentrate on the meaning |
| DEVELOPMENT OF THE SPIRITUAL HEART | Once a week, work with some religious or charitable organization, or lend your help in some similar way |

| | |
|---|---|
| *Agni Sara Kriya* (breathing and abdominal manipulation), page 21, three rounds, and *Uddiyana Bandha* (abdominal contraction), Positions 1, 2: Plates 7, 8, three times each | Same as in Lessons I and II, plus *Nauli Kriya* (manipulation of abdominal muscles), Positions 1, 2: Plates 9, 10, three to six times |
| *Soorya Namaskar* (sun exercises), Plates 20 through 31, twelve times each; *Dhanurasan* (bow pose), Variation 1: Plate 84, two times; *Trikonasan* (triangle pose), Plates 135, 136, 137, 138, two times each | Same as in Lesson II, plus *Dhanurasan* (bow pose), Variations 2, 3: Plates 85, 86, three times each; *Trikonasan* (triangle pose), Plates 135, 136, 137, 138, three times each |
| Ten to fifteen minutes | Ten to fifteen minutes |
| Fast once a week. Avoid fried foods, excessive coffee and tea and other liquid stimulants. Drink lots of fresh fruit and vegetable juices | Become a total vegetarian; live on a natural diet (read chapter on diet) |
| Same as in Lesson I. Other cleansing exercises may be practiced under the guidance of a competent teacher | Same as in Lessons I and II |
| *Kapala Bhathi* (diaphragmatic breathing exercise), page 20, three to four rounds, and alternate breathing with retention, fifteen to twenty rounds | *Kapala Bhathi* (diaphragmatic breathing exercise), page 20, four to six rounds, and alternate breathing with retention, twenty to forty rounds—ratio 1:4:2 |
| Avoid smoking and drinking alcoholic beverages completely | One by one, try to eradicate all of your bad habits, with steady progress |
| *Tratak* (gazing exercises), Variations 2, 3: Plates 5, 6, five to ten minutes; meditation and chanting of OM, fifteen to twenty minutes. Read chapter on OM | Meditate on OM, or on God, in conformity with your religious beliefs (thirty minutes or more) |
| Same as in Lesson I. Try to find time to devote additional help | In your own way, seek more opportunities to help people as a means of heart purification. See God in all human beings at all times |

# TRAINING TABLE 5

Yogic Exercises for Children of Normal Health

*It is the duty of all parents to provide their children with home education, emphasizing physical, mental, and spiritual aspects within a framework consistent with the religious background of the family. It is also the duty of parents to establish a constructive pattern of deed and action, so that their children might benefit from force of example. If parents themselves do not give evidence of self-control or self-discipline, their children cannot reasonably be expected to make adequate progress in their physical, mental, and spiritual development. There are, unfortunately, some parents who subject their children to excessively strict control, in the name of religious belief, blocking completely the young individuals' spiritual development by denying*

| Yogic discipline of body and mind | **Lesson I**—2 to 6 weeks, or more |
|---|---|
| PHYSICAL EXERCISES | *Soorya Namaskar* (sun exercises), Plates 20 through 31, three times; *Sarvangasan* (shoulderstand), Variations 1, 2: Plates 42, 43, two minutes; *Paschimothan Asana* (head-knee pose), Plates 55, 56, 57, 58, three times; *Bhujangasan* (cobra pose), Plates 76, 77, 78, three times each |
| BREATHING EXERCISES | Abdominal deep breathing, five to ten minutes. (See chapter on Breathing) |
| RELIGIOUS READING | Read aloud and explain stories from religious books of your preference, fifteen to thirty minutes daily |
| ERADICATING BAD HABITS | Make daily efforts to understand the problems confronting your child and act upon them constructively. See that he selects wholesome and stimulating companions |
| RECREATION | Devote thirty minutes or more every day to open-air recreation with your child. Visits to a zoo or active play and swimming tend to relieve tensions created in the home and school |
| STUDY | Allot a certain time for his homework or study. If possible, arrange study periods during the morning hours, the best time of day for this activity |
| PRAYER | Have your child recite his prayers before retiring and before his meals, approximately five minutes each time |

them sufficient time to develop naturally in this sphere as they grow physically and mentally. Parents should make every effort to bring forth all the hidden knowledge that lies dormant in the subconscious minds of their children, by encouraging them to think freely and constructively and to keep them free of the stultifying fears of hell, destruction, death, etc. The following simple home exercises will help a great deal to awaken the young subconscious and bring forth the hidden knowledge contained therein. These exercises and instructions do not conflict with any religious beliefs. They are formulated to provide proper methods of eating, exercising, breathing, and thinking. Good habits formed in early life have a lasting, beneficial influence, just as bad habits in eating, drinking, etc., developed at an early stage, have deleterious effects, even over one's destiny; happily, however, destructive habits may be removed by constant Yogic practice.

| Lesson II—2 to 6 months, or more | Lesson III—1 to 2 years, or more |
|---|---|
| Soorya Namaskar (sun exercises), Plates 20 through 31, six times; Sarvangasan (shoulderstand), Variations 1, 2: Plates 42, 43, three minutes; Paschimothan Asana (head-knee pose), Plates 55, 56, 57, 58, three times; Bhujangasan (cobra pose), Plates 76, 77, 78, three times, Dhanurasan (bow pose), Plates 84, 85, 86, 87, three times; Padmasan (lotus pose), Plate 13, two minutes | Same as in Lesson II, plus Sirshasan (headstand), Plates 32, 33, 34, 35, 36, two minutes; Ardha Matsendrasan (spinal twist), half spiral, Variation 1: Plates 101, 102, three times; Trikonasan (triangle pose), Plates 135, 136, 137, 138, three times each; Pada Hasthasan (foot-hand catch pose), Variations 1, 2: Plates 133, 134, three times each; Chakrasan (wheel pose), Plates 95, 96, 97, 98, 99, two times each Same as in Lesson I (if time permits) |
| Same as in Lesson I | Kapala Bhathi (diaphragmatic breathing exercise), page 20, three to four rounds, and alternate breathing, ten to twenty rounds |
| Same as in Lesson I | Same as in Lessons I and II |
| Evaluate the extent of improvement in your child's habits | Same as in Lessons I and II |
| Same as in Lesson I | Same as in Lessons I and II |
| Same as in Lesson I | Same as in Lessons I and II |
| Same as in Lesson I | Same as in Lessons I and II |

# TRAINING TABLE 6

Advanced Training in Yoga for Quick Development of the Body and Mind, and to Awaken the Spiritual Force in Man

*The exercises in the following table should be practiced only after having mastered those in previous lessons, according to your age group. In this table, the physical portions of the Yogic exercises have been omitted. The difficult Yogic positions given in this book may be practiced by young, healthy, advanced students along with the positions in the table that follows, with*

| Yogic discipline of body and mind | **Lesson I**—1 to 6 months, or more<br>preparatory stage for the purification of the *Nadis* (nerve centers) |
|---|---|
| KAPALA BHATHI<br>(*diaphragmatic breathing*) | Three to eight rounds. Number of expulsions in each round starts with thirty, gradually increasing to fifty. Do not practice excessively in the event of congestion or pain in the chest |
| ANULOMA VILOMA PRANAYAMA<br>(*alternate nostril breathing*) | Twenty rounds. Proportion 4:8:8. Gradually increase the proportion until you reach 8:16:16 (within six months). CAUTION: Never increase to higher proportion unless you have mastered the lower proportion perfectly |
| UJJAYI PRANAYAMA<br>(*Hatha Yoga breathing*) | Five to ten rounds |
| SURYA BHEDA PRANAYAMA<br>(*a light variety of Yogic breathing*) | |
| BHASTRIKA PRANAYAMA<br>(*a light variety of Yogic breathing*) | |
| MINOR BREATHING EXERCISE | *Sitali* (Yogic breathing), pp. 249–250, and *Sitkari* (Yogic breathing), pp. 249–250, ten to twenty rounds each |
| RHYTHMIC BREATHING EXERCISES | Fifteen minutes. Proportion of inhalation to exhalation 4:4; four seconds inhalation, four seconds exhalation |
| DIET | Abstain from meat, alcohol and smoking |
| RELAXATION | Ten to fifteen minutes |

*consideration to your nature and available time, and under the guidance of a competent teacher. Do not rush from one exercise to another. To achieve perfect discipline of body and mind and to derive all of the benefits described in these pages may require years of practice. Patience, regular and systematic practice, faith in God and your teacher, are the keys with which to open the inner chambers of your heart, wherein lie all knowledge and power.*

| **Lesson II—1 to 2 years, or more** awakening the *Kundalini* (psychic forces) | **Lesson III**—until perfection achieved |
|---|---|
| Six to ten rounds. Number of expulsions, fifty to one hundred. Keep within your capacity. Take several normal breaths between rounds | Six to ten rounds, one hundred expulsions per round |
| Twenty to forty rounds. Starting proportion 4:16:16. Work gradually up to 8:32:16. CAUTION: Attempt the higher proportion only upon the advice of your teacher | Thirty rounds, twice daily: morning and evening, on an empty stomach. Proportion 8:32:16, increasing 12:48:24. CAUTION: Do not attempt the higher proportion until you are able to do the lower one easily. Stop exercising for a time, in the event of discomfort |
| Ten to twenty rounds, with *Bandhas* (locks) | Ten to twenty rounds, with *Bandhas* (locks) |
| Ten to fifteen rounds, with *Bandhas* (locks) | Ten to fifteen rounds, with *Bandhas* (locks) |
| Three to twelve rounds. Achieve a minimum of ten expulsions at the start and a maximum of twenty-five in each of the rounds. The desired effect is a sensation of heat in the lower spinal region. CAUTION: Keep within your capacity | Same as in Lesson II. At the end of each round, hold your breath, using *Bandhas*. Various sensations may be felt during this exercise. CAUTION: In the event of painful sensations, stop exercise pending advice of teacher |
| Same as in Lesson I (if time permits) | Same as in Lessons I and II |
| Twenty to thirty minutes | Twenty to thirty minutes |
| Abstain from meat, alcohol, smoking; do not eat fried, putrescent or bitter foodstuffs. Also observe a salt-free diet for a considerable time | Same as in Lessons I and II. In addition, observe a liquid rather than a solid diet, and drink milk and fresh fruit juices. Do not fast completely or, conversely, overload stomach |
| Fifteen to twenty minutes | Twenty to thirty minutes (more, if required) |

| ETHICAL, MORAL DEVELOPMENT THRU YAMA AND NIYAMA | 1) Clean your body daily by means of Kriyas<br>2) Make an effort to remain happy constantly<br>3) Seek contentment (*Santosha*) with what you have |
| --- | --- |
| MEDITATION EXERCISES | Candlelight gazing, Plate 4 (or meditate upon a picture of your religious God). Repeat OM, ten minutes |

Practice non-violence. Do not harm or kill any living creature. Be honest and straightforward in all your dealings. Read from the Gita, Bible, or other religious books

"Simple living and high thinking" should be your motto. See the presence of God in all things and beings, from mineral to man. Develop compassion and sympathy for the poor and ignorant

Meditate on the *Chakras*, or the plexus in the spinal column, fifteen to thirty minutes; repeat OM for ten minutes

Meditate on the *Chakras*, thirty minutes, or more. Repeat OM, ten minutes. Do not be unduly proud of your spiritual achievements. Even after climbing the highest spiritual ladder, you may fall to the bottom. Only God's grace brings complete perfection. OM

# List of Asanas (Postures)

*(The figures after the colons are plate numbers)*

# GLOSSARY–INDEX

LAVA—A period of time, according to Hindu calculation. 284

MAHARLOKA—Mental plane of consciousness. 16

MALA—Impurities of the mind. 220, 315

MANIPURA CHAKRA—The bird plexus situated in the spine. 296–297, 299

MANOMAYA KOSHA—The mental sheath. 15–16

MANTRA—A mystical syllable or holy name for God which Hindus chant or repeat mentally. 298–299

MANTRA YOGA—A branch of Raja Yoga. 220

MAYA SAKTHI—The illusory power of God which veils the consciousness and brings individuality. 260, 287

MODA—Great joy. 17

MOOLA BANDHA—Anal contraction. 234, 247–249

MOOLA SODHANA—Rectal irrigation. 21, 26

MOORCHA—A light variety of Yogic breathing. 248

MUDRAS—Hatha Yogic postures which produce electrical currents or forces. 13, 247, 296

MULADHARA CHAKRA—The lotus or pelvic plexus located in the lower spine. 230, 233, 251, 289, 294, 296–297, 299

NADIS—Physical and astral nerves. 230, 234, 240–245, 250, 295

NAGA VAYU—A manifestation of *Prana*, or vital force. 232

NAKSHATRA MANDALA—In ancient Hindu scriptures, man traveling to the stars. 282

NAULI KRIYA—Manipulation of the abdominal muscles. 39, 44–45

NIMESA—In relation to time, the twinkling of an eye. 284

NIRMANU—The Yogic method of cleansing the body in order to achieve perfection in breathing exercises. 240

NIYAMA—Religious observances, such as cleanliness, contentment, mortification, study, and worship of God. 61, 221

OM or AUM—The sacred syllable of Hindu philosophy. 227, 228, 242–244, 249, 255, 298, 314–321

PANCHA PRANAS—Five vital forces. 232

PARAMA SIVA—Supreme being. 295

PARAMANU—The subdivision of an atom. 283, 285

PARARDHA—The time measurement to denote the creation and dissolution of the cosmos by Brahma. 285

PARARTHABHAVINA—Where the external things do not appear to exist. 322

PINGALA—A subtle tube; an astral counterpart of the sensory and motor fibers in the spinal column through which the nerve current (*Prana*) moves. 230, 242, 295

PITRS—Manes or spirits of the dead; gods of the lower world. 284

# SELECTED

# BIBLIOGRAPHY

*Bliss Divine* by Swami Sivananda
*Concentration and Meditation* by Swami Sivananda
*The Hatha Yoga Pradipika* by Swatmarama, commentary by Swami
     Vishnu-devananda
*Kundalini Yoga* by Swami Sivananda
*Meditation and Mantras* by Swami Vishnu-devananda
*Mind: Its Mysteries and Control* by Swami Sivananda
*Raja Yoga* by Swami Sivananda
*Sadhana* by Swami Sivananda
*The Sivananda Companion to Yoga* by The Sivananda Yoga Center
*The Sivananda Upanishad*, compiled by Swami Vishnu-devananda

# ABOUT THE AUTHOR

Swami Vishnu-devananda was born in Kerala, South India, in 1927. In 1947, he came to the Sivananda Ashram in Rishikesh, in the Himalayas. There he lived and worked with his Master, Swami Sivananda.

Swami Sivananda saw in his young disciple special tendencies toward Hatha Yoga. With his training directed toward this discipline, Swami Vishnu-devananda became an expert, mastering many of the most difficult and advanced Hatha Yoga techniques (asanas, pranayamas, mudras, bandhas, and kriyas). He was appointed the first Professor of Hatha Yoga at the Sivananda Yoga Vedanta Forest Academy.

In 1957, Swami Vishnu-devananda was sent to the West by his guru with the words, "People are waiting." Vishnu-devananda founded several Yoga centers in the United States, then settled in Canada, where he established the Sivananda Yoga Vedanta headquarters in Montreal. In 1960, his best-selling book *The Complete Illustrated Book of Yoga* and his respected periodical *Yoga Health Digest* were first published.

Swami Vishnu-devananda's innovations in Yoga instruction have reached millions through his Yoga centers, which are now found in five continents; his popular "Yoga vacations"; and his Yoga teacher training courses, which thousands have attended.

Swami Vishnu-devananda has also committed himself to the cause of world peace and brotherhood. To demonstrate his concern and the importance of the individual nonviolent struggle for peace, Swamiji has flown around the world dropping leaflets and organized peaceful demonstrations at designated trouble spots. He is especially known for his peace mission to Belfast with the late Peter Sellers, his flights over the Suez Canal, and his "bombing" of the Berlin Wall with leaflets and flowers.